Dementia: Love's Bittersweet Journey

ROBERT E. SKEELE

ISBN: 978-0-578-12816-0

LCCN: 2013916824

Printed by Gorham Printing,

Centralia, Washington USA

Front Cover: Entitled *Two Lovers,* this image of an older man and woman walking along a beach or pathway was painted by Vincent Van Gogh in Arles, France in 1888. The author was attracted to the painting because it depicted something essential about the nature of love. Lasting love between a man and woman is always a journey, overcoming differences with constant affection and support, as they make their way.

Books by Robert Skeele

Dementia: Love's Bittersweet Journey
Love is Like That
Side Show
Blue Cow
Whittling (with wife, Joan)
Whistling

This book is dedicated to
the staff, nurses and attendants at
the Birchview Memory Care Community
Sedro-Woolley, Washington
Caregivers All

Acknowledgments

It takes a village to raise a book. That's the conclusion I came to after putting together my last book and it became even more evident with this one. While the writing of it was done in isolation in my study, I was, even then, drawing on the community's resources to give shape and direction to what I thought and wrote about. Caring for a loved one with serious memory loss required the help of others, often in the form of advice and counsel. Dementia is a terrible disease, puzzling as it is mean. Visits by nurses from Island Hospital, telephone contact with nurses from the Group Health Cooperative, visits from the Northwest Regional Council concerning my respite care, visits to the Alzheimer Support Group in Anacortes led by Ann Giboney, appointments with Dr. Allen Horesh at the medical center in LaConner, connection with the Gentry House and its director, Christy Marx, the weekly contact Joan had with neighborhood friends Janet Saunders, Cynthia Rowe and Jean Kleyn, and later the staff and employees at Birchview Memory Care in Sedro-Woolley, all served to help me understand and write more cogently about what was going on as well as to help me be a better caregiver.

The critical job of actually reading what I wrote and evaluating it for publication fell to Jim and Anne Airy, Janet Saunders, Jean Mac-Gregor, Rob and Tricia Longworth, Rebbeca Powell, Cynthia Rowe and Kevin and Chelsea Dacres-Andrews. Tom Winn was there always on hand to provide the technical support. I can't thank them all enough for the time and effort they have put into this project. I want to thank as well the staffs at The Next Chapter Bookstore and

LaConner Weekly News for the encouragement they offer, selling my books and publishing my poems. I'm grateful, too, for the skilled staff at Gorham Printing in Centralia, WA for the high quality of their design and production. As I say, it takes a village, a big and diffuse one, to raise a book.

Contents

Prologue

The words in this book were forged in the fire of caregiving. Sometimes the fire was red hot, other times the red coals were banked to an even heat. Often, the coals, worn gray, offered only small warmth. Whatever the level of heat, I wrote about our journey as things were happening, trying to capture the moment, trying to get me and now you, the reader, to feel something of the pain and joy of caring for someone you love whose memory is slipping away, and with it the close companionship of six decades.

The journey described in this book is not an easy, level walk into the sunset. It is more of a circling, downward spiral, repetitive each time around, but with slight, worrisome differences confirming dementia's progressive nature. It never gets better. There were, however, in our spiraling journey together, many beautiful, sweet times that offset the bitterness of it, meaningful memories which served to numb the pain, at least for a little while.

To get a better grasp of what is going on, it helps to have a full picture of our journey, not just the last few years. For this reason, I consider what I have written in *Dementia: Love's Bittersweet Journey* as a complement to my previous book, *Love Is Like That,* which describes all 61 years of our married life. While each book stands alone, the two books belong together. I have used the same picture (Van Gogh's *Two Lovers*) on the cover of both books to underscore their connection.

Most of us have read the figures. As many as six million people in this country are currently suffering from Alzheimer's disease or some other form of dementia. The number of people with memory loss issues is expected to reach 16 million by the middle of the century. The need to understand dementia in all its devastating configurations has never been greater. *Dementia: Love's Bittersweet Journey* is one step in that direction.

There's much to be learned from following my journey with Joan but it is not an instruction manual. For specific guidance, one of the most practical books available is *The 36-Hour Day* by Mace and Rabins. Another helpful book is *Alzheimer's 911* by Frena Gray-Davidson. To gain understanding of dementia through the novel, none offers more insight than *Still Alice* by Lisa Genova.

Being a caregiver is both perilous and a privilege. It's a privilege because you have the opportunity to express your love and concern for your beloved in a multitude of practical ways right through to the end. It's perilous because you may become a victim of that love, putting your own health in jeopardy. My first warning of such a possibility was from a visiting nurse who told me, after visiting Joan, that I was in for a long haul. It was going to be arduous and demanding. In too many cases, she pointed out, the caregiver, vowing to carry on, has succumbed before the one being care for.

Blind as I was to my own limits, I wouldn't, I couldn't, believe her. As a result, I put Joan's life in danger, too tired late one night to care what happened to her. Love of the beloved, I realized finally, doesn't mean you have to do it all; that, in fact, others are quite capable of caring for your loved one with great skill and tenderness. The last lines of the poem *Compassion's Threat* come to mind…"What's the point, we ask, if in pursuit we lose our own way?/ Can it be that within compassion there lurk the seeds of our own destruction?/ Unless in reaching out we reach in, a compassion toward self,/ Love thy neighbor, left to linger over compassion's red coals, soon dries up, putting life in peril./ Only with its counterpart, Love thy neighbor as thyself, is compassion seen whole, love made holy."

Bob Skeele

2010

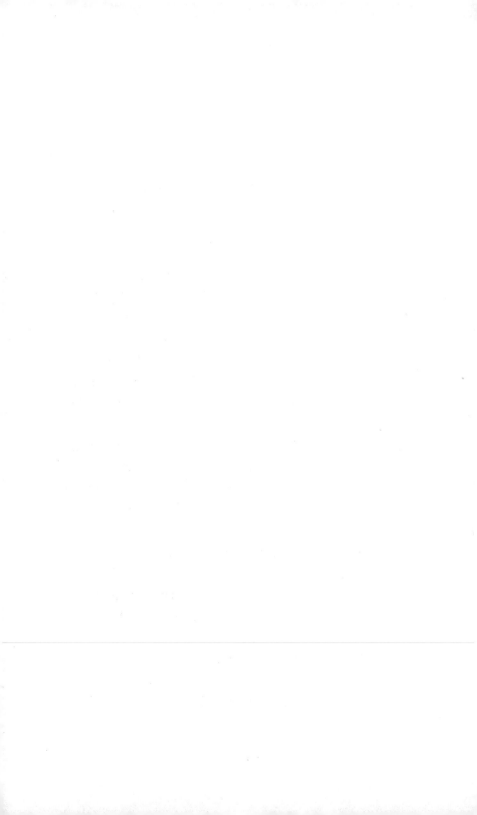

"What do I do now?" she asked. It was five-thirty in the morning on the first of June, 2010 when I heard the light tap on my study door. I had been writing for an hour or so and had just begun to don my sweats for a workout at the fitness center nearby when I heard the knock. I opened the door to find Joan standing there in her floral pajamas and tousled gray hair. Too thin and frail, Joan was still beautiful to my eyes but the look in hers convinced me of her sincerity. She really wanted to know: "What do I do now?"

The question did not completely surprise me. Sadly, Joan's ability to remember anything for long—both long term and short term—was deserting her. This was the first time, though, that she was unable to recall her usual morning routine of showering and dressing before breakfast. I suggested she go back to bed and assured her that I would awaken her when I returned in half an hour. Joan was only too happy to comply. She seemed to covet the warmth and comfort her bed provided. Most evenings now she retired early, usually around six o'clock or so, too tired to read or watch television, while I did the dishes and cleaned up the kitchen. Once an avid sports fan, baseball and tennis now bored her, she said, and the evening news was no better. Recently she confessed that she did not understand what they (the newscasters) were saying. They talked too fast.

How could such a thing happen to a woman who had managed to avoid unhealthy habits like smoking and drinking and had been so bright and mentally active? In her memoir, Joan wrote with justifiable pride about her academic ability. Even though her father required her to take the commercial rather than the college track in high school, she became a member of the National Honor Society and, when she got to the university, passed the required college math course with flying colors. An English literature major, she went on to work, among other things, as a school teacher and, after bearing and raising four children, was employed as a paralegal in a public defender's office. It was then that she studied the law and—without the benefit of attending law school—passed the Vermont Bar and, at age 59, opened her own law practice.

Later, after the move to Washington State, Joan exercised her literary talent by completing two novels and writing extensive letters to Seattle newspaper editors as well as poetry, some of which appeared in the book *Whittling* which she co-authored with me. I read portions of the two novels several times and remember being impressed with her character development and the complexity of the plots. It was only later when it was Joan's turn to write the annual Christmas letter bringing our friends up to date on our activities that I realized she could not do it. She was not pleased with my interference but at least I was able to piece something together and get it in the mail during the Christmas season.

Even then I was not aware how serious Joan's memory loss was until much later when she was writing her memoir. To get it ready for publication required more editing than would have been necessary in an earlier time. Slowly I became aware of other problems such as a lessening ability to play gin rummy, our favorite card game, mainly because she could not recall the rules and procedures. There soon followed a decreasing interest in the daily *New York Times* cross word puzzle and the newspaper's editorial page. And then came the knock on my study door. Slowly, our familiar world was changing. It was only a few days later that I was shocked into the realization about just how dangerous that new world could become for Joan and how worrisome for me.

On this particular day I came home for lunch at noon, the usual time, and could not find Joan anywhere inside or outside the house nor did she leave a note for me which she normally did. When I wrote the poem that follows, I was thinking primarily of physical absence or disappearance. The question took on new poignancy as I realized that Joan might be lost to me in other ways. Dementia, I soon came to learn, went only one way: down. I already knew I was going to be walking with her on the journey, holding her hand and singing, but what more must I do as her lover and spouse? The answer came as I asked the question. I must be alert and watchful, learning everything I could about cognitive impairment. For this reason I closely tracked our journey, day by day in many cases, so that I might be in a better position to determine my next steps. I also wanted others to learn from what Joan and I were experiencing and so kept to the original record, starting with the knock on my study door.

Joan, Where Are You?

I came home from work at lunch time to find
the house empty. I ran upstairs and outside
calling your name, just to make sure.
You said you would not walk anywhere alone.
Are you taking a late walk with one
of your walking pals? Unlike you, though,
to leave no note telling me your plan.
A half hour goes by, still no sign.
Where are you? Where have you gone?

In our camper, I cruise First Street and
the Marina, following your usual walking
trail. Did you decide to walk by yourself
after all and fall somewhere, tumbling down a
channel bank or off a dock? You're not
sitting on a bench, catching your breath.
Oh, dear, dear Joan, where are you?
Where has my lover, my sweetheart, gone?

Frantic now, I return to the house and
begin phoning. No one has seen you
walking today. You were not visiting
a friend. You did not stop at the Town Hall
to say hello to your friends there. Some
begin looking and inquiring on their own

trying to find you. You seem to have
disappeared, vanished. Where are you?
Where have you gone?

As a last resort, I return to the Museum
where I had been working most of the
morning, out front tending the plants.
Has anyone seen you? Yes! You had come
to the Museum looking for me! Of course.
I should have known. But how could we have
missed each other? I begin walking around
the building, checking the steep drop-offs
and rocky terrain, more worried than ever.
Oh, dear, dear Joan, where are you? Where
has my lover, my sweetheart gone?

I peer down into the thick brush beneath the
fir trees and into the blackberry bushes,
calling your name. I walk around the south
end of the building and down the slope where
I know you would never venture, still calling,
and then, do I hear a faint response? I keep
walking north toward the Museum's East Wing
and the Observation Deck, once more calling
your name and then I hear you "Please, someone
help me" and there you are, collapsed on the
gravel down slope, unable to move but unhurt,
and with help from a neighbor and me, able to
stand and make your way, unsteadily, to water
and rest.

You were lost to me, Joan, for a terrible moment
but now you have been found, love finding love,
this time around, my cry, my frantic questions
seeking answers and, thankfully, finding one,
barely heard, in your desperate and lonely
response. My only plea to you now, my only
prayer is to never again let me have to ask:
Where are you? Where have you gone?

June 1, 2010

For many years Joan set out each morning on her own to walk a vigorous three miles out to the north marina and back. Now she seldom ventured out on her own. Two younger women who lived a few blocks away walked with her three days a week. The rest of the time she preferred to wait and walk with me in the afternoons following work and lunch which was just as well. She had become less stable on her feet, misjudged curb heights and dips in the sidewalks. Lately, she had become entranced with cloud formations, constantly looking up to exclaim on this or that color or shape—the skies out here were dramatic to be sure—and when she was not looking up, she was looking down to collect this pebble or that pine cone. A gravel pit was growing right in the center of our dining room table with pine cones for trees. It looked like a landscape design. Because she was constantly distracted, I no longer tried to engage her in any detailed conversation.

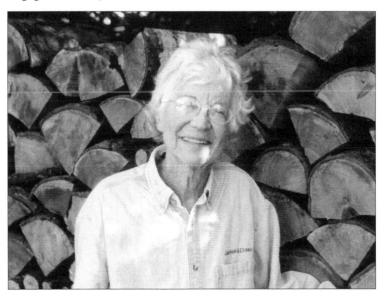

Joan always liked the pattern and texture of the stacked wood. LaConner, 2006

How the Public Works Best

The loud, whining noise from the gas-powered trimmer
fills the air, forcing my walking partner to hold her ears.

The operator, a Public Works employee, seeing her distress
turns off the engine, and knowing me, walks the few feet

to join us on the sidewalk, to say hello and to apologize.
The trimmers are noisy machines, we all agree. In response,

Joan rewards him with her warmest smile and presents him
with a small stone she has collected along the way.

Holding the piece of gravel in his hand, the operator looks
at it and then at Joan and thanks her as if he'd just been

given a nugget of pure gold. For me, standing there, it was
an exquisite moment, the simple exchange between two

human beings, an old silver-haired lady and a vigorous
young man, so rich in understanding and respect that I

know it set the angels talking. I can hear them still. "See,"
they say," this is the way it should be in all civic discourse."

It's how the public works best.

June 2, 2010

This morning about 1:30 am, Joan called to me from her bedroom down the hall. She had heard me, she said, call to her to answer the phone. I reassured her that the phone had not rung and that I had not called to her. A short time later the hall light flicked on. When I asked what was happening, Joan said she thought there were prowlers trying to get into our cars. (The camper and the Saab were parked in front of our house and were visible from Joan's bedroom window). She turned off the hall light but I could hear her continue to move around her bedroom. When I investigated, she was standing at the window, peering down at the cars. I urged her back to bed. She was cold, she said. Yes, I could see why, I told her, after standing at the window in pajamas for half an hour. "I keep thinking Bill (her brother) wants to get in the house." I told her that Bill had been dead for several months now. "I'm confused," Joan said.

This time Joan stayed put but, of course, I was unable to get back to sleep. Oh well, I got up at 3:30 most mornings anyway so it was not a big deal. This night time activity occurred several times each week. Most of the time Joan heard the phone, people talking outside or a bee buzzing around the bedroom. On several occasions she was bothered by the small red security light flashing from just below the Saab's windshield which I remedied with a small patch of black tape. What worried me most was that Joan, in her wandering, might fall down the steep stairway. In her frail condition I did not think she would ever survive it.

One of the consequences of retiring so early each night was that Joan would sleep for an hour or so, then get up, dress and come downstairs thinking it was morning already. She did it again last night. Only this time she sat with me watching television, thoroughly enjoying a concert with Carol King and James Taylor entitled *Live from the Troubadour.* We went upstairs to bed about 9:30 pm. There was not a peep from her the rest of the night.

June 6, 2010

Each time Joan rejoined me downstairs at 8:00 pm or so, I tried to get her to eat something. Once in a great while she would have a cup of warm milk or a small bowl of dry cereal, most of which she would not eat. Getting Joan to eat was an ongoing battle. I had become quite at home in the kitchen and by this time was doing all the cooking and, in the process, had developed some good recipes that appealed to her.

But no matter how much Joan enjoyed looking forward to this or that new concoction, she ended up eating only a fraction of what she served herself. Her eyes were always much bigger than her stomach. As a result, she was not getting adequate nutrition. The only food items she really seemed to enjoy were my muffins for breakfast, ice cream and chocolate chips (which I kept in a handy jar for baking purposes), although not at the same time. Her doctor had said that she was one of a growing number of elders with an eating disorder. I did not believe it until I researched it on the Internet. Sure enough, anorexia was a widespread phenomenon among seniors with few coping strategies. As I had told Joan, she was slowly starving herself to death. She disagreed and tried to make herself eat more, but she simply was not hungry and only nibbled at her food. Although no substitute for whole foods, daily intake of multivitamins seemed absolutely essential in her case. Noting her increased difficulty with swallowing capsules, I switched to a liquid equivalent and made sure she took it each morning along with a small vitamin D capsule (1000 i.u.) and her usual prednisone tablet (5 mg). I made an appointment at the medical clinic for her to have a blood draw the next week before seeing the doctor.

June 7, 2010

This morning she came quietly into my study at 6:00 o'clock while I was at the computer typing these very sentences, kissed me on the head and asked if she had to be at school today. I told her no, she had already been through all that and did not have to go anymore. She said she thought so and, relieved, ambled back to bed. The high point of the day had come Sunday morning. As we were returning home from our walk we passed by the yellow caution sign along the road which read: "Slow. Children at Play." Without pause, Joan said, "I wonder where the fast children play." We both had a good laugh over that. Happily, Joan's wit seemed very much intact at this point.

For Joan's lunch Sunday noon, I prepared a small slice of ham, two quarters of a small, browned potato, half of a single egg omelet and a slice of whole-wheat toast cut in half diagonally. She ate the three bites of ham all right, but only one of the two potato slices and very little of the omelet. She noted that she would never be able to eat all the toast I had given her (and she did not). At the same lunch hour she wanted a glass of wine. I told her the bar was closed until 4:00 o'clock. A few minutes later she was looking for a wine glass to help herself. Within a short space of time Joan consumed three four-ounce glasses of the stuff and I urged her to slow down. (We had had many previous conversations about how her wine drinking worked against her health. She would become sleepy which, in turn, would affect her appetite, not to mention her balance). With my caution, she only got angry and told me to go to hell. Sunday afternoon, as expected, she slept on the wicker sofa in the dining room and was barely able to wake up for the evening meal. Much to my surprise, she actually ate a small slice of meat loaf, a few bites of mashed potato and all of her candied carrots. As at the noon meal, she enjoyed a small bowl of vanilla ice cream. Within a half hour of eating (about 6:45 pm), she was ready for bed and made her way, unsteadily, upstairs. She seemed to sleep well until 2:00 am when she wakened me. "Will someone help me!" she yelled. I ran to her bedroom. She said her face was bleeding. I turned on the light. There was no blood. All appeared normal. With my reassurance, she was quickly asleep again.

June 8, 2010

Surprise of surprises! Joan did not ask for a glass of wine or go looking for one herself. Happy hour came and went and not a peep. You can bet I was not going to say anything. Joan did not eat anymore than usual for supper which meant she barely touched her food except for a small dish of ice cream for dessert. She did, however, take a short walk with me around the block to take in the sun and enjoy the light breeze (and pick up too many pebbles), after which she watched with me the final innings of the Mariners game against Texas. How about that! We went up to bed about 8:15 pm and I read to her for a half hour or so (as was until recently the custom), staying in bed with her for a little while afterward. I could only hope that we would keep to last evening's healthier, pleasanter, pattern.

June 9, 2010

The pattern held for a second day. Around 4:30 pm Joan asked if she did not usually have a little wine about now. I said nothing but gave her a small glass of orange juice which she accepted without protest. She only took a few sips but there was no mention of wine the remainder of the evening. One direct result of not having wine appeared to be less restlessness at night. As yesterday, we retired early and I read to her. To my knowledge, she was quiet from that point on. I thought I might see a change in her appetite as well, at least for the evening meal. No such luck. Last night I placed before her an attractive platter consisting of a small piece of meat loaf (the equivalent of three small forkfuls), two small slices of well seasoned potatoes, six green beans with lime juice and almonds and a hot dinner roll. Joan looked at it and could only shake her head. It was way too much food. She could not possibly eat all that, she said. And she did not, leaving most of it. She did eat a small bowl of ice cream immediately afterwards.

Pebble-picking was becoming a boulder issue. Yesterday afternoon as we crossed the street, Joan spied a pebble she wanted and darted back into the street to retrieve it. A driver who was just turning the corner at the time stopped and waited for her to get back on the sidewalk. I told Joan, once more, not to do that, that it was dangerous. At this point she got angry, telling me that I could not tell her what to do and that she had a much better notion of what was dangerous than I ever would have, and proceeded to walk on ahead of me for several blocks.

Today was one of those rare times when Joan walked up the hill to the Museum to see me, not once but twice, during the morning. Both times I was engaged with contractors and could not stop to talk to her immediately. She seemed hurt and mad at my apparent rebuff. When I finally did get a chance to talk with her, she seemed only somewhat mollified, then walked carefully back down the hill to our house. How lonely and vulnerable she seemed as I watched after her. It brought tears to my eyes even later as I sat at my desk recalling the scene. Was it now time for me to quit my job? Would it help to employ a companion for Joan during the mornings at least? She had said "no" to both so far.

June 10, 2010

The pattern held for a third day. No mention of wine. Again, happy hour came and went. After watching the Mariners fall behind 2 -11, we called it a day and went up to bed where I read to her until about 8:30 pm. After two hours of fitful sleep, I moved to my own bed in the study with its more comfortable mattress (a Tempur-pedic). At 12:30 am, Joan awakened me, concerned about the running water she was hearing. I listened but heard nothing, went down stairs to check all the faucets and listened again. I reported my finding to Joan and returned to bed. She was unconvinced but after a few minutes I heard nothing more until I arose at 3:30 am to begin my day. I had hoped that Joan's night time activity would stop when the wine stopped but apparently not.

Usually, breakfast was the best time of the day for us. After writing for an hour or so and a good work out, I was happy to be in the kitchen listening to Classic King Radio or the jazz station while mixing and baking a batch of muffins for Joan and others. Normally, Joan made her way downstairs by 7:00 am, freshly showered and dressed in her running attire, greeting me with a kiss and a quick embrace. The last few mornings, however, had been far different. She had appeared yesterday, for example, in her bathrobe, stating that she did not feel like showering and proceeded to curl up on the wicker sofa. She obviously was not feeling well. I asked her if there was any pain anywhere. No pain. She just felt tired and not her usual self. At that point, I decided to take the day off from the museum and stay home. Eventually, with fresh muffins, hot coffee and orange juice, Joan began to perk up and, after a brief rest, showered and dressed. I was glad I had scheduled the blood draw. What followed anorexia, I wondered, anemia?

June 13, 2010

Two more days and no wine. Yesterday Joan said she would like some wine but was quite willing to forego it when I said I thought it was the worst thing she could do and cited her more restful nights among other reasons. She said she could do without it. Five minutes later she asked me to get her a glass of wine, having forgotten our previous conversation, apparently. I was busy cooking and did not respond. She did not ask again, only stating over the dinner of sautéed shrimp and asparagus how good a glass of wine would taste. She was right there. Last night we stayed up until after 8:30 pm, watching a biography of Pavarotti.

The pebble collecting continued, which slowed down our walks, but so far seemed harmless except when she stopped in the middle of the street to inspect or pick up a little rock that caught her eye. Much more worrisome now was Joan's hearing loss; it seemed to be getting steadily worse judging by the number of times I had to repeat myself during the course of a day. I had asked her numerous times to get an appointment to have her ears checked out, but she always insisted it was not a problem.

June 18, 2010

Joan and I met with her doctor as scheduled. The blood test results were normal—no anemia—but her glucose level was high. With her slight increase in weight from 82 lbs. (last October) to 87 lbs. now, the diabetes seemed to have returned. Another blood test, taken right there in the office, revealed a dangerously high glucose reading of 476. The doctor was alarmed and put her on insulin therapy immediately. The nurse administered the first shot (15 units per) to her stomach. I was to follow the same procedure beginning tonight after supper using a prefilled pen and gauge with a short, sharp needle. There seemed to be no other alternative at this point. Joan's glucose reading this morning before breakfast was a comfortable 115 but by lunch time had shot up to 370. The glucose reading after lunch was still high. Obviously alcohol of any kind was taboo. There was no argument from Joan. She seemed to understand the seriousness. Then, we were off for an afternoon walk.

That evening after supper, I administered the insulin (15 mg) using the Levemir Flexpen we had been supplied with, a fairly simple procedure with only a short, sharp needle to tolerate. Joan still did not like it anymore than I did. As was our custom, I read to Joan in her bed until about 9 pm. At 10:30 pm she awoke complaining how warm she was, her hair damp from sweating. After checking her blood sugar (it read a scary 36), I got Joan to drink six ounces of orange juice. Within 15 minutes or so, she was feeling normal once again. Her blood sugar read 67 and was presumably increasing. She slept the rest of the night without incident. It was some hours before I could sleep.

June 21, 2010

A new preoccupation: monitoring Joan's blood sugar level 3-4 times a day and trying to regulate her diet with her sugar and carbohydrate intake in mind. Some of the morning was spent researching diabetes and looking for good recipes. Between my usual Saturday chores, she and I squeezed in a couple of walks around town, collecting the mail at the post office along with an assortment of pebbles. She was hungry by four pm, so I heated up spinach ricotta pie, added a side dish of green beans (laced with lime juice and chopped almonds) and whole wheat bread. Because she had eaten little of the earlier meal and few, if any, of the green beans, by 6 pm

Joan was hungry again. I fixed her a bowl of hot oatmeal and buttered toast at her request but she ate very little of it.

After an entertaining program on PBS featuring Chet Atkins, we watched the Mariners baseball game against the Cincinnati Reds for several innings and at 8:15 pm or so called it a day. The insulin injection had gone smoother this time, although Joan still winced her dislike. I did not blame her. Following our evening routine, I read to her for awhile, turning off the light around 9:30 pm. In a repeat of last night, she awoke at 10:20 pm complaining of feeling hot and sweaty. I immediately went downstairs to get her a glass of orange juice. Upon my return however, she started shaking uncontrollably, her back stiff and thrashing around, crying in alarm "Bob... Bob... Help me... Help me... I'm dying... I'm dying..." No one was more alarmed than I. Getting her to swallow the orange juice was out of the question. I tried to keep her on the bed but she was convulsing so rapidly that she slid, with me holding her as tightly as I could, to the floor between the bed and dresser. Leaving her there for just a moment to grab the phone, I was finally able to dial 911. "Keep her on the floor," the operator insisted, "Keep her free of objects... Don't let her injure herself..." By the time the medics arrived, the seizure had ended and Joan had managed, though weak and limp, to swallow the orange juice. The medics followed it up with an IV of sugar water. And with her blood sugar back up into the 300s, concluded that hospitalization was not warranted. Their recommendation: Cut insulin dosage in half and notify her doctor of the action Monday morning. Our neighbor from across the street stayed behind to help me get Joan comfortable and to clean up the kitchen. Such a sweet, timely gesture by a neighbor.

As I was writing up these notes at 1:20 am, Joan called from her bedroom, complaining of feeling hot and sweaty. How could that be? I checked her blood sugar (yet again) to find it had plunged to 39! Quickly I brought her two glasses of orange juice which she drank thirstily and began almost immediately to feel better. Another blood sugar reading at 76 confirmed the improvement. In another hour I would check her blood sugar again. She said her fingertips were getting sore from all the pricking. No wonder!

Joan called to me again at 2:15 am complaining of a cramp in the arch of her left foot and a few minutes later of a cramp in her right calf. I rubbed both without bringing any noticeable relief. Applying a hot water bottle to the left foot (at her suggestion) did not seem to help either, but she soon eased into regular breathing and what I hoped was a gentle sleep. Should I wake her to take another blood sugar reading, I wondered. I thought not. Instead I slipped into bed beside her to better monitor her condition.

I awoke at 5:30 am, Joan breathing normally. Reassured, I got out of bed to shower and dress. Just as I turned off the shower and pulled back the curtain, I heard a quiet knock at the bathroom door. I told her to come in. As Joan passed me on the way to the toilet, urination being her morning's coronation (that is to say, thank goodness she was alive and able to pee), we touched hands. I felt like Adam, without a fig leaf of course, doing just the opposite of the biblical story, that is, returning to paradise after being kicked around in, if not out of, hell. Last night was for me the mother of all nightmares. She said she was tired enough to sleep all day. I told her to do just that. It was Sunday after all, God's day of rest, and I would be home all day to cook and care … and recover.

After lunch I checked Joan's blood sugar level which was now 424, too high for me to ignore. I explained the situation to the doctor on call that weekend at our medical clinic. She confirmed the medic's recommendation: cut back the insulin—but to even less,

5 units per shot. Meanwhile, in the doctor's experience, the higher sugar level was much less worrisome than the lower one of 30 or 40 mg, so we should "hang in there" until we met with the doctor again the following Tuesday. "Hang in" we would, but once in a while we might lose our grip in other matters associated with memory loss.

When Joan asked me what I wanted for Father's Day, I said I would like to go to Christianson's Nursery to get plants for a butterfly garden. Did she want to come with me? No, she said, she was too tired but indicated she might like to go later in the day. When I asked her again in the afternoon, she declined, saying she really did not feel like driving in the camper. I said okay, I would drive to the nursery myself then and be right back. And I would consider the time it took as part of her gift to me. With that understanding, I departed for Christianson's, selected 16 plants recommended and collected by Andrew at the nursery and headed directly home, pleased with both the little time it took and the selection. I was finally going to have my butterfly garden!

I walked in the door excited to show Joan the array of plants I had lined up next to the garden space. I was surprised to be met by an angry wife who wanted to know why it had taken so long and why I had not asked her to accompany me. She denied I had ever asked her and said that in fact I had pulled this same trick on her last Father's Day. I had no idea what she was talking about and after an exasperating five minutes of shouting charges and counter charges, I told her I was going upstairs to read and write. A half hour later, she was calling upstairs to ask if I was hungry and wanted to eat. I came down and began putting together the lunch items she had heated up in the oven but not before she came up to me, hugging me and tilting her face up for a kiss. She seemed to have forgotten our recent brouhaha which was all right with me. I showed her the plants eventually. She was even more pleased when, a few days later, I had them all in the ground arranged according to Andrew's instructions. Oh yes, I did kiss the proffered cheek, gladly.

June 23, 2010

The doctor, after listening to my recount of all that had occurred over the weekend and reviewing the glucose record I had been keeping, concluded two things: we should continue with the five units per day of the Levemir insulin and try to control the higher glucose levels with a fast-release insulin called Novolog. The ideal glucose level was between 100 and 200 mg. Whenever Joan's level got higher than 200 mg, I was to inject Novolog according to a certain formula. Neither she nor I liked the injection routine but I was getting better at it and, under the circumstances, it made good sense. I had recently learned from another diabetic that there were two kinds if insulin, slow-release and fast-release, and that he took both with satisfactory results. It worked.

June 24, 2010

At 1:00 am Joan came into my room to report she did not feel well. How was she "not well?" I asked. "Weak, sweaty," was her response. With those last words I quickly ran downstairs for orange juice and blood draw equipment. After she drank six oz. of juice, I checked her glucose level. It was low as expected: 44 mg. I gave her part of a second glass. Within five minutes she said she was feeling better. Within ten minutes she wanted additional covers. I would check her again in another 30 minutes or so. Why the low count, I wondered. She was 309 after supper. I had injected her with the usual 5 units of Levemir before bedtime. At 1:50 am Joan's blood sugar was back up to 110 mg and she said she felt fine. I turned off her light but would check her again in another half hour when I finished this report.

Last night was the museum's annual Volunteer Appreciation Supper at the nearby Civic Garden Club. I rearranged my schedule, working in the afternoon instead of the morning. During the course of the afternoon, Joan phoned me numerous times, asking where I was and at one point apparently set out to find me but was confused (about where the Civic Garden Club building was) so returned home. It was becoming clear that I must either quit my job at the museum and stay home or find someone to stay with her during my absence. Our daughter Susan was researching the Veterans Affairs website for information on their Home Care Program that might provide some coverage for a caregiver.

Two observations: the Novolog seemed to work well. Yesterday morning, Joan's glucose level had been 275 after breakfast. I gave her a 3 unit injection. One and a half hours later, her blood sugar had dropped to 187. I had started to feel more confident about controlling her glucose level. But after this morning's experience, I was less confident though thankful for what I was learning (and for orange juice!). The other observation: she was hungrier these last few days. I no sooner would finish cleaning up after a meal and begin one project or another that Joan would say she was hungry and needed to eat something. However, she would eat only a few bites of what I fixed. Before long, she would feel like she wanted something more to eat but she was not sure what. It was not surprising that she was craving chocolate drops from the jar that I kept on the counter for baking purposes as well as her favorite desert, ice cream. So far she had resisted temptation. It may have helped that I removed the chocolate chips from view and easy access. Occasionally she would ask for a glass of wine but did not pursue it after I mentioned what it would do to her glucose level.

July 6, 2010

At our next visit to the doctor, a new strategy was decided upon: eliminate the use of the slow-release insulin (Levemir) altogether using only the fast-release insulin (Novolog) as needed. After each meal and before bedtime I monitored Joan's blood sugar and injected her with insulin based on a certain scale: the higher the blood sugar count, the more insulin units. The strategy seemed to be working—producing fewer extreme glucose readings and, in some cases, not requiring insulin injection at all. It had probably helped too that Joan's diet was veering away from higher glycemic carbohydrates while eating more oatmeal and cinnamon in muffins and as a snack before bed. Last night she had weighed herself on the bathroom scale. For the first time in many months (years, even) she hit 90 pounds! A good sign surely but it did not seem to translate into increased strength or stability. On our walks her tolerance for walking on gravel or any slightly uneven surface was less and less. At a July fourth gathering we were invited to, she seemed to feel threatened by the presence of a big, friendly dog as well as several smaller dogs who were constantly underfoot and she had even less tolerance for the noise and confusion of a large number of kids and adults in the small living room and kitchen. We stayed for an hour and made our excuses. Although challenged by having unexpectedly to prepare a meal at home, I shared Joan's pleasure at arriving back to the peace and quiet.

July 10, 2010

Driving alone to Haggen's, a supermarket in Burlington, was admittedly pleasant, although unintended. Joan had been agreeable to getting groceries late on Saturday afternoon but just before we departed the house a most unusual thing happened. A young deer, a three-point buck, showed up in our backyard, curled up and relaxed (as much as an alert deer could) in full view out our dining room window. After a 30-minute delay while we were totally absorbed in deer-watching, we reluctantly headed for the car. At the last second, just as Joan was getting in the front seat, she changed her mind and decided she did not want to leave the deer and urged me to go ahead and get the shopping done.

Joan did okay most mornings during the week when I was at the museum so I took her up on her suggestion. Shopping without Joan was much easier, less distracting, in that I did not have to worry about her whereabouts. Several times we had gotten separated within the store and had spent anxious minutes looking for each other. It was also the case lately that she tired quickly and wanted to leave before I had completed the shopping.

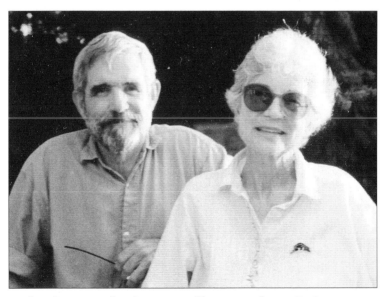

Bob and Joan seated at their picnic table enjoying the sun. LaConner, 1988

Hiking

Hiking up and down the smooth, well-marked paths,
looking left and right as we go, along the lardered aisles,

identifying some of the things that line the steep hillocks,
colorful and varied in size, a safe way—no bears for miles—

to stretch our legs, and fill our minds, for an hour or so.
For in this walled world where the sun perpetually shines,

glinting off the abundance it holds, and the temperature
is always constant, slightly bold—just a little short of cold—

there are no wilderness regulations, no rangers to contact,
no prohibitions to staunch our free will, here we can

pick and choose, keep and covet, or if we decide we don't
like something we can shove it, put it back, without complaint.

We can even stop, now and then, to rest and bivouac,
gathering around the deli fire to sip coffee and munch a

trail side snack and get our bearings for the final leg of the
morning's spree, then, finally, wheeling our backpack

carward, to the trailhead, relieved, but surprised, too, after
paying, what seems, each time, like a higher user's fee.

After arriving at Haggen's parking lot, I phoned Joan. She was surprised that I had only just arrived there. I explained to her I had taken an extra 20 minutes to get her car (the Saab) washed. I used my cell again after I completed the shopping (another 40 minutes) to let her know I was on my way. She could not understand why it had taken so long. Upon arriving home, Joan was visibly upset, angry that I had left her behind. I explained what had been the case, that she had decided to stay behind. She argued that I had intentionally driven off without her. On top of that, she said, several strange men showed up in the back yard and she had been frightened. She could not remember what they wanted. I had no idea who the men might have been or whether in fact there had been any men at all. Additionally, she had been drinking wine, forgetting how that worked against her glucose battle. My conclusion: do not leave Joan alone again for that length of time.

July 12, 2010

Our life together was not always so bizarre or off-centered. There were times, particularly at night after we had climbed into bed (aboard our "nightship," I liked to think), we often had some normal conversations, pillow talk at its finest, times when memory was not an issue. Other times there was no conversation at all, when passion for each other simply took over, consuming us for a brief burst of time. Afterwards, we rested contentedly, naked against one another, totally amazed (and proud too) that there was still this sizzle between us in our mid-80s. Who would believe it? We did not even believe it ourselves.

Love Is Like That: Union

Forgetting to forgive, forgiving to forget,
neither is the lover's way.
Was, is always there, between,
to counter any final say.

In intimacy's tight embrace,
dark memories race
to disappear,
squeezed to dust
by passion's redeeming power.

The particles draw upward, cloud bent,
only to gather and fall gently
upon the spent,
wet as rain, cooling the lover's brow.

Like pebbles worn smooth by the ocean's rhythm,
yesterday's sharp-edged images,
friction prone, are rubbed round
by nature's universal beat.

The crashing surf, lapping waves,
the pounding flesh, gentle after strokes,
both polish the past,
gleaming it to manageable proportion.

July 16, 2010

Joan's follow-up appointment with her doctor at his La Conner office was a further effort to fine-tune her insulin injections. The first step had been to eliminate the Levemir (slow-acting) insulin and use only the Novolog (fast-acting) when indicated an hour or so after meals and at bedtime. Now I was to give Joan the insulin immediately after meals (when glucose levels required it) pretty much on the same scale as before. The idea here was to prevent the peaks in glucose levels by injecting the insulin earlier, the peak in the insulin's effectiveness matching the glucose's peak ninety minutes after eating. I did not think the doctor had ever tried anything like this before but I liked the creativity he brought to it. Joan's situation was unique (no obesity issues, to begin with) and demanded an unique solution. I liked as well his intention to monitor closely her progress. She had another appointment next week.

July 21, 2010

At the next appointment, I described to the doctor my alarm when I tested Joan's blood Sunday after lunch. Having given Joan two small pancakes and low-sugar syrup for Sunday breakfast, I expected the blood sugar reading to be in the 200s. Instead, the monitor read "Hi." I referred immediately to my instruction booklet for an interpretation. It was hardly a friendly greeting. Quite the opposite. It was a warning! "Hi" meant that the glucose level was at 600 mg or higher and a physician needed to be consulted without delay. The clinic doctor on duty listened to my explanation of her colleague's strategy and calculated accordingly. I immediately injected Joan with 8 units of insulin. The insulin did its job all too well. At the next reading, an hour or so later, Joan's glucose had dropped to 96 mg! I quickly gave Joan two ounces of orange juice and her glucose soon leveled out and remained more or less even since. The doctor did not think Sunday's breakfast would cause such a radical jump. I did not either but it made me even more cautious about carbohydrate intake.

Last night proved to be another one of those moments when Joan became acutely aware of her condition. She was tired so we headed upstairs to bed about 8:30 pm where I read to her for some time, eventually moving to my own bed in the study. About 10:30 pm the hall light startled me awake. Joan stood next to my bed and asked where her mother was. I told her that she had died many years ago as had her father.

Obviously restless and upset, I returned to her bed where I rubbed her back and shoulders while she asked a series of revealing questions. Her first one was to ask who I was. She thought I was her brother. She was relieved to know that her sister, Patti, was still alive and living in Salina, Kansas. Did she have any children? As in all her questions, I answered in detail, naming the children, their families and where they lived. Where did the money come from that allowed us to live so comfortably? Who managed the house and cooked the meals? Was she ever in the WAVES? After my answers, she could only conclude that she was really losing it, that she felt increasingly like she had landed on a strange planet. How had it happened that she was experiencing memory loss? I said it had been gradual which was not unusual among the elderly. She wanted to assign the memory loss to some specific cause and was sure that at some point she had cracked her head against the car's windshield or dashboard. Didn't I remember her being treated for it? What can be done about memory loss? Not much, I said. There were a few medicines on the market but they did not sound promising. Joan needed little time to recognize how critical I was to her well being and expressed her gratitude for sticking with her even if she was ruining my life. This notion I quickly dispelled. She was not "messing up" (her word) my life. We were in this together. We were going to love our way through it wherever it took us. Before long Joan's sense of gratitude translated into wanting to be close to me, physically. At 1:00 am, against all reason, we were wide awake, her hands alerting me once again to passion's soaring power. Frail and forgetful? Not Joan. At that moment she was queen of the universe, focused and intent. By 2:00 am we were in our pajamas once more, bed clothes rearranged and able, for a few hours, to forget what was out there ahead of us.

July 28, 2010

Over the past four days Joan had been preoccupied with concern about her brother Bill, at various points asking where he was living now and wondering if he might be able get out here to La Conner for a visit. Each query I met with the fact that Bill had died some months ago now (before his 90th birthday June 1, 2010) and that Terry Lee, his adopted daughter, had seen to funeral arrangements. He was buried with full military honors at the cemetery at Fort Snelling in Minneapolis. Still the questions persisted. Shouldn't she call her sister, Patti, to let her know that Bill had died? I told her that Terri Lee had already done that, notifying Patti at the same time she had notified us months ago. Still Joan tried several times to phone Patti but she was never home. At one point, she had once again dialed Patti's number and then turned to me to ask what she was calling her about. At another time Joan wondered why Patti couldn't take care of Terri Lee now that Bill had died. I explained to Joan that Terri Lee was older now, happily married with adult children of her own. Joan seemed relieved but an hour later was raising the same issue again concerning Terri Lee's welfare and how Patti, a little younger, might be able to take care of her. Was Bill no longer living? What about her brother Don and her oldest brother Jack, were they dead too? Again, I repeated the facts. Don had died a few months before Bill and Jack a number of years before that. I really did not mind being the bearer of bad news repeatedly but the devastated look on her face each time I did, made me extremely sad, wishing I had the power to overcome her discomfort.

Joan's discomfort soon took another turn with increasing pain in her lower stomach. After a day of that, we were able to get to the clinic. A urine test revealed infection somewhere in the bladder or urine tract and an antibiotic (Cipro) was prescribed. Within 5 days the pain had subsided to be replaced the last several days by lower back pain, sometimes severe and immobilizing, at other times only faintly bothersome. I made an appointment to see the doctor to check it out. And so continued what appeared to be the dominant domestic rhythm of old age, moving from one doctor's appointment to another, the pattern broken only with trips to the grocery store.

July 31, 2010

After repeated discussions with Joan, I canceled the appointment. The fact that the back pain came and went seemed to rule out internal organ problems, a major concern, and it seemed that with rest and Tylenol Joan would weather the spasms, waiting them out until the pain lessened and normalcy returned. That was how it had worked out in my case in any event. Not Joan, however. Friday the lower back pain became worse. The doctor, at my request, prescribed a relaxant (Cyclobenzaprine), a half pill (5 mg) at bedtime. The half seemed to have no effect. Last night she tried a whole pill on top of the half pill and still no relief. As a result, Joan (and I) were up often during the night, with me helping her out of bed and back into bed (after frequent trips to the bathroom), each effort so painful that Joan ended up in my lower twin bed with the Tempur-pedic mattress. I slept, or tried to, in Joan's old bed, with one ear cocked to hear Joan's slightest groan. After a decent breakfast, Joan returned to the sofa in the front room and, like yesterday, slept through the morning. I was looking for signs of change, some easing of the pain. So far I had not seen it.

I completed today my application for health benefits from the Department of Veterans Affairs in the hope I could get help for Joan during my mornings at work. Joan had done well most mornings so far but I had begun to see changes, her sense of loneliness and growing inability to entertain herself among them. Her confusion around the kitchen continued but I was not going to worry about it as long as she stayed away from our gas stove. But would she?

August 1, 2010

Last night went much better. Getting settled in her big bed was painful but after a back rub, a very gentle one, she slept until about midnight. At that point, she took two more Tylenol, and with another soft rubdown, slept until 3:30 am which fit nicely with my morning schedule (I usually would arise around 3:30, shower, do floor exercises and then write until 5:30 or so, followed by a good walk/run or workout at the fitness center). Another gentle backstroking and Joan went quickly back to sleep. So it seemed like she may be on the road to improvement. I hoped so for the lack of sleep really knocked me out these days.

I made a huge decision yesterday but it seemed like the right one: I decided to begin notifying my neighbors that I was shutting down the Buns of Skeele Home Bakery effective immediately. I realized I needed more time to write in the mornings before work and I had been putting myself under a lot of pressure trying to bake and deliver a dozen or so muffins to friends every morning along with one of my own poems of the week. I planned to keep baking, of course, but at a much more leisurely pace, my attention focused now on getting one last book completed and published. I would miss the satisfaction derived from knowing how much many of my "customers" enjoyed and appreciated the high quality muffins, warm from the oven, for their breakfast along with a poem to read and, in some cases, to actually discuss.

August 2, 2010

I had anticipated that Sunday would bring improvement but, instead, Joan's lower back was even more painful and immobilizing. The Cyclobenzaprine did not seem to help whatsoever and the Tylenol did little if anything to limit the pain. She felt most comfortable lying on the leather sofa in the front room, but getting in a prone position on it was, each time, obviously excruciating and accompanied by involuntary cries. She compared it to the pain at childbirth. With each move during the day, Joan needed my help, holding her arm, easing her into a chair. Her appetite disappeared sometime after a breakfast of Belgian waffles and coffee. Joan could only nibble at the food at lunch and supper except for ice cream, the one food she always seemed to enjoy. All in all, a terrible weekend. It seemed obvious now that a serious painkiller was in order. It was equally clear that Joan's back needed careful attention beginning probably with a scan. I had winced at the thought of getting Joan in the car to see the doctor if in fact he could see her today.

August 4, 2010

Although Joan's doctor was not on duty, his wife, a physician's assistant, was available, but it meant traveling to Anacortes for a 2:30 pm appointment. Joan had said she never wanted to have to drive to Anacortes again but of course we did just that the next morning. The physician's assistant did exactly what I had hoped she would do: took a urine sample (which showed the presence of white cells, but I wondered what kind of white cells), authorized a back ex-ray (lumbar/thoracic area) and blood work, then gave Joan prescriptions for back pain (Vicodin) and the urinary infection (more Cipro) until she got the lab results. With the painkiller in her veins Joan did really well, although I was struck once again by how frail she had become, walking ever so slowly and gingerly, holding my arm or hand every step of the way. Helping her to disrobe and redress for the x-ray procedure at the hospital put an exclamation point on her degree of dependency now. By the time the hospital visit had concluded, she was visibly tired and complained of feeling weak. She did not want to eat at the hospital cafeteria, The Island Bistro, preferring to get home for lunch. My intermediate solution was to stop at Bob's Chowder House for some of his excellent New England clam chowder on the way out of town. Joan enjoyed the soup soon after our arrival home but ate very little. I, on the other hand, had two bowls of the delicious stuff. Perhaps, I thought, Joan would want the rest of it tomorrow for lunch. I kept hoping against hope she would begin eating more one of these days but it did not seem likely.

Joan said she enjoyed the evening out, literally, as we were invited to a five o'clock barbecue in the backyard of a neighbor who was one of my appreciative muffin customers. She had purchased the house of John Pedersen, my old friend, from his estate and closed the deal on my birthday. She had been making improvements on the property ever since, starting with landscaping and the creation of a beautiful round, flagstone patio where we ate a meal of grilled pork chops and slices of marinated sweet potatoes and big juicy chunks of watermelon. Joan ate about half the serving which was good for her, but enjoyed the rose wine most of all in spite of my cautions.

After the full day we retired early (About 8:00 pm). I read to Joan from Ivan Doig's newest book *Work Song* for awhile, turning off the light about 9:00 pm. An hour later, Joan was awake; a pattern of sleeping and waking through the night followed. At one point, she was certain she heard voices downstairs, at another, she wondered where Beth (our daughter-in-law) and her child were sleeping. A third time, she came into my back bedroom to ask where Bob was. At 4:00 am she was taking a shower, thinking it was time to get up. Obviously a confusing time. She opted to return to bed and slept a little longer, but before she did she asked me to tell her what was going on. She said she felt totally lost. I explained that we were in La Conner, in her favorite old house and that she was having trouble remembering. Like many of us as we grow older she was experiencing dementia but that right now she should not worry about it since I was going to remember for both of us. Is there anything that can be done about it, she wanted to know. Not much, I thought, but I said I was going to look into it.

Joan got up and joined me for breakfast but she ate only a single muffin (usually she would have 2 or 3) and did not look or feel well with a lot of back pain. She did not mind if I went to work at the museum for an hour or so. I promised I would keep in touch by cell phone and would notify her walking pal that she did not feel like walking today. Her pal, who lived just two blocks from us, was happy to change her plans and ended up stopping by for a visit which Joan told me later she really enjoyed.

I had talked with the museum director and would take the rest of the week off. It was becoming clear that I would need help caring for Joan whether or not I was able to continue at the museum. She indicated to me that she would not mind having someone else in the house to be with her if it meant I could continue working and earning the extra money (which, given the economy, was a lot less "extra" than it used to be).

August 5, 2010

Joan spent the remainder of the morning and most of the afternoon resting on the couch in the front room. In general, she seemed preoccupied, even listless, due, I suspected, to a combination of the drugs and not eating. At lunch she could not eat the clam chowder because the bits of clam were too tough so she removed them from her mouth and lined them up around the rim of her dinner plate. I then made a (turkey) bacon and lettuce sandwich which she said she would like, but then ate only a bite or two. Later, for supper, thinking to entice her, I made a scalloped oyster dish but before I could get it on the table, I realized Joan had double-dosed inadvertently, on the Vicodin which alarmed me for fear that she might, due to her small size and lack of food, move from drowsiness to a complete shutdown. To counter the Vicodin she drank some milk and ate a few saltines. She became too drowsy to eat, of course, but eventually she revived enough for me to put her to bed where she slept soundly until about 2:30 am. Concerned about her glucose level at this point, I drew some blood from her finger. With relief, I read 104 on the monitor. The back pain had returned so I gave her a single pain pill (I did not dare give her two pills with so little food in her stomach) and then crawled carefully into bed to rub her back which seemed to help. She is sleeping easily as I write this.

August 6, 2010

The Friday appointment with the doctor revealed nothing special. The urine infection was not internal, i.e., not in the urinary tract, so the Cipro was no longer necessary. The blood test revealed only a slightly elevated liver reading, otherwise it was normal and the x-ray confirmed what we already knew: the spine, due to osteoporosis, was continuing to degenerate. The pain was likely to continue, the only counter was to increase the Vicodin from two pills every four hours to 3 pills up to a maximum of 12 daily. I was surprised that Joan did not react at all when the doctor prodded none too gently the length of her spine and the lower right side under the ribs.

Joan seemed today even more confused and unable to track conversation. Part of it had to be her poor hearing, but so far she had refused to have her hearing checked. Physically, she looked unwell, pale and hardly able to move around and then only when I held her hand or arm to steady her. As usual, she barely ate the sandwich and soup I prepared for her but enjoyed a small cup of vanilla ice cream. She would now probably sleep away most of the afternoon on the sofa in the front room.

The writing was on the wall: it was unlikely that Joan could be home alone during the five mornings I was at work. Getting someone to cover my work hours at $12/hour amounted to about $250/week which was about what I earned. I might as well quit my job and stay home unless the VA could take up the slack. I had thought it would be a while yet before we reached this point but here we were suddenly with few options.

August 7, 2010

Yesterday afternoon seemed particularly worrisome. Joan rested until about 4 pm and then moved into the dining room as I began meal preparation in the kitchen closeby. She began reading to me aloud from the La Conner Weekly News and during and after every article would comment on how "crazy" it was. Neither the articles nor their juxtaposition to each other seemed to make any sense to her. At one point she read the article I had written ("How the Town Turkeys Led to Good Music") pronouncing the author's name as if I were a stranger, a third party. At some point, she concluded that she was the "Joan" referred to in the story and was upset, informing me that she was going to sue me since I did not have her permission to use her name. I had read the article to her earlier (which she had said she liked) and after I told her Sandy, the editor, had liked it and was going to print it, she had raised no objection. Just the opposite, she had seemed pleased. But, of course, she was unable to remember any of that and appeared to cling to the suspicion that I had made the whole thing up.

When Joan decided to rest on the sofa some more, I asked again how she was feeling. She said she was not feeling well, that she felt "used," and "played with" by me. I tried to reassure her otherwise but she was not buying it. Later, at supper, the animosity seemed to have disappeared, replaced with her effort to eat at least a few bites of the meat loaf and baked potato I had prepared. A few bites was about it. She did not touch the string beans and took only a nibble or two from a cooked carrot. As the chef, I despaired. I kept thinking that there were some meals out there that Joan would like if I could just find the right combination. I decided I would try some halibut cheeks for dinner, compliments of our son in Alaska. She sometimes ate more of her meal when I served fish fried or in the form of fish cakes.

This morning at 5:30 am Joan was awake which gave me the chance to give her some Vicodin and rub her back with an analgesic balm which she found soothing, her anger of yesterday forgotten or buried. It was clear that the management of her back pain would need to include a lot of massage with effective ointments and heat.

August 11, 2010

Joan's eating was not improving in the least. The halibut was excellent but she ate little. I followed it the next night with one of her favorites, spinach ricotta pie from the *Moosewood Cookbook*, but no luck. She just ate a few bites of the filling and maybe half of a small fruit salad, ignoring the lettuce altogether as something specifically to avoid. I had told her that her poor eating habits were going to lead to a peck of trouble. She said she could not help it. She just was not hungry, period. I noticed with surprise that she was even cutting back on vanilla ice cream. I had served her the usual modest bowl full, and, as she had been doing lately, she had me put half of it back in the ice cream container. Again, I asked myself, was Joan unconsciously starving herself?

August 16, 2010

For a few days. I thought maybe Joan was recovering a little lost ground. She seemed to be eating a little more and was sleeping well through the night. Then, the night before last, she was restless again, thinking Susan, our daughter, was staying at the house with her son and worried that they had not returned for the night. My efforts to reassure her that Susan was safe in Santa Fe never were accepted. She was also experiencing severe dry mouth where even gargling with Biotene and drinking plenty of water was uncomfortable. The restlessness seemed to have abated once again and as hot as it was at night (We were in the midst of a record heat wave), she slept through it. The eating had gotten worse however. She managed to eat one of my muffins in the morning along with a cup of coffee but that was it. At noon, today (by way of example) she could not eat even a bite of a hot pizza slice or take a spoon of black bean soup. It was all I could do to get her to eat a small dish of ice cream. Meanwhile she said she was very tired and spent most of the afternoon sleeping. She looked terrible, her face was pale and drawn and I had told her as much. She simply had to eat. If she was unable to, then it seemed I had no choice but to put her in the hospital so that she could be fed intravenously. It seemed at this point that the vicodin she was taking for her back pain plus the insulin to fight her slightly higher blood sugar count complicated her condition. Surely both medicines were formulated assuming a normal intake of food. I had a call in for the doctor. Alarm bells were going off in my head and my heart rate was up. Joan continued to sleep on the sofa in the afternoon heat. Was I losing my sweetheart? I wondered if she would even make it to our 59th wedding anniversary on September ninth.

August 18, 2010

Neither the nurse nor the doctor phoned back. I learned later that the doctor had hospital duty this week and was not available even for consultation. During the course of the day, Joan seemed to feel increasingly bad which was not surprising. She had not touched her breakfast and lunch. At her request, urgent now, I was able to make an appointment at our clinic with a physician's assistant. I alerted her through the staff nurse that I hoped she would see the wisdom of urging Joan to admit herself to the hospital.

Joan weighed in at the clinic at 83.6 lbs., down about 4 lbs. from two weeks ago. The assistant did her part. First, she analyzed a sample of Joan's urine to see if the infection had returned (This could cause loss of appetite) and then she urged hospitalization. As expected, Joan's reaction was a vehement "No." She was not about to go to the hospital and pick up somebody else's disease!

Upon our return home, Joan retired to the couch and I began supper preparation, thinking foolishly that she might eat a little something this time. Just after we sat down to eat, however, our son, David, phoned from Slippery Rock. Interestingly, Joan reported to him that she was feeling okay and still doing her daily walk (neither of which was true). By the time the phone conversation ended, the food was cold and she had eaten little. Joan did manage to eat a small bowl of ice cream. Before long (around 7:30 pm), Joan said she was ready for bed. I joined her soon after, finding pajamas for her and reading aloud to her in bed (Ivan Doig's book). My strategy was now clear: When Joan next expressed the need for medical attention, I was going to take her directly to the ER at Island Hospital. It was the only solution. I expected that to happen today (if she did not collapse from malnourishment first). I also intended to phone David (and Matt) to update them on the seriousness of Joan's condition.

It should be noted for the record that the urine analysis was negative and that Joan's blood sugar level for the day was in the low 100's (123 and 107 respectively).

August 20, 2010

Today was not one of Joan's better days. She spent the morning and afternoon in her pajamas and oversized sweatshirt, too shaky and unsteady to shower and dress. It was when Joan was moving to the wicker sofa to rest that I suggested we go to the ER to begin the process of finding out what was wrong; with no appetite and losing weight, the issue was getting serious and needed serious attention. Joan concurred, reluctantly. By 4:00 pm we were on our way to the Island Hospital in Anacortes after notifying the medical clinic of our plan.

With minimal procedure, Joan was admitted to the ER and was soon gowned and in her mobile bed. Eventually, the ER doctor appeared and the questions and testing began—chest x-ray and blood draw—and, at the doctor's request, an IV (sodium chloride solution) was hooked up. Then began a long, torturous wait for the private room Joan had been assigned. Apparently, four new patients had been admitted to the hospital at about the same time as Joan. It was not until 9:00 pm, some four hours later, that Joan was finally wheeled to her room on the second floor of the new wing. The wait had seemed longer due to Joan's repeated questions and my repeated efforts to reassure her. She wanted to forego this whole tiresome business and return home. By this time I did not blame her. I departed for home at 9:30 pm with Joan and the pleasant young duty nurse talking and getting acquainted.

Arriving home to the empty house, I warmed up a small piece of leftover pizza, ate a few chips and a slice of a friend's homemade chocolate cake which she had left along with a note at our front door. Just as I was climbing into bed at 10:45 pm, the telephone rang. It was Joan. She wanted me to come and get her right away. There was no need for her to remain in the hospital overnight, she reasoned, since her doctor would not see her until the next morning anyway. I told her that I was simply too tired at this point to do any more driving and, besides, the doctor may want to continue the IV through the night. Obviously disappointed and unhappy, Joan hung-up, the anxiety in her voice ringing in my ears. In the hope she would settle down, I fell asleep the minute my head hit the pillow.

I awoke at 3:30 am, as I most always do, to write. Five minutes later the phone rang. Oh no, I thought, another false alarm at the museum. Wrong. It was not Dictograph but the night nurse. Joan was restless, agitated, disoriented and would not allow her to reattach the IV which she had pulled from her arm. Could I come to the hospital now? Joan's doctor, whom she had apparently phoned first, thought my presence might calm Joan down. It did not take me long to shower and dress. By 4:30 am I was at Joan's bedside once again. She was pleased—relieved would be the word—to see me and, at my urging, was soon resting, even sleeping for an hour or two. Now, at 7:30 am, she did not recognize the room or remember why she was there rather than at the hospital in Mount Vernon. I explained that we had always had a preference for Island Hospital and it was also the hospital that her doctor worked out of.

Our son, David, phoned on my cell. His home line had been down yesterday which was why I could not reach him after repeated tries. David encouraged his mother to stick with the plan. Soon thereafter, the doctor came in, sat down and tried to get Joan to focus on what he saw as the issue. First, the test results were all negative. He could order some further tests but they did not seem warranted. Secondly, Joan was at a crossroad which he did not feel she really appreciated. He could understand that she might not want to use a feed tube in her side but it would be a way to obtain the necessary nourishment. Joan was adamantly opposed to a feeding tube. The only other alternative was to continue as she was, understanding that she would continue to lose weight until her organs began to fail and that would be that. He urged us to consider pulling Hospice into the planning at some point soon. He agreed that home care through Veterans Affairs or some other agency which would allow me to keep working was a sensible intermediate step, but he wanted to be sure Joan understood the inevitable result of continuing as she had been. Another friend whose wife was now under the care of Hospice echoed the same sentiment. Joan's predicament was irreversible. The few things I had read regarding anorexia among the elderly suggested the same thing.

Joan was relieved to be back home in the old, familiar surroundings. She was able to eat half of a tuna fish sandwich and a little soup for lunch and ate even less for supper with the promise to do better tomorrow. I continued to be perplexed. Joan seemed to have the will to eat, she wanted to eat, but her body just seemed to shut down after a few bites. I was planning now to meet with close friends, together with our son, Matt, who would be visiting here over the weekend, to develop a strategy for the next months that would help Joan and allow me to work.

August 25, 2010

The meeting with my friends never materialized. Sunday morning, Joan awoke feeling nauseous with severe chills but no fever. After consulting the weekend duty doctor, I decided, with Joan's agreement, to readmit her to Island Hospital, grabbing the last bed that morning. A CAT scan that afternoon revealed a distended bladder which a catheter soon solved. Almost immediately Joan looked and felt better and even ate a little beef stew and peas. She would not, however, consent to stay overnight at the hospital to follow through with more IV and the continued use of a catheter and, in fact, became extremely agitated at one point, insisting on getting out of bed to urinate (which was unnecessary of course), threatening to pull the IV tube and catheter with her. When I attempted to restrain her, she slapped away at my hands and arms repeatedly, saying if I did not let her go she was going to leave me. I told her to go ahead and do that but right now she had to remain still. Shortly thereafter, she was once again discharged from the hospital, this time with a prescription from the doctor for home care services. By 8:30 pm Sunday evening, she was back home, tired but seeming to feel somewhat better judging from a return of her appetite, slight though it was.

By the next night, however, she was back to her "normal," eating very little of the baked salmon and the special side dishes her son had created—Portuguese potatoes with mint and a tossed salad. She slept soundly Monday night but felt bad, extremely tired and listless upon waking with no enthusiasm for showering, dressing or eating.

Two nurses from Island Hospital met with Joan and me for an hour or so to evaluate Joan's situation and to acquaint us with the hospital's other home services such as physical therapy. They said they were going to see that Joan got more frequent visits during the next weeks and might consult with Hospice to see if an informational visit from them would be beneficial at this point. Meanwhile, Group Health phoned to offer their advisory services. An RN, they informed me, was on duty all the time to answer questions that might arise during Joan's care. Many suggestions were made about how to get Joan to eat, which all recognized was the main issue and challenge. So far I have had no luck. Last night, for example, I baked a Russet potato and fried some bacon, both of which she identified as favorite foods, but to no avail. She ate only part of the half potato on her plate and less than one strip of the bacon. She was able to eat a small dish of vanilla ice cream. It was when watching her across the dining room table in one of those rare, stark, unadorned moments of truth that I concluded, with an unspeakably profound sadness, that Joan was not going to make it. She was bent on starving herself. "I can't help it," she said, "I'm not hungry. I just can't eat." We went up to bed after 8:00 pm. I fell asleep rubbing her back. She awakened me an hour later; she felt unsteady and needed my help to make her way to the bathroom and back.

The initial nurse visit was followed by two more. These nurses would be Joan's case nurse and our primary contact. Both nurses were attentive and savvy. They saw the need for a physical therapist and the need for a walker to avoid any falls. They were equally concerned about the steep stairway leading to the second floor. It was the case nurse who suggested we move both twin beds downstairs soon to the front room and purchase a baby monitor to use when I was upstairs writing. It was the case nurse, too, who said privately to me that Joan's decline was apt to go on a long time which made it harder for me as her primary caregiver and cautioned me to make sure I did not get consumed by it. At this point, Joan insisted that she wanted no one else in the house watching over her. Until yesterday, Sunday, I had been inclined to go along for awhile, letting her manage alone while I was at work during the morning hours. Sunday, however, Joan awoke feeling bad and did not improve during the course of the day. She slept in her new (twin) bed in the front room a good bit of the morning, getting up only to have tea with a concerned neighbor who visited for a pleasant hour. After a meager lunch she returned to sleep a good bit of the afternoon as well.

I am indebted to a close friend who came over to our house for a couple of hours Saturday afternoon to help me move the twin beds downstairs and the marble top chests of drawers upstairs. At 6'3" and several hundred pounds, my friend made quick work of the whole project. Our reward afterwards was to sit down to mugs of cold draft Guinness and some cheese and chips, a pleasant interlude. Joan joined us with a cup of tea. She was as excited as I was by the new furniture arrangement and slept well the inaugural night with me in the twin bed right next to hers and no steps to worry about. The following night, however, was a nightmare. At about midnight,

Joan awoke complaining that she was cold. I put a comforter over her, the same one she used upstairs, and she said it would not do. It was too heavy. Then a whole series of complaints followed—her head pillow was too large, the pillow she used between her knees was too big, the sheet was too wide, etc. With each complaint I tried other remedies but nothing seemed to work. Joan was clearly distressed and wondering what was going on. So was I. Finally, after repeating various combinations of covers and pillows and giving her a mild sleeping pill, she settled down. So eventually did I, thinking that I could not, after all, let Joan manage by herself for any length of time.

As I wrote this section it was 7:15 am and Joan was still asleep. No way was I going to be able to get to the museum today. I would need others to help Joan manage if I was to continue employment. Joan's home care nurse was due today. Perhaps I needed to consider making use of Hospice's services earlier rather than later.

August 31, 2010

The morning did not begin well. I had been upstairs writing at about 7:30 am waiting for Joan to awaken. She surprised me by coming up the stairs and joining me for a few minutes. Since she had not showered the day before, she decided to shower this morning. She managed to get in and out of the shower by herself but complained of nausea. A few more minutes and she began vomiting, dry heaves really, since there was no food to eject. I helped her get dressed and walked her downstairs to the dining room and the wicker chair while I made her breakfast starting with liquids, water, orange juice and coffee. Later she ate most of two muffins.

Both the restlessness during the night and the vomiting in the morning were worrisome. As to the former, the home care nurse recommended to Joan's doctor that she have available a mild sedative to reduce her anxiety when necessary. And regarding the latter, the nurse thought it would be better, starting now, for Joan to shower only after she has had something to eat, which made perfect sense. Joan seemed to suffer no ill effects from either episode and, as the day wore on, could not recall anything about either one. Getting her to eat enough to sustain her remained the key goal. Ice cream remained a favorite food along with chocolate pudding. At lunch Joan rediscovered Jell-O and at the same meal managed to eat almost 3/4's of her BLT sandwich. At supper, Joan did not do nearly as well, eating very little of the fish and chips (the fish, fresh frozen cod delivered by our son John from Alaska).

In the course of one of our telephone conversations during the day, the home care nurse reminded me of our objectives in Joan's case: keep her comfortable. Hospitalization was not an option and her health, due to lack of food, would decline over time. I hated looking too far into the future but I had to, enough at least to make sensible plans which Hospice could help me with. When should I call them in, and how, without alarming Joan?

September

September brings us the first day
of autumn and the start of school,
its ember the hint of color in the
pin oak leaves on the tree next door
and, after a few days of summer's
lingering return, the promise of
cooler, crisper air.

It is within this ember of similar
splendor that we wed, my wife
and I, so many years ago. To the
music of Bach, we went forth,
bowing to fate,
vowing to date,
in perpetual romance,
whatever the circumstance,
be we sick or healthy,
poor or wealthy.

September 25, 2010

I was surprised it had been more than three weeks since my last entry. There was a reason for it: Joan seemed to have hit a plateau with nothing much to report. On the upside, I began giving Joan a single pill (.5 mg) of Lorazepam at night which completely eliminated the restlessness at bedtime. She had also begun eating a little better from time to time which showed in her weight gain. Two days ago the scale read 83 pounds. On the downside, her blood sugar occasionally spiked. Last night, for example, it skyrocketed to 393. I reacted by injecting her with 5 units of insulin. An hour and a half later, her blood glucose read only 87 which I countered with 4 ounces of orange juice. I hated these flare-ups partly because I could not entirely account for them. I would think I was on the right track dietarily and then, whammo! The solution was obviously in the direction of a low-carb diet. I had started with recipes from Rabnitzky's book by the same name.

The diabetes really complicated an already complicated problem. Joan was unable to recall the rationale for controlling diabetes so I found myself frequently re-explaining the arguments. One of the big issues was wine drinking. About the same time every afternoon, she "wanted something," meaning a glass of wine, and every afternoon I had told her to hold off until supper time but it was always a fight, a source of tension. At supper I would pour her one small glass to sip with her meal but she would usually insist on a second one and would often get up from the table herself to pour it.

The visits from the home care nurse from Island hospital had tapered off to a weekly telephone call. The visits and calls were scheduled to end next week with an exit visit. The nurse had concluded that I was doing all the right things at this point. Meanwhile, the physical therapist came to the house to evaluate Joan's situation. Joan was not a cooperative patient and could not understand why the therapist bothered coming. Joan had forgotten completely her sense of things just a few weeks earlier when she was feeling unsteady and had felt that having a walker to move around the house and the side yard might be a good solution. While the prescribed home visits would expire soon, I was still in touch by phone with the RN assigned to us by Group Health. I could call there at anytime, night or day, for medical advice. I had a feeling that this home care program with Group Health would prove a primary resource for me in the days ahead. The Group Health nurse, like the home care nurse, was knowledgeable and helpful.

September 28, 2010

Suppers had been getting more creative and therefore more fun for me. Two nights ago I tried for the first time a dinner of roasted vegetables. Joan and I both enjoyed the meal. I followed it up last night with a smoked fish chowder which we liked equally well. I simply took the vegetable leftovers, added a little more onion, skinned and cut up the small vacuum pack of fish (from our son John), heated it all up in a little water and butter and added whole milk. Both nights we accompanied the entree with a small fruit salad of pineapple and seedless grapes with a sprinkle of shredded coconut and a few pecans on top. It was music to my ears to hear Joan exclaim how hungry she was and how good it tasted. As distinct from lunches when she ate little, the evening meals of late ended with consumption of at least one full helping of everything!

I continued to worry about Joan being at home alone mornings while I was at work. For four days last week, none of her usual friends were able to visit or walk with her and I had not yet found anybody for Mondays. I was reassured that Joan remembered how to contact me on my cell phone and would call several times a morning.

It was the afternoons when I was home, however, that were proving most challenging. She was restless and bored with nothing to do, she said, which put pressure on me to find activities for her. We might take one or two short walks and that helped. I tried to involve her in household tasks such as cleaning windows etc., but she was not up to it physically, often complaining of her back and had to sit down. We read poetry to each other and that was enjoyable. Getting to my computer upstairs to write or work in my study on other projects was out of the question. Joan would go shopping with me but she quickly tired and sometimes did not feel up to getting in the car for any reason. Consequently, I did not get many errands done. She read the newspaper during the morning at breakfast but did not seem interested in the several other magazines we subscribed to and, as I had mentioned before, television was out of the question.

Two nights ago I awoke at about 2:00 am to find Joan trying to get dressed to go outside. She was having trouble finding her clothes. When I turned on the bed lamp, she was trying to fit her arm into her pillow case. I could never determine why she wanted to go outside other than she thought she heard a voice or voices outside calling to her. This was the first time there had been even the slightest inclination to go outside in the dark. Needless to say, this propensity for "night walking," if that was what it was, bore watching. I had heard of too many scary cases of friends' elderly mothers getting up in the middle of the night and disappearing into the dark in their nightclothes. Ruth, Joan's mother, was a case in point. Even with a caregiver residing overnight, Ruth was able to slip outside unobserved. She was found a little later, wandering the streets, totally lost and confused. Needless to say, the caregiver was fired promptly. Only later did Joan's brother, Don, discover that the caregiver had made off with most of Ruth's valuable jewelry.

Sleeping in the same room was obviously important at this point. Last night after I had finished reading to her and had turned out the light, Joan suggested another reason: physical closeness. She would like me in the same bed with her so we could touch, i.e., so I could rub her back. I intended to measure our queen-size guest bed today to see if I could make the swap. There were disadvantages to twin beds, that was clear.

September 29, 2010

A few days back, I made a change in the breakfast menu, switching from fresh homemade muffins and coffee to oatmeal and homemade whole wheat bread (toasted) and coffee. Joan seemed to like the change and it was probably better for her. I would bake muffins for Joan now only on special occasions or when I was baking a batch for others.

I measured the queen-sized bed yesterday. It was only 5 feet wide so it would fit in the front room downstairs just fine. Next question: could I squeeze the twin beds in the upstairs guest room? It looked like it might be a little tight with all the other furniture we had in there. Possibly I could move the sewing table into my study as extra work space.

October 7, 2010

A measured look at the upstairs bedroom left too little space between the twin beds to make the switch workable. So I guess we leave the twin beds where they are for the time being at least.

We had an appointment with our doctor yesterday. He was pleased with Joan's weight increase. On their scales, she weighed in at a hefty 87 lbs (fully clothed). The doctor reviewed my efforts to manage Joan's blood sugar. In response to my difficulty in keeping the blood sugar below 200 (our prearranged goal), he suggested I increase the insulin dosage by one unit to see if that might bring the blood sugar count down. I intended to start that first thing this morning. I noted that Joan's hands were always cold which worried me in terms of what it might indicate: poor circulation, blood not getting to the extremities. He said for diabetics, it was the feet that were the first to indicate a circulatory problem. Joan's feet were warm to the touch so circulation was not an issue at the present time.

Not mentioned to the doctor was my ongoing concern about Joan's memory loss and hearing loss. The combination of having to repeat things both because she did not remember and because she could not hear was an exhausting business, a real challenge for me to remain patient and relaxed about it and accept it as part of what was required at this stage. I was hopeful that Joan, at some point soon, would acknowledge that she had a hearing problem and would do something to remedy it. So far she only continued to scoff at my suggestion that we see an audiologist.

I knew Joan was worried about her inability to recall things when from time to time she uttered "What's happening to me?" or "Am I going crazy?"in response to the experience of disorientation or another situation where memory had deserted her. But, of course, she soon forgot what had upset her and so there was nothing to build on, no accumulation of experiences to make a case for change.

October 8, 2010

I was reminded anew of the memory problem. Both David, our youngest son, and Susan, our daughter, phoned at different times during Sunday afternoon with the happy news that they would be visiting us in La Conner, flying in Wednesday evening, October 20, and departing Sunday morning, October 24. For some reason, Joan thought they were arriving sometime over the next several days. On Tuesday morning (10/5) I discovered a note she had written and apparently had attached to the front door, welcoming David and Susan and explaining she was on her morning walk and would be back soon. Later, during the course of the afternoon Joan would ask repeatedly when David and Susan were arriving. At one point she asked who was arriving, thinking it was Don, her deceased brother, and Patti, her sister who lived in Salina, Kansas.

One of the most obvious signs of memory loss was with respect to dressing and undressing. It was not that long ago that Joan had required no assistance, but now she seemed confused by the process. In the mornings I found myself selecting her clean underwear and other clothing items (usually these days it is just running pants and sweat shirts) and placing them on the bed for easy access. At bedtime she seemed even more confused, unable to distinguish her floral pajamas from her printed long johns and even seemed unsure where the "tub room" was, a common designation for the room at the back of the house where she usually brushed her teeth.

On that Tuesday morning when she thought David and Susan were due to arrive, Joan was able to take a shower and find her own clothing without any assistance from me, much to my surprise. Does this mean that I was creating her dependence on me and, if I were not around, she would do just fine? I did not think so.

October 9, 2010

Did our relationship to the world really change as we got older? This question was triggered by an incident at the post office yesterday afternoon. I was waiting for a customer to complete her business with the postal clerk. Joan moved up near the customer apparently to make sure I was serviced next. As the customer turned to leave she backed slightly into Joan. Joan said something like "Hey, watch what you're doing!" The woman immediately turned to Joan and apologized in what I thought to be a kind and courteous manner saying she was truly sorry and walked toward the exit. Joan turned and yelled after her, "Yeah, well, you would be a lot sorrier if you had knocked into me any harder!"

Joan's reaction upset me because it was totally uncalled for. First of all, Joan had no business crowding the counter on my behalf or for any other reason. Post office protocol dictated that we stand back and provide a modicum of privacy for the conduct of business. Secondly, the customer had no way of knowing Joan was standing behind her when she turned to leave. Thirdly, that the customer actually stopped and offered Joan an apology was a gracious act, exhibiting some level of respect for the elderly.

As Joan and I walked down First Street, I tried to make sense of Joan's reaction in the post office, concluding that, in fact, her world was changing, becoming much more threatening, less controllable. Noise, for example, was a threat nowadays. Twice on our walk she had to stop and cover her ears as a motorcycle rumbled past, followed soon by a diesel truck. A child running down the sidewalk also posed a danger as did any dog, leashed or unleashed, lest they knock against her. She was equally upset by the strollers who did not make room for her to pass on the narrow sidewalk and often let them know with a curt, even belligerent, remark.

Odd Month Out

In the final quadrant
of the year
like four sausages
linked in a row,
there is October,
tied to September
on one side,
and on the other,
November and December,
an ober among the embers,
odd month out.

October 12, 2010

Gauging change as we get older was difficult. I thought Joan's memory loss was getting worse but was it? I did not know. All I knew was that it was bad enough, serious enough, to effect relationships. Our eldest son, John, made an unexpected visit over the weekend, staying overnight and taking a few meals with us. At one point Joan took me aside and asked who the young man was who was at our dinner table. But then Joan had asked the same question of me when Matt visited last August. For several months now she had confused me with one of our sons, speaking to me about "Bob" or "Dad" who was at the museum or out shopping. She told me that she did not recognize me when she saw me mowing the side yard Sunday afternoon. Was this a precursor to the inability to recognize me at all? I suspected it was and accepted the fact that I must be prepared for that. I guess I was really answering my own question. If Joan's memory was not getting any worse for the time being it soon would be, and much more so. I continued to help her get dressed in the morning and undressed and ready for bed in the evening; what to wear and where to find it were ongoing problems.

Meanwhile, I had to do a lot of double-checking to determine what had and what had not transpired. For example, a former colleague at the museum and good friend, phoned me yesterday to say she would walk with Joan at about 10:30 am. At noon, when I got home from work, I asked Joan how the walk went. Joan could not remember taking a walk or that my friend had, in fact, visited. Today I would phone my friend for confirmation.

October 14, 2010

My friend confirmed that she had walked with Joan and reminded me that she would walk with her again Friday morning (today). I wondered if further memory deterioration was occurring when I noticed now that Joan was retiring earlier in the evenings. For the last several days she had complained of being tired and had started undressing for bed (with my help) by 6:30 pm. Up until a month or so ago, I could cajole her into staying up until 8:00 pm. Then she began folding earlier at about 7:00 pm.

Now it is 6:30 pm and I had wanted Joan to watch the evening news with me but it was evident that she simply could not follow it even when it was something as gripping as the mine rescue in Chile. Television, unquestionably, was out for Joan as a form of early evening entertainment or stimulus at this point. I would have to do something else with her—cards, poetry reading or walking around the block—but she seemed too tired to want to do even that. I knew I was tired at that time of the evening too, having cooked supper, done the dishes and cleaned up the kitchen. It was a difficult time of day to think creatively about anything, at least for me.

Part of the problem of retiring early was that Joan would then wake up about 8:00 pm and think it was morning and was ready to dress and eat breakfast. Last night I made her some hot cereal (cream of wheat) and chamomile tea and then coaxed her back to bed. She insisted she would not be able to sleep but she soon did.

October 20, 2010

Joan's last few nights resulted in less restful, broken sleep for me. For some reason, Joan's breathing the first night was erratic and noisy, sending me searching for my pair of ear plugs. I could not find them and settled for a cotton ball, torn in half and stuffed in my ears which only slightly muffled the sound. I got no sleep the next night and retired last night about 8:30 pm after reading aloud to Joan, totally bushed. Fortunately, Joan's breathing was normal, i.e., quiet, and I got four solid hours of sleep. At 12:30 am or so Joan awoke to pee and, as usual, I turned on the bed lamp so she could find her slippers and I could tuck her back in bed upon her return (The condition of Joan's back and shoulders made it difficult for her to pull the pile of covers back over her. She also used a pillow between her knees and another smaller one to support her arm). I never knew getting in bed could be so complicated. Last night, however, she could not get warm and wanted me to move in with her. The twin bed was too narrow but I slid in beside her for awhile, barely able to keep from rolling out. However, she was unable to settle down, fidgeting with the covers, pulling at her pajama sleeves and pants to get them just right. After a while I told her I needed to get some sleep and returned to my bed. It took her another half hour to quiet down, complaining of the heavy covers. I finally ended up removing the top comforter altogether. It was exactly this same kind of restless fidgeting with the covers that she first experienced a month ago or so upon retiring. The medication (Lorazepam) had helped in that case but what about the middle of the night? More medication? I hoped not. I had no idea what to do about the cold. Joan felt cold most of the time and it was just the beginning of the winter season. Was an electric blanket the answer? It might well be.

David and Susan arrived late tonight. Joan had been expecting them every day since Sunday; with every car door slam, she heard a trumpet announcing their arrival.

October 26, 2010

It was a quick visit. David and Susan arrived at 11:00 pm Wednesday and departed at 7:30 am Sunday, but it was a rewarding time nevertheless. For one thing, just to catch-up with their lives at a leisurely pace around the dinner table brought much pleasure.

David was still doing creative stuff at Slippery Rock and with his own writing and wanted to do more. With her involvement with Red Rock Films and now the Storydance project, Susan's work was finally taking an exciting direction to match her ability and interest. Even more impressive was her physical change. Through a strenuous fitness program (kettle bells) and non-gluten diet, she had slimmed down, her body taut and tough with an attitude to match. I now refer to her as a warrior princess. Both did long runs together through Pioneer Park every afternoon, happy and sweaty after the exertion. (I had been only a few years older than David when I began running seriously.)

It was also good that David and Susan could see for themselves how their mother was faring. The reality of the situation really sank in when they realized that there were moments when Joan did not recognize them. We had time to talk about the future after Joan had retired for the night. Susan had been in conversation with the VA and was informed that I made too much money to be eligible for the Veterans Home Care program. Apparently Congress set an income limit (some years ago) of $39,200.00. Anything over that and you do not qualify even though most of our income was from pensions and social security, not earnings (I read in the newspaper recently that the average yearly income nationally was about the same, $39,269).

It appeared that I would soon have to retire from my job at the museum to be with Joan, a fact which struck home after David and Susan's departure. I never felt quite so isolated and alone. The next morning, yesterday, I felt the same way, particularly after Joan's blood sugar was alarmingly high and I had to, wanted to, stay with her to see how the heavy dose of insulin would affect her. As suspected, it brought her blood sugar down all right, from 478 to 57! I quickly supplied Joan with 4 ounces of orange juice and within a half hour her blood sugar was back within the normal range (120). I got up to the museum at 11:00 am and, at that point, discussed my situation with the director who also happened to be a good friend. As an interim measure, I would cut my work time down to 3 mornings a week and see how that went. With regular morning visits from Joan's friends, it might work for a time, but ultimately I saw myself at home full-time, probably by the first of the year if not sooner.

The VA had asked me to resubmit my application, listing income minus job, medical expenses and estimated home care costs— which would be considerable at 20 hours per week for the fiscal year or a portion thereof. Around here, caretakers receive around $15/hr. so the yearly cost would amount to $15,600.

October 28, 2010

I really disliked nights like last night. I was used to Joan getting up about every two hours to pee but last night around midnight I was awakened by Joan fumbling in the dark with the small clock radio on the bed stand. When I asked her what she was doing, she said she was looking for an aspirin and apparently thought the radio was a box of some sort. Even when I turned on the light so she could see the knobs and dial, she still tried to open the top of it as if it were a lid. I was unpersuasive until she inadvertently switched on the radio and heard music emanating from it. She finally desisted and settled back down. Just as I was getting relaxed enough to sleep, the radio alarm sounded and woke us both up, forcing me to turn on the light once more to reset the radio. I vowed to get rid of that little radio first thing in the morning. We never listened to it anyway. I had a smaller digital clock next to the guest bed upstairs that I could replace it with. Joan had not remembered any of this and was sleeping soundly downstairs now as I wrote at my computer upstairs with the listening monitor geared to pick up the slightest noise.

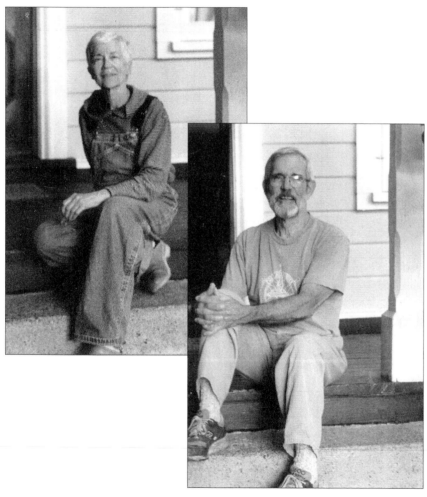

Joan and Bob sitting on the porch steps on a July afternoon. LaConner, 2000

October

October, with its odd ober,
turns us cold sober,
the tasting of the vintner
slowly overcome
by the warnings of winter.
Trepidation in the gut
and leaves in the gutter,
we shutter in the warmth
as best we can and
use All Hallow's Eve to
play dead and to scare away,
in masked merriment,
the gray days ahead.

November 4, 2010

Yesterday was Joan's 86th birthday but we did little in the way of celebrating. I had a card and a small wrapped present—a book she had picked out at the bookstore –awaiting her at the breakfast table and I prepared special morning fare—fresh coffee and her favorite buttermilk waffles—but other than that, we spent a good deal of the day walking.

It was a beautiful day and Joan wanted to spend it outside. Usually a single morning walk to the post office would suffice but this day she seemed much too restless and could not sit still to read or talk. Our first walk (to the post office) was pleasant and we had a lot of mail to haul home (happily no campaign brochures). Within an hour, she wanted to take another walk, having forgotten already about the first walk. Shortly after lunch the same thing. She was unable to remember either of the earlier walks so we took another one. Admittedly good exercise but I had some other domestic things I wanted to get done—assembling a new bookcase was one—but never had a chance because I suddenly had to think about the evening meal. Originally I had planned to take Joan to supper at the Rhododendron Cafe but had finally settled on the pub at Nell Thorn's. However, she decided she wanted to do neither, preferring to stay home in familiar surroundings and avoid the whole process of ordering food and waiting for it in a crowd of other diners. Fortunately, I had some oysters and onion rings I was going to prepare later in the week so I hopped to, upped the schedule and we had what I thought was a fine birthday supper with candlelight. Joan, however, ate little, hardly touching the oysters though she said she enjoyed them.

The highlight of Joan's birthday was always the telephone calls from our children. All of them did phone except for Matt. Instead, he and Annie sent a beautiful bouquet of roses with an equally beautiful note that brought Joan to tears. We naturally called them and Joan had a good talk with Matt at that time. Joan was able to identify Susan and David by voice, but did not recognize her sister Patti's voice when she called nor John's when he called later.

The most pleasant surprise of the day was a phone call from the daughter of good friends of ours in Alexandria, Minnesota. Her birthday was also on November 3rd. The daughter recalled her fourth birthday party which we celebrated with her at their home on Bryant Street in Alexandria fifty years ago. How I have enjoyed our Minnesota connections. They never seemed to end.

November 13, 2010

For the last several days, Joan seemed to be preoccupied with her family, thinking at one point that her brother, Bill, was still alive and staying at our house, that her father was nearby and her mother was working up at the museum. Her last question to me at bedtime lately had been to ask if everyone was home for the night and safely abed. Instead of explaining that no one else was in the house, etc., now I just say that everyone is home and safe and let it go at that.

Joan seldom alluded to their presence in the morning at breakfast, but then, later in the day, she would wonder when her mother was coming back from the museum. At those times during the day I attempted to set the record straight, putting the fact that her parents (and mine) had been dead for some time now in the most gentle of terms. Yesterday she began wondering about our children and where they were and, at one point, asked when Bob was getting back from the museum. Then, as we were at the stove preparing supper yesterday evening, she said she was "lost." When I asked her in what way she was "lost," she reverted to an old term (which I do not even know how to spell) "discombobulated" to explain her state of mind which, in my understanding, had always meant "confused" and "disoriented" which certainly seemed to be the case.

I wanted to go into town to do some shopping yesterday for underwear for Joan and furniture, but she preferred to stay home, spending part of the afternoon resting on the small dining room sofa, the shopping postponed. She did drive with me to the local grocery to get a few supplies, helping me to pick out a handful of apples, but was easily put off by the crowd of shoppers, the cars and carts and the fast-moving youngsters. We ate a small pizza (that I made from scratch) and salad about 4:30 pm and by 5:30 pm Joan was in bed. The change from Daylight Savings had not helped with the evening's earlier sunset.

It was becoming more and more evident that Joan derived little pleasure from her usual occupations. She may have read a magazine article for a time or tried the daily crossword puzzle at my urging, but her interest soon flagged. The same held for playing the piano or watching television. The news anchors, she confessed, made no sense to her. "I don't know what they are saying," she continued to complain. As I mentioned before, she was clearly bored to tears by most everything, the only holdout being card games such as solitaire and gin rummy with me. Her sense of loneliness had to be fierce even with me at her side. It was becoming increasingly urgent for me to spend every available moment with her, but I also felt the necessity for time away by myself; my writing time in the early morning was essential to my own sanity now. It helped to be writing about Joan and me from time to time as I was doing now. I worried about the repetition but, in a way, that was the experience I was having, the spiraling circle of decline, where much was the same but getting continually, frighteningly, worse. I was sad. I was sad for Joan. I was sad for me. I was sad for us.

The shared life was completely dependent upon shared memory. Without memory, the exchange of thoughts and ideas, so vital to our relationship, disappeared and we were left with the only fallback there was: habit. The habit of eating together, walking together, being together was a small anchor keeping us from floating away from each other entirely—and even this I could not expect to last. The separation, the quiet withdrawal and floating away, had already begun. "Don't leave me, Joan, don't leave me!" I shouted to myself. But she already had... she already had.

November 15, 2010

Still, every time we started out for our daily walk to the post office, Joan would grab my arm and say "I love you." The warmth and sincerity expressed at these times I could not dismiss as simply "habit." When getting supper or attending to some other chore, I made it a point to stop what I was doing to embrace and kiss Joan lightly to remind her of our love. Lighting candles for the evening meal was part of the same ritual—habit on my part by now, but invested with passion. So we continued to play out our days.

November 22, 2010

Randy Williams and Lucie Reiderer, Joan's nephew and his wife, were expected for supper Friday evening at 5:30 pm so I turned to, getting a good start by baking the crescent rolls yesterday. Today, after work and lunch, I focused on cleaning up the kitchen a little (I could not believe how the dust accumulated on the open shelves!), making the coleslaw and preparing a big side of sockeye salmon. These simple culinary tasks turned into one of the most exhausting afternoons in my entire married life. For some reason, Joan was constantly restless, agitated, nervous about the upcoming dinner, asking repeatedly who was coming and when. At one point I got her clothes together and helped her put them on, thinking that might calm her down some which it did for awhile. But then, she began again to worry whether they were going to arrive and wanted to know why they had not called if they were going to be late even though it was an hour before their expected arrival. I kept stopping each time to answer her repeated questions with repeated answers (to the point where I was almost too tired to respond) assuring her all the while that Randy and Lucie were always very prompt and would be this time. Joan was not at all convinced, insisting that she was not going to wait long after 5:30 to eat. As luck would have it, Joan was right! Randy and Lucie never arrived. Joan and I sat down to eat at 6:00 pm, Joan not caring, and me wondering what had happened to our guests.

The next morning I phoned and found out. Lucie, who had arranged the scheduled dinner with me, had only mentioned "Friday" which I assumed meant the next Friday. All the time she was thinking of the Friday after Thanksgiving Day. They were, of course, upset and felt bad about all the work I had gone to. We agreed to get together some other time but not for supper. I had concluded that Joan and I could not have guests for dinner anymore. Our own kids yes, but anyone else, a restaurant was the only solution. Too bad, really, since I enjoyed cooking and the company but I could not put myself through that experience again. Having said that, I already had arranged a supper party for December 2 with three former museum colleagues. I could not bring myself to cancel it so could only hope that the preparation for it would go more smoothly.

There were plenty of other issues to worry about, that was for sure. When I came home from work recently, the overhead light in the kitchen was not working. Then I noticed the refrigerator light was out and the hall lights in the utility area as well. Checking the electric panel, I discovered all the circuits on one side had been shut off. I asked Joan about it but, of course, she could not remember doing it. That noon after lunch, I placed the kit of diabetes stuff on the table along with the plastic bottle of rubbing alcohol (to clean the injection area for the insulin shot). While I was clearing a few items from the table, she poured a good bit of the alcohol into the last of her soup and began eating it, then dashing by me after the first swallow to spit it out in the kitchen sink. These two episodes, put together, were clear danger signals. When was she going to drink something else mistakenly or light a burner on the gas stove and forget to turn it off with disastrous results? (She has already scorched a few sauce pans of food.) The Group Health nurse had alerted me to begin thinking about locking away medicines and cleaning supplies. Until this last episode, I had not thought it necessary.

November

November reminds us
in the Northwest
that winter is here,
the fallen leaves,
maybe raked and burned,
or maybe not,
give way with frosty breath
to the mountain drama
of falling snow.

November's ember, though,
is not found in the Olympics
or Cascades
but in earlier escapades
on the other coast,
the Pilgrim's landing
and later, with the natives,
banding together for the very
first Thanksgiving roast.

November 24, 2010

Yesterday afternoon was pleasant enough. During the morning I took a brief break from work and helped Joan get dressed for the cold day—20 degrees last night after a light snow and now icy roads. After lunch we ventured out, going to the post office, the bank and back. I was impressed again about how skittish Joan had become on even the most dry, walkable surfaces (between the icy patches). She seemed to live in constant fear of falling, getting knocked over by an exuberant child or friendly dog. Everyone, it followed, must seem like a threat and may account for her belligerence toward other pedestrians. Pedestrians as enemies. I really hadn't carried the logic of her fear to that point before.

The worst afternoon had occurred a day earlier when Joan decided she wanted to leave on her pajamas for the day and was quite prepared to slip on her jacket over them for our afternoon walk. I urged her to reconsider, offering to help her get dressed. She was offended by my efforts, just another example of my treating her like a child or, even worse, like an idiot. This was a frequent accusation these days as my role as caretaker expanded. I was beginning to think I did not, after all, have the patience for the role. Plus, the reality of the change in Joan's perceptions was hard to keep up with. In bed the other night, she looked over to me as I was reading to her from the other bed and asked where Bob was. Was he still at the museum, she wondered. I asked at that point who she thought I was. She was not sure. Part of the problem getting her to change from her pajamas earlier was the fact that she did not see them as sleepwear but as normal day wear, clothing that others would not notice as inappropriate. She seemed to see my effort to persuade her to change clothes as yet another example of my worry about what others would think. This criticism harked back to a perennial complaint of hers: I always put the welfare of others before her welfare. She simply dismissed my argument that you had to see everything in context, the individual within community, ourselves in relation to others. Her welfare was uppermost in my mind, of course, but I could never get her to believe it, particularly when we were out driving and I hit a pothole or manhole cover (either jolt would cause her pain) rather than trying to avoid it and risk a collision with the car behind or beside us. Safety first was viewed with suspicion by my dear spouse. "Safety first" was just a cover for "others first."

Joan spent the day in her pajamas and we even managed a pleasant candlelight dinner, the tears in her eyes daubed dry by then but it had been a difficult, trying afternoon for both of us. The evening was pleasant. I started a new book, reading aloud to her, until the words began to blur. The book, incidentally, was *Border Songs* by Jim Lynch and was proving a delightful way to end the day.

December 1, 2010

Thanksgiving Day came and went. I roasted a pair of Cornish game hens with the usual side dishes of dressing, mashed potatoes, cranberries and homemade rolls, all of which settled well on our palates and stomachs while we fielded phone calls from our children. I missed having others around the table but it was pleasant enough. Among other things, I read aloud President Obama's Thanksgiving Proclamation which was a dandy with its emphasis on the importance of the Native Americans to our survival and success in those early years.

The remaining days of November were of the same caliber, quiet, uneventful with only the usual aberrations to mark the days. For several nights running, Joan had been worried about the whereabouts of the young woman who was supposedly staying with us, sleeping upstairs at night. One night, some time after Joan had retired, I crawled into my twin bed, the creaking sounding to her like someone knocking at the front door. She thought it had to be the young woman wanting us to let her in. I had been unable to figure who that "young lady" might be other than some reference to our daughter, Susan, who had visited us some weeks earlier. Joan had not mentioned the young woman for several days now.

Other night noises would also get a fearful response from Joan. Most any car door slamming, or the sound of our neighbor starting his truck would set off alarm bells. She was certain that someone was trying to steal one of our cars. If we had a garage you can be sure I would keep the cars in it just to minimize that fear but, of course, we did not and continued to park the cars along the street in front of the house.

Marsh, our grandson, and his girlfriend, Molly, drove up from Seattle to see us yesterday for lunch. I made pizza and cooked pinto beans with ham which were big hits. It was a delightful visit with Marsh and Molly bringing such energy and zest with them. Joan kept interjecting herself into the conversation, stating that she could not understand a word any of us were saying. Marsh would then turn to her, recap the conversation, and then we would continue talking for awhile until the next interjection. The vision of Joan pale, withdrawn, unable to hear (or follow?) broke my very heart; tears well in my eyes as I write these words. I can not help it. On the other hand, how sweet Marsh's reaction to his grandmother's plaint, stopping to update her as he did. Molly, too, was ever solicitous and tender, seeming to understand Joan's difficulty. It was altogether a pleasant three hours tempered, of course, by Joan's reaction to our conversation around the table. By now I would be surprised if she were even able to recall the visit or the pain of it.

December 2, 2010

Dilution the solution. There was a place for deception under the circumstances—or at least a healthy deception. It suddenly occurred to me the other afternoon to dilute Joan's wine at supper with sparkling water. It seemed a perfect solution. She thought she was having her usual two small glasses of wine when, in effect, she was drinking half that, which was all to the good in terms of her diabetes, particularly as I (we) attempted to avoid spikes in the blood glucose. The deception was harder to pull off when we ate out, but as long as we dined locally, I could arrange the deception by having the waitress pour our wine elsewhere before delivering it to the table. Since Joan drank red wine and I white, there was no chance of getting the two reversed.

December 6, 2010

I awoke at 3:30 this morning to cries of "Mom! Mom! I'm sick. Hurry!" I told Joan her mom was not around any longer. She could not help. "What can I do?" I asked. When Joan was fully awake she realized she was okay, but there were a few minutes there when she seemed to be frozen in time, eyes opened, staring into space, unblinking. I actually thought she had died just that quickly. Then her eyes blinked and she was back with me, feeling normal and ready to sleep some more while I got up to shower and write.

This episode bothered me because Joan felt unwell most of yesterday which had something to do, I was sure, with her high blood sugar (over 600 mg) at noon and the extra shot of insulin (6 units) I gave her which, in turn, dropped her blood sugar too low. I then countered this by giving her a slug of orange juice, the usual remedy, which worked but left her tired and ready for bed at 4:30

pm. Nevertheless, we had been able to get in two long walks in the brisk, sunny weather. Although she was not hungry after the tiring day, she ate a small serving of a plain egg omelet and half a piece of multigrain toast with a little butter.

I was busy rethinking Joan's diet. She certainly needed to consume more vegetables. The challenge for me was to make them attractive and tasteful so she would eat them. I was again researching for more meal ideas for underweight diabetics. So far my search had led me to some good low carb recipes, but right now I needed more breakfast ideas that would appeal to Joan who was not a big breakfast eater to begin with. So far, she had seemed content with a small bowl of oatmeal and my whole wheat muffins along with coffee. But what was triggering her high blood sugar reading after lunch?

December 13, 2010

Last Saturday morning, I encouraged Joan to take a shower. She would not believe it when I told her she had not showered since the previous Sunday. We got as far as the upstairs bathroom, standing by the tub, when she decided that she could not do it, stating that she felt much too weak and unsteady. What she felt like doing was going back to bed (after 11 hours sleep) which she did for an hour or so. I wondered to myself if this did not in some way mark the beginning of the end. Joan had always been meticulous about her personal grooming, showering every day and washing her hair. That her loss of memory would bring change is one thing, but when she was too tired and too weak—after sufficient rest—to shower suggested a serious physical decline that I did not like to see or accept. I am happy to report that a couple of hours later she did shower and seemed better for it. I resolved to try very hard to get her to shower at least once during the week. My target date was Wednesday morning, the first of my two weekdays home from work.

To offset the threat of another boring weekend, Joan and I braved the rain to get to Haggen's supermarket. Here, at least, we could get a little exercise in a pleasant, dry atmosphere. I had hoped to get to the nearby shopping mall to pick up a few things for Christmas, but Joan seemed too tired after the grocery shopping to attempt it. My thought then was to drive to the mall the next morning when the mall first opened and do the Christmas shopping. The next morning, however, she showed little interest in such a jaunt so we stayed put, she reading the Sunday paper while I did a little biblical research on the use of the extensive genealogy at the beginning of Matthew's Gospel (in connection with the Christmas story). Why would Matthew, brilliant story teller that he was, begin his story with something as deadly as a genealogy? Luke included a genealogy too but not in the opening lines.

December 19, 2010

I could not persuade Joan to take a shower on Wednesday, but she finally consented to shower and wash her hair on Saturday, yesterday. She said she saw no reason to take showers every day since she washed herself daily with her wash cloth (standing before the downstairs wash basin presumably)—which would be fine if, in fact, she did. I knew she did not give herself a wash before dressing since I helped her to get dressed every morning and I could not imagine her disrobing, even partially, to bathe herself during the day. It was also true I was not around for portions of three mornings every week so she could get it done then but she certainly did not dry bathe any of the other four days. Should I settle for Joan's showering once a week and let it go at that? Good hygiene tells me "no," push for twice a week at least.

Joan's rebellion against her normal rituals was matched by the oddity of new ones. Recently, her annoyance at the ugly ends of the bananas had broadened to include other fruits. I brought home some fresh pears the other day and before long I saw the stem ends dug out leaving divots which, of course, would hasten the rot. The next time I looked, she had completely cored them. The same was true with the apples. I now store all the fruits out of sight in the cupboard or refrigerator. Recently she started after the garlic and, in spite of my protestations, peeled each bud. All I could do was preserve the skinned pieces by covering and placing them in the refrigerator with the other victims. I am now using garlic in everything except the breakfast cereal.

So our curious life continued, getting odder and odder, mixed with moments of deep pleasure and sustained aggravation, the latter occurring usually during the afternoons when Joan would become hungry and restless and could not find anything to do and I was tired and less patient. It did not help that she ate little at lunch and she often refused my snack suggestions for fear it would spoil her supper. This forced me to begin meal preparation before I had even digested my lunch, or so it seemed. It was at this period of time that I had to become more creative for both of us. Joan wanted to help me prepare and cook and that was a good thing, but she had forgotten how. Yesterday, I gave her a ripe cantaloupe to cut up for a side dish but she could not remember how to do it. The two small bowls were filled all right, but only with slices of the green outer section. Any attempt to help at that point failed. She would just walk away and lie down on the sofa where she continued to spend too much time.

Concerned about Joan's frequent urination during the day (and night) and at the higher blood glucose in recent weeks, I decided it should be checked out at the local clinic. The urine sample proved negative so the whole thing was probably related to diabetes. The results of the blood draw should be known by Joan's next medical appointment, January 4th. She had not gotten up to urinate as much these last few days, but I had no idea if that was significant. Probably not.

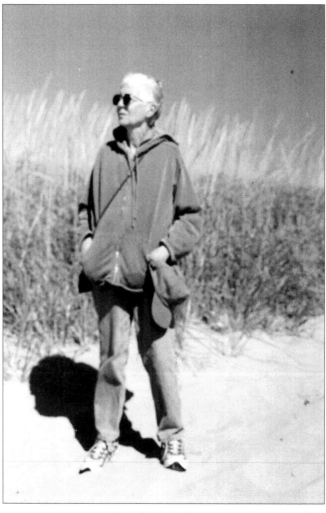

Joan, scanning the coast for seabirds. Del Ray Beach, Oregon. Fall, 2001

December

December finds us seeking
warmth and light
as we make our way
to the year's shortest
and darkest day.
I swing my axe, splitting
wood for two stoves,
an old Vermont notion,
my body's generating motion,
no match for the fire's
eventual heat.

Opening the fire box door,
the hot light within,
now loose,
flickering and
bouncing off
the white kitchen walls,
recalls the innocent potency
of December's ember,
the mythic light of
an infant birth,
guiding the magi in us
to quiet and unexpected
places.

2011

January 3, 2011

Joan has asked my name several more times now, the latest last night, adding a second one: "Where do you live?" I told her I lived in La Conner in this very house. I did not hear a response but there may have been a soft "Oh" in acknowledgment.

Friends asked how the holidays went and I replied, with as much enthusiasm as I could muster, that they were fine, quiet but fine. And they were. The children had all visited in the fall at different times for short stays. No, that's not entirely accurate. Susan and David visited at the same time for three full days which was great at several levels. They had a chance to visit with each other as well as with us. There was no expectation that we would have any family with us over Christmas. I thought I might try to gather a few neighbors together for Christmas Day dinner, but all had other plans which was probably just as well.

Joan and I did get out on two occasions. Our next door neighbor invited us to join him and his woman friend for supper at Nell Thorn's restaurant one night. Joan barely touched her food and with only a little wine fell gently asleep at the table. Our neighbor and his friend understood the situation and we continued our conversation for a while. Joan just as gently awoke and we all shared one of the restaurant's luscious desserts before our short walk home.

The other occasion was the annual museum staff party this year at La Conner Seafood and Prime Rib Restaurant on First Street. Joan and I sat at the end of a long table with the eight other staff. It was a festive occasion with Christmas music playing in the background, good food and the hubbub of exchanging and unwrapping presents (under $20). Joan was included in the exchange of presents which seemed to please her, but here again the background noise, the loud talking (to talk over the music) and the general activity was too much for her. Several times during the two hours she leaned over to say she could not understand anything that was going on. We left as early as we could with her doggie bag full of the good food she was unable to eat at the table. I thought, too late, that we should have seated ourselves in the middle of the table instead of at the end but I was not sure that would have helped much. I concluded from our two restaurant excursions that eating out was out. It would be much better for Joan, it appeared, if we invited people to our house and, to keep it simple, ordered take-out food from the local Thai restaurant or the Mexican one. That was what I proposed to try next anyhow. I might also try having folks for breakfast, as I once used to do. Or lunches—simple ones with soups and sandwiches—might work too. Evenings are just the wrong time of day for her, even with an early dinner. In fact, someone mentioned to me recently that she had read that afternoons and evenings were the worst times of day for most dementia patients and had earned them the name "sundowners." It was certainly the worst time of day for Joan.

January 1st, New Year's Day, was a beautiful beginning to the year. The sunrise over the Cascade Mountains was as intensely orange and red as I had ever seen it and was matched, even surpassed, by the sunset which treated us to a constant change of

vivid colors, starting with deep orange and changing to reds and blues as darkness enfolded us. The weather between was clear, cold and sunny. Altogether, a memorable day. It was pleasant in other ways too. Joan and I walked several times and in the course of them had many good laughs—nothing involving memory, just plays on words of one silly kind or another. I asked her at one point what she knew about the origin or meaning of "curiosity killed a cat and satisfaction brought it back." She could not remember, of course, but she started launching into this wonderful story about a Mr. Cur. I had not laughed so continuously for a long time. What fun! She was good, too, at giving a new twist to the old road signs we walk by every day.

Stopping

My wife, Joan, is at it again,
looking at a street sign
and seeing something I don't.
This particular sign reads:
  STOP
  4—Way
Are there four ways to stop?
My dear wife wants to know.
Sure, I answer, trying not to
miss a beat, starting at the top:
you can put on the brakes or
you can coast to a stop or
you can give an old boat
anchor a throw (as Rochester
did on Jack Benny's comedy
radio show years ago) or
you can simply do an illegal
U-turn on a dime and head
back home to consider other
signs of the time.

January 4, 2011

Joan's frequent trips to the bathroom were interruption enough since every time she got up, I turned on the bed lamp and made sure she found her way back and was tucked in. But last night added a new twist. I had finished reading to her at about 8:30 pm. At 10:30 pm I was awakened by kitchen noises. I got up to find Joan cooking a couple of eggs. I got out the toaster and toasted her some flourless bread to go with her snack. That she was hungry surprised me because she had eaten more than usual for supper (halibut steak, potato cakes and peas with coleslaw on the side and a small dish of ice cream for dessert). Amazing to me, she ate most of her eggs and the toast. Where did this appetite come from so suddenly?

Joan has an appointment with her doctor this afternoon. We may learn something from her blood test results. He may want to adjust her insulin intake. Her glucose readings still tended in general to be higher than we wanted, averaging in the mid-200 mg with occasional spikes up to the 600s.

January 13, 2011

This was much too long a gap between entries but I was trying to spend what little writing time I had in the morning producing poetry. Last night, however, required me to stop and take note.

At about midnight, I heard Joan get up and, as usual, I turned on the bedside lamp. She seemed more disoriented than ever before. She had no idea where she was and needed help in finding her way to the bathroom. When she came back to the bedroom she wanted to get dressed and leave the house. We were in danger but she could not tell me what the danger was. I finally coaxed her back to bed and we talked for another 45 minutes about her fears.

When I offered to turn off the lamp she said to leave it on; the dark was too scary. I never did determine the source of her fear. She just kept asking if there was not some organization that could help us, arrange for food, take over control of things. At another point, she wanted to know if relatives could come here and get us and drive us elsewhere (out of danger, I gather she meant). I kept matching her illusions with reality but she had a hard time grasping it. I explained several times that we did not need an organization, we owned our house and maintained it ourselves; we drove to the grocery store ourselves and purchased our own food. She worried then if we had any money to pay for it. She was also surprised that we were the only ones living in our house and had been the only ones for the last 25 years. Her mother and our daughter Susan were mentioned as the most likely live-ins.

Joan finally dozed off to sleep with the light on. At 3:30 am she awoke, alert and ready to get up. I told her the time, tucked her back in bed, turned off the light and turned up the heat. She seemed content to sleep some more while I came upstairs, showered and began writing this segment. I had the impression that she remembered none of what occurred last night, but I planned to ask her at breakfast to confirm. Any little inkling of what she feared or was worried about might be helpful regarding future strategies.

The visit with the doctor did not reveal anything new. The urinalysis and the blood work were negative. The doctor agreed that it might be time to reintroduce Levenmir, the long-acting insulin, to see if that helped to reduce the high blood sugars. So far, the results have been inconclusive. In one case, it created a problem. The evening before last, Joan's glucose reading was 182 mg. I then injected her with insulin according to the scale the doctor and I had agreed to. It turned out to be too much insulin, dropping Joan's blood sugar to the point where it triggered convulsions and another of those frightening episodes where she was shaking so hard it was all I could do to hold her on the bed. Fortunately, I saw the beginnings of the trembling this time and was able to get some orange juice in her. As a result, the episode was not as prolonged as the previous one, but it was still traumatic.

Joan's desperate cries of "Help me, help me. I'm dying, I'm dying!" (along with the fear in her eyes and uncontrollable convulsions) continued to ricochet off the walls of my memory two days later. However, she said she remembered none of it. Thank goodness for that. To avoid such a reoccurrence, I intend to reduce the insulin levels back to the earlier or original levels when we were using both insulins—at least when the blood glucose reading was below 200 mg. I will, of course, check this all out with the nurse and doctor. Joan's glucose reading last night was only 124 mg so I gave her no insulin in accordance with the prearranged scale.

January 31, 2011

Joan's nephew, Randy Williams, and his wife, Lucie, joined us for lunch last week. They wanted to see "Aunt Jobie." We had missed the usual connections over the holidays (because of the schedule mix-up) so it was pleasant catching up with each other over a spinach ricotta tart and fresh fruit salad I had whipped up for the occasion. Lucie, always a good baker, provided a plate of homemade cookies for dessert. Before they left, Lucie took note of our plans to celebrate our 60th wedding anniversary on Saturday, September 10, 2011 at the Garden Club. They intended to be there. I wondered if we would.

For the last five or six mornings now, Joan had gotten up later than usual, complaining about how terrible she felt. Only one morning did she attempt to specify, stating that she felt nauseous.

She has had no appetite for a long time but she seems now to be eating even less. At the same time her weight, if anything, increased the past few days from 86.2 lbs. to 87.8 lbs. Whole wheat bread, butter and jam and plain vanilla ice cream are the only foods she genuinely seemed to enjoy, although she did eat most of a small salmon patty last night for a change.

Joan's blood sugar continued to run higher than I liked. I had increased the Levenmir from 2 units each morning to 3 units and adjusted her Novolog accordingly, but the blood sugar level was not leveling out as I had hoped. Perhaps it never would with her small size and lack of appetite.

I tried to get some work done on my computer upstairs last night after I tucked Joan into bed at 7:00 pm and cleaned up the kitchen. I carefully explained why I needed to use the computer (book layout) and that I had the monitor on to pick up the slightest sound from our bedroom downstairs. But it did not work. About every 15 minutes, Joan would be at the bottom of the stairs, wondering when I was coming to bed. Like her glucose level, her anxiety level was high, especially at night with worries that the doors were not locked or that someone was stealing our cars. When I finally shut down the computer and joined her in the other twin bed, she spoke to me as if I were a guest, explaining how her name was pronounced. She asked me if I had a nickname. I said I did not. I asked if she did. Yes, her family gave her the nickname of "Jobie"—all of which I knew, of course. I had often called her by that family nickname myself.

My guest status was further established when she turned down my bed covers as a gesture of hospitality. Sweet, really, and considerate. I did not recall Joan ever doing that before. Once I was in bed and the lights were off, she started asking about her family. She was unable to remember that they were all deceased except for her younger sister,

Patti, so I was the conveyor of the sad news once again, but focused on how lucky we were that Patti was still with us and that we had each other. Joan concurred and, finally, slept for a few hours. And that was all it was, a few. These days Joan's trips to the bathroom seemed to be increasing. I was totally astonished at the amount of toilet paper and Kleenex she would go through in a day and I was left wondering what the connection was between the frequent bathroom trips, her feeling unwell in the morning, and another emerging pattern: during the course of most meals now, she complained of feeling uncomfortably hot to the point where she would practically tear off her clothes to get some relief. She has an appointment with the doctor in a few days. This will be one issue to raise with him certainly.

February 7, 2011

"May I ask your name?"

"Sure. It's Bob."

"That's my husband's name."

"I am your husband."

"Oh yes, of course."

So the confusion continued. I was writing upstairs at 3:45 am when I heard (on the monitor) Joan moving around. I dashed downstairs to find her standing in the dark of our front bedroom, unable to find her way to the bathroom. She thought she was upstairs. I added to the confusion by having partially closed the bedroom door to keep the light out of her eyes while I adjusted the thermostat; but then failed to open it again. It was just after I had walked with her to the bathroom and back and tucked her in that she asked me my name. She was happy to learn she did not have to go to school today and could stay snug in bed until I told her it was time to get up. An hour later now and not a peep from her. I hoped she had fallen into a restful sleep. First the raccoons frolicking on the porch and then the winds had made for a noisy night.

The appointment with Joan's doctor was amiable. He took plenty of time to talk and listen. He reviewed Joan's blood test results. Everything was normal so no clues there. We agreed that I would increase Joan's Levenmir dosage from 3 to 4 units each morning to see if that would help to keep the blood sugar down within the 100 to 200 range. He speculated that increasing the long-term insulin beyond 4 units was probably not a good idea, given Joan's size. Incidentally, she weighed in at 87.2 lbs. Saturday before her shower.

February 12, 2011

Joan's hearing continued to be a problem. I thought maybe we might have had a breakthrough recently when we received a card from All About Hearing, a clinic in nearby Burlington, inviting us to a free hearing test. At Joan's urging, I made an appointment for the two of us, all to no avail as it turned out. We arrived on schedule and I volunteered to be tested first. It was a simple procedure. I stepped into a small booth and, fitted with earphones, listened to repeated series of sounds at various pitches, indicating with a clicker what I could and could not hear. Result: My hearing was within the normal range for both ears. A previous peek into my ears with a video camera revealed no abnormalities either. So I was home free.

Next. Joan? No! She was adamant. She did not have a hearing problem. No need to be tested. She only wanted to get out of there. The clinician was understanding and sympathetic, reassuring her at every turn that she was not about to be forced into doing anything she did not want to do. We left under amicable terms but I was, of course, disappointed. Joan was only relieved and happy to go on to the grocery store to do some shopping. Parenthetically, I phoned the clinician later, out of Joan's hearing, and thanked her for her professional manner in dealing with Joan. She said she ran into this problem all the time. People were often in denial, reluctant to admit they had a hearing problem. I was impressed. If I did develop a hearing problem, I knew where I would go (that is, if I do not lose my voice first trying to get Joan to hear me).

Loss of hearing. Memory loss. What next? I'll tell you. The loss of eye glasses. I had been looking for Joan's glasses throughout the house now for two days and had not been able to figure out where she might have put them, her only pair of clear lenses. The last time this happened she had been fitted for a new pair, only later to re-cover the first pair. I suppose we would have to go through the process once again. Oh well. This is how we old folks often spend our days: chasing after forgetfulness. I could think of a lot of things I would rather be doing.

Recycled Love

Sometimes I carry my heart on my sleeve
but today, the day before Valentine's Day,
I carry my heart in my hand,
heading west, down the hill to
La Conner's First Street,
the small red heart-shaped box,
unlike my own, empty,
yet, like my own, longing to fill,
and be filled, with sweetness.

I make my way through the crowd
standing inside the Cascade Candy
store waiting for ice cream, to place
my order for the usual—dark chocolate
truffles—extending my box over the
counter. "It's funny," the confectioner
says, "We were just talking about you,
wondering, if again this year, you'd
stop by."

How many years have I done this now?
Not many, three or four,
but the red sweet-holding heart,
with its delicate, faux-cloth cover,
remains unmarked, pristine,

its only patina, the imagined finger-
prints of the loved and her lover.
It may be that you would never put
new wine in an old wine skin
but is there anything wrong with putting
a new sweetness in an old heart?

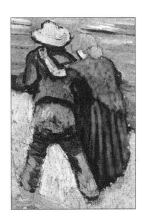

February 21, 2011

I found Joan's eye glasses! I was vacuuming the downstairs bedroom and there they were on the floor at the foot of her twin bed. I had canvassed the room earlier, including a thorough scan under the beds so the eye glasses must have been lodged in the bedcovers and fallen to the floor after I had done some rearranging. Now the challenge would be not to lose them again. Several times since finding the glasses they had been lost momentarily because Joan, without the ability to remember and recall, had no way of establishing a set routine for keeping track of them. How else could you explain it?

My biggest concern now was the way Joan felt in the mornings. For the last two weeks she had told me upon arising, that she felt terrible and wanted only to go back to bed. Some mornings she had done just that. When I asked her if she could describe the feeling more specifically she was unable to. It was a general malaise described by such words as "tired", "unsteady" and her most common word "shaky." Twice over the 14 days she mentioned feeling "nauseous." There had been two or three times in the last week or so that she had complained of chest pain but it seemed to disappear after a short while. One night at bedtime around 8:00 pm, as I may have mentioned earlier, she experienced sharp chest pain on her left side which persisted to the point where I phoned the duty doctor, who properly said Joan should come to the ER for tests if she wanted to pursue the matter. Otherwise, there was nothing she could do. After Joan and I talked about it some more, she opted not to go to the ER and settled for a pain pill.

A high point: Sunday morning! Joan and I were able to watch live the worship service at First Community Church in Columbus, Ohio, where I was raised and where we were married. Joan was as thrilled as I with the splendid music and strong sermon, humorous and compelling. We had rejoined FCC as full members of the cyberspace community. Joan did not remember our new affiliation but she thoroughly enjoyed the hour's time together in our sunlit dining room worshipping, joining in the prayers and singing. My thought for that time: religion, the worship of God in this church, brought out the very best in me. It was that simple. It had always been the case. It had always brought out the best in me. It was such a wonderful thing to rediscover at this point about myself.

February 23, 2011

This morning at 6:00 o'clock I was still at the computer writing when I heard Joan calling up the stairs. "Hello, hello!" she called with some desperation in her voice. I quickly ran to the top of the stairs where she could see me and told her where I was and what I had been doing, identifying myself—I'm not sure why—but I said, "I'm Bob, your husband." She said, looking up the stairs, "No you're not. I don't have a husband named Bob." At that point, I came immediately down the stairs and looked at her squarely nose to nose. Astonishingly, I saw no recognition in her eyes whatsoever. I was a complete stranger. I tucked Joan back in bed but still no hint of recognition. I reassured her that I would soon be getting breakfast. She seemed content to stay in her warm bed. I did not dare leave now to work out at the fitness center which would normally be my next move. I no longer felt confident that she would stay put or that if she decided to get up, what she might do. My usual morning exercise time may not be feasible unless I moved it to an earlier hour and wrote after my return. Today the issue was suddenly moot. Looking out the study window in the morning's slow light, I discovered that it was snowing heavily, six inches predicted, which would stop everybody in their tracks.

Winter Sun

Like the young woman instructed by her mother
to avert her eyes when meeting an older man,
we avoid looking directly at that old summer sun,
the flirtation much too dangerous.

It's enough to feel the heat burning our arms,
and working its way through out Tee shirts.
No need to look up. Better to look down,
there to see our shadow.

However distorted, the figure following
us or, depending on our direction, leading us,
belongs solely to us, its dark presence confirming
our being, for good or bad.

The winter sun offers no such problem. We can
look directly up at it, flirting outrageously if we desire,
with no damage to eye or heart. Glancing around,
looking down, is another matter altogether.

Though weakened by gray, moisture-laden skies,
the winter sun, scattering its diffused rays against
the fresh snow, is yet strong enough to force a squint
from our red-cheeked faces.

Not only that, but a search of the litter-free, glitter-white street, fore and aft, at our feet, offers, disconcertingly, no shadow at all. With no confirming presence under the winter sun, no shady company during our cold solstice, we are, it seems, very much on our own.

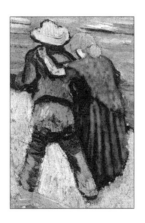

February 28, 2011

Joan continued to wake up not feeling well but was unable to point to anything specifically. She did not look well either. Her face had taken on a puffy look, particularly around the eyes. And her stamina was short-lived. The other day, she wanted to drive to Burlington with me to develop some film for the book I was trying to finish and get to the printer. Within minutes of arrival, she was too tired and needed to find a place to sit and wait. I had planned to do some other shopping while we were close to other shops and the supermarket, but did not, could not, with Joan as tired and unstable as she was. It was all I could do to steady her as we negotiated the slush, the parking lot and shopping carts, every little noise, every quick movement of others around us, a threat. It seemed her instability and vulnerability were creating a life of fear and I felt helpless to do much about it except to hold her, to try to keep her from falling and me with her.

To complicate matters, I was not feeling as well as I should. Arthritis had hit my shoulder joints which was only aggravated by my weight-lifting program at the fitness center and it had been too slippery and cold to walk or run in the early morning. Limiting myself to a set of routine floor exercises and the Health Rider seemed a sensible substitute. I was also experiencing some difficulty swallowing and would need to look into that soon. Meanwhile I was being very careful what I ate and had almost given up trying to swallow my handful of vitamin pills each day. I suspected this might be an old problem. It acted a lot like the hiatal hernia I had back in Santa Fe days. We would see. I would make an appointment with my doctor soon. He would no doubt order tests at the hospital which brought up the question of Joan's care in my absence. Did it ever!

March 1, 2011

Joan awoke early this morning when I did, the house cold and still dark outside. I asked how she had slept. She said okay but then added "I just don't feel well." When I asked if she could be more specific (I'm always looking for a specific area that might yield a clue) she said "No. It's just that I feel tired." "Tired" is the term that seems to describe her present state as well as any. Joan did seem without energy, needing to lie down often during the day (to rest her back). I noticed last night that while she wanted to help me with supper preparation, she could not, cutting up the onion too much. She had to lie down. A degree of self-awareness was beginning to set in it appeared. Sunday afternoon, after resting for awhile on the sofa, Joan sat up and said "I've got to do something. I need to go back to school or get a job." Totally unrealistic, of course, but it may spur her to make more social contacts. Joan, for the first time, expressed interest in getting involved with the Senior Center here in La Conner if I would go with her. I said I would and later realized that it was the one morning a week that I could not. The museum's weekly staff meeting occurred on Tuesday and that I must attend. Perhaps I could get someone else to go with her or simply quit my job which I was planning to do before long anyway. June (2011) had now become my tentative retirement date.

March 3, 2011

My swallowing issue seemed to have subsided. Slowing down before eating, taking deep breaths, drinking lots of fluids all seemed to help. Joan's "tiredness" had not subsided. She accompanied me to the grocery store in Burlington (a 20-minute drive via Hwy 20) and about halfway through the aisles she was ready to fold. I cut the shopping short. Upon reaching home, she collapsed on the sofa (and was quickly asleep) while I hauled in the bags of groceries from the car. I was tired, too, having gotten up at 3:00 am to write, but I was way short of Joan's level of exhaustion.

My other ongoing concern was her lack of appetite which I had mentioned many times now. Joan was simply not eating enough to provide the nutrition she needed to get through the day. She was simply not going to be able to make it over time The small portions I served her she saw as enormous, too much to eat although she wanted to eat more and she tried but it was the same most every meal. I gave Joan half the normal serving and, at best, she ate only half of that, bread and ice cream the exceptions. Last night she complained of stomach pain but passed it off as gas.

To be noted, too, were her frequent trips to the bathroom. They continued without let up. I tucked her in bed at 6:00 pm. She was restless for the first hour and finally settled down. At 9:30 pm she found her way to the bathroom, again at 10:03 pm and 10:18 pm and at 11:15 pm, followed by several other trips during the course of the night. I knew because I turned on the bed lamp each time to make sure she could find her way and to tuck her in again upon her return. Once in a while, Joan could not find her way and I had to walk with her through the living room and kitchen to the half bath. At one point (at the 11:15 time) she said she was hungry but refused my offer to fix oatmeal, my usual menu for that time of night.

March 5, 2011

Joan felt bad most of yesterday. She slept later than usual, complaining early on of her stomach hurting. She felt even worse when she learned she had forgotten it was my birthday and had not gotten me a present. I kept telling her she had given me a present, the new

MacBook laptop I was typing on much of the day, but, of course, I had purchased it online and thus it had little meaning to her as any kind of personal gift. She thought for awhile that we should do something special like go out for supper, perhaps at Nell Thorn's, but in the end we opted to buy take-out at the Thai restaurant. At the last minute I baked a gluten-free chocolate cake from Betty Crocker and bought some ice cream. About the only thing Joan ate for our birthday supper was the dessert. She barely touched the pad thai or mixed vegetables saying they were too difficult to chew. The new, tapered candles cast romantic light and the wine was good and I thoroughly enjoyed the food but watching Joan unable to eat, feeling unwell, almost constantly these days, stole the romance away, replacing it with worry.

My 84th birthday was a depressing day for the most part, offset some, thank goodness, by our friend's usual Friday morning visit and my friend's technical help in installing some new software so Joan and I could once again watch worship services live from First Community Church in Columbus. It also helped that we talked to our daughter by phone and that a colleague of mine at the museum gave me a birthday card and a book of poetry by Don Blanding called *Vagabond's House* which she said her mother read to her when she was a child. I spent a pleasant half hour reading some of it aloud to Joan. Another new colleague at the museum added color by leaving a decorated mason jar full of young daffodils and a nice note at our front door which was now the centerpiece of our dining room table. I was moved to write a poem about the daffodils and because Joan liked it, I included it here:

Daffodils

When we first got the daffodils, they were green, the 18
stems standing together in water in a ribboned canning jar,

top to bottom the shade of the Emerald Isle which I would
not have thought to say had it not been early in the

month's march to Saint Patrick's Day but as the weeks
went by and the gray sky gave way to blue, the yellow

blossoms emerged from their green hold, slowly to unfold,
the delicately-petaled heads all bending just so slightly

forward and tilted up as if listening for the dreaded
sounds of the tulips' festive approach, the worry showing

all too soon, the crop of heads turning brown around
the edge and beginning to droop and drop, signaling

change. I want to say to them clustered there so sadly,
not to despair for, again, they have done their job, preparing

us for a greater glory, baptizing us with the promises of
spring and the renewed hope that warmth and color bring.

Joan, as usual, was tired and went to bed before 7:00 pm. I followed a few hours later when she called up the stairs where I was typing, asking me to come to bed. She did not like being alone. I gladly joined her, turning off the lights and slipping into the adjoining twin bed. We both seemed to drift off to sleep eventually after she was reassured that all the doors were secured as if asking about the doors (and cars) three or four times in the course of a few minutes would make them all the tighter. At 10:30 pm she awoke to go to the bathroom, soon returned, and after I had tucked her in, said she felt terrible; "scared" was the word she used—a panic deep within about which little could be done, it seemed. When she said the bedcovers were too heavy, I realized I had failed to give her her nightly Lorazepam which was designed to ease anxiety. I quickly supplied it and then crawled in the narrow bed with her as carefully as I could to rub her back and legs, the old remedy for the "spooks." It worked. Eventually she began to relax and fell into a deep sleep. Never had I relied on a pill more to bring peace to the evening's end. I could not believe I had forgotten it!

March 14, 2011

The chilling refrain continued with Joan's first words each morning being those of not feeling well, "tired" and "shaky" and wanting to go back to bed. The other night they were her last words as well before I turned off the bed lamp. The downward spiral seemed to be accelerating in some way. Her hearing seemed worse so I sometimes found myself shouting to make certain she heard me. She read less and less of the newspaper each morning although she looked forward to its arrival. There was now little conversation at the dinner table and even major happenings, such as the recent tsunami disaster in Japan, she was unable to recall.

On the other hand, Joan was almost constantly preoccupied with what she saw out the dining room windows as we sat for meals. She insisted the ugly bare branches should be cut back. I kept telling her that they would soon bear buds and leaves but she did not believe me. She worried constantly about the big fir trees as they swirled and swayed in the big winds and kept asking when we were going to move the racked firewood onto the porch. I repeatedly told her we didn't want to do that because of bugs, termites, etc. but she wanted to get out there the next day to start moving it since it was my idea to begin with (which, of course, it was not). Also, she often thought she saw the residents out on the porch of their house up on the hill across from us. I would often find her waving to the "grandmother" or "grandson", or saluting them with her glass of wine. When I followed her gaze, I saw no one there. Furthermore, it was unlikely they could see us at such a distance. I had no idea that it was a "grandmother" and "grandson" living there, but Joan told me she overheard the grandmother shouting to the grandson not to take the car (parked in front of their house) and demanding that he get back in the house.

I was able to draw Joan's attention from the outside for a few minutes yesterday morning as we watched a video from First Community Church. It was a beautiful service called "Winter Song" with a full choir and instrumental music. We followed the music from the program that I had gotten earlier. Joan seemed to enjoy the program but had great difficulty following the printed words.

Later in the day we took our usual walk but, upon our return, she complained that it was too long and she did not want to go that distance again. She was obviously worn out by the walk which was as good a measure as any for what was happening to Joan physically. She was not able to maintain her strength. Complaining during the course of the walk was noticeable as well. Everything was wrong to the point where it was becoming unpleasant to walk with her. The cars were driving too fast; the sidewalks were wet or dirty; the road had too much gravel on it; people were crowding the sidewalks, etc., all of which I saw as part of her physical decline. How you felt affected how you saw.

March 16, 2011

A new development: the last two days now Joan had shown visible anger because I had been at work at the museum and not home with her. Both days I had to remind her what my morning work schedule was. She seemed to be losing track, as well, of the time of day, confusing mornings and afternoons. One Monday she walked up to the museum a little after noon searching for me. I had been just preparing to head for home when I saw her and greeted her pleasantly. Her unpleasant response was to wonder, indignantly, when I was ever coming home, that seven or eight hours ought to be long enough to be away. It was much the same response when I arrived home the following noon. She greeted me at the door sullenly, perturbed at the time I was spending at the museum, unable to remember that I had made a special point of coming home at mid-morning to spend a few minutes with her and brew her a cup of tea. She was unable to remember her walk with a walking buddy earlier in the day either. It may be that I would soon need to retire and give my full attention to Joan and her needs. Originally I was going to hang up my security keys this month, but decided to stick with it until June, assessing the situation week by week to see if I really had that much time. I don't think I do.

March 17, 2011

Joan's life now seemed to be mostly comprised of confusion with moments of clarity. So often these days, usually at night, she would ask me who I was. When I told her my name was Bob, she responded with "Oh, that's my husband's name." When I, in turn, asked where her husband was, her usual answer was "I don't know" or "He's at the museum." This time she paused for a long moment and said something like "Wait a minute. You're my husband, aren't you?" We both laughed. A break through the clouds, momentary but welcome. My question was suspect, a trick question, and she ferreted it out.

Actually I was not certain she knew who I was most of the time except that I was there and caring for her. Several times during the day she would come up to me and tell me how much she loved me and I responded accordingly. When I ask her exactly how much she loved me, she still responded with our stock measure: "a bushel and a peck and a hug around the neck." I was never certain, though, that there was any memory, any sense of longevity, behind the declaration. Sometimes Joan asked if we were in fact married. When I told her that yes, indeed, we were married and told her how long, she was incredulous. On the other hand, there seemed to be little confusion when she asked me to crawl in bed with her and rub her back. At least she was confident that whoever I was, I knew all the right places to rub and that she was perfectly safe in my hands. Some of the time, the rubbing led to more intimacy and sexual arousal which she seemed to enjoy immensely, letting herself go with abandon. On this point, nothing had changed in our 59 years together. Given her frail frame and lack of stamina, I was impressed with the energy she brought to these occasional (and delightful) encounters. I would not have thought she had it in her to reach such an intense level and to sustain it over such a surprisingly long period. Was this saying something about sheer animal instinct and power, the one characteristic that never seemed to fail us as human beings?

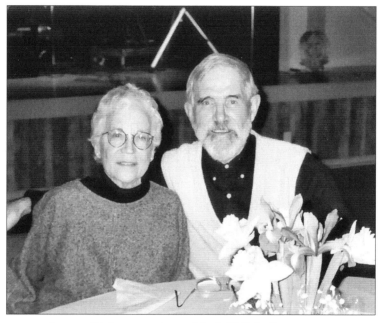

Joan and Bob at an outing at Maple Hall. LaConner, 2004

No Parking

I don't know what it is with Joan and street signs
but the spin she puts on them sometimes
leads me to whole new avenues of thought.
Yesterday on our walk
a common one caught her eye: NO PARKING it said,
the letters against white an unmistakable red,
with no space to impose or compose,
one's own correction or direction.
But Joan does,
on the spot."I'd like the sign better
if there was the letter
'S' before Parking." "Sparking?" I asked,
"No Sparking?" "Yes," she says, "that
makes for a much more interesting prohibition."

I had to agree with her. "Sparking," an old fashioned
term for "necking" or "making out," has a
passionate nuance and fame
that mere "parking" can never claim.
But can you imagine the reaction if suddenly
all the NO PARKING signs in La Conner read
NO SPARKING instead?
The hilarity and laughter would shake every rafter
and rattle every window to Seattle.

Yet rumor and innuendo has it that one time
in the sixties, the town fathers,
apparently dusted by pixies,
considered doing just that ... almost.
Desperate to keep the kids and their cars away
from the water tower and View Hill,
and to avoid the parents' constant criticism
and ill will, the town came close,
figuratively, to planting
"No Sparking" signs.

Instead, with relief, View Hill was sold
to the Historical Museum.
"Sparking" became an artifact,
stored and cold,
we think with a nod and wink.
Ever since, kids and cars
have managed, somehow,
to find other places to park
and new words for "spark."

March 18, 2011

Our trips to the supermarket in Burlington were always determined by our supply of toilet paper and seltzer water. Joan needed a lot of both these days. Our trip was pleasant enough but she tired rapidly once the shopping started. This time I escorted her to one of the benches near the check-out counter where she sat while I hurriedly finished the shopping. Not a bad solution, but I worried now about leaving her alone, even for a short period in unfamiliar surroundings for fear she would wander away. In this instance she had stayed put and was waiting patiently for me, much to my relief. Her level of exhaustion was such that I decided, then and there, to only do "supershopping" in the mornings when she was most rested.

Once home, I urged Joan to lie down on the sofa while I hauled in the groceries from the car. As tired as she was, she still wanted to help unload in some way, but I persuaded her that the best thing she could do was to stay where she was and relax. Finally, after I was through storing, we fell into a conversation we have only been able to have on rare occasions: a frank talk about her condition, her loss of memory. What led to it was the usual problem of her not being able to recognize me.

As we often did, we had embraced and held each other for a moment as I was brewing tea. Joan then stepped back and asked, "Are you my mother?" For a second I thought she was joking but she really was not. Seeing my puzzled expression, she asked, "Are you my father, then?" I replied, identifying myself by name and relationship, and, after observing the concern, the fear, in her face, I walked her back to the sofa.

I then described to her some past instances where she had failed to recognize me, particularly at night, after I had been reading to her in bed. Joan was aghast that she would do a thing like that. I told her it no longer bothered me, that it was just part of what many older people had to put up with in themselves as they got to be our age. And then, I stressed something I had been emphasizing a lot lately—that even though she might not be able to recognize me, I was always going to recognize her. A good friend in Columbus had sent me a story via email about an elderly man who had visited his wife every day in the rest home for six years even though she did not remember who he was. When asked why, he said "Because, while she doesn't know who I am, I know who she is." Such a powerful notion I welcomed and was only too happy to incorporate.

Joan was obviously reassured by the notion but she was still astonished, shaking her head in disbelief. It should come as no surprise that later that night, last night actually, after I had read to her and turned off the lamp next to the bed, she again asked me my name. When I told her, I got the typical response: "Oh, that's my husband's name too." After I told her I grew up in Columbus, Ohio, in response to her question, she told me about growing up in Portsmouth and attending Ohio State University on the GI Bill. She made no connection with me in her recounting even though OSU was where we had met and dated. She was able to remember the name of her Greek sorority without prompting.

An amazing day in some ways, but devastating in its direction. Downhill we go. If only it could be on a Flexible Flyer sled, Joan's body atop mine, coasting down a snowpacked hill on a bright winter's day.

March 21, 2011

Saturday Joan awoke as usual feeling unwell and wanting to go back to bed for awhile, which she did, while I prepared breakfast. Eventually she perked up after some coffee and a couple of my fresh muffins—enough so that she consented to taking a shower, washing her hair and putting on freshly laundered clothes. Joan obviously felt better by this time but later when we got back from our morning walk she was totally exhausted. It did not help that she was battling a sore arm and elbow from a fall on the hard road surface the afternoon before. Fortunately, I was walking with her and was holding her hand when she tripped and fell, softening the hard landing at least somewhat. By late afternoon Joan was feeling worse, chilling and shaking occasionally which began to alarm me since they reminded me of the slight convulsions preceding hypoglycemia. I checked her blood sugar level but it was a safe 95 mg. Finally, Joan got to the point where she was truly frightened by the feeling of being cold inside, at her core and, after more discussion, decided that the only recourse on a Saturday was a visit (again) to the Emergency Room at the Island Hospital in Anacortes.

We arrived at the Emergency Room about 5:30 pm. After Joan underwent blood and urine analysis and diagnostic imaging of pancreas, liver, kidneys etc., without any positive findings, she was eventually discharged at about 11:00 pm. There was a lot of waiting around in the small treatment room where she rested due to the large number of emergency room patients. The RN pointed out that the Emergency Room was always more crowded on nights when there was a full moon. And the moon was clear and full this Saturday. I would like to report that Joan was a good patient but she was not, becoming more and more agitated as the night wore on. She felt neglected understandably but the ER doctor could do little until he got the tests results from the laboratory. Meanwhile, Joan, upset, more and more vocal, threatened to get dressed and walk out. I realized, after a while, that I had forgotten all about the Lorazepam pill I normally gave her at home to relieve her anxiety. Once the RN supplied Joan with the medication, she began to calm down some and the threats ceased. In some ways, I was disappointed that no specific cause for Joan's malady could be found. But, of course, he did find from personal observation and discussion what I already knew and so wrote on the discharge papers: dementia and anorexia. The ER doctor's last words of advice to Joan were to try to find ways to eat, consulting a nutritionist if necessary, and discussing with her doctor the possibility of further tests of the upper and lower intestines. Her doctor had already suggested such tests, but she had refused. Too much was too much. Talking with her later about the possibility of further testing reconfirmed her opposition. She was not interested. I was prepared to think that no abnormalities would be found that would result in a better appetite anyway.

We drove home Saturday night under the light of a full moon in a cloudless sky, had a bowl of oatmeal and piled into bed after midnight. At 1:35 am the telephone rang. It was Dictograph calling about an alarm being triggered at the museum. There was nothing to do but get dressed and meet the police there. As usual, it was another false alarm. One of the new staff had forgotten to latch an interior door and it had swung slightly open, separating the contact points. Some nights were more restful than others; this one was not. Nor was last night but I had no excuses to offer. That Joan again asked me my name just before turning off the bed lamp did not bother me. It was becoming a nightly feature. Would it eventually become a daily feature as well? Probably.

March 25, 2011

Joan's evening of shaking and feeling cold continued. If I had not already taken her to the ER, I would have taken her again several evenings ago. It was that bad, and terribly upsetting for her. An unscheduled visit to the doctor's office confirmed my opinion that her sense of feeling cold and the shaking was directly due to not eating enough to maintain strength and produce any protective fat. The doctor had no suggestions for increasing her appetite. He did adjust her insulin intake, suggesting I inject her with only three units of Levemir (instead of four) to reduce the danger of hypoglycemia. Yesterday represented a shift of some kind in Joan's condition. She experienced no feelings of being cold or shaking. Instead she was tired and listless, not feeling at all well, either lying down or sitting up and, of course, not eating much. Over the last several days she had eaten small milkshakes with ice cream and chocolate protein powder (Carnation's Breakfast Essentials) but unable to eat much of my homemade vegetable soup (which I put in the blender to make it easier for her to swallow). She did eat a few crackers with almond butter and a slice of multigrain bread and butter and she managed to eat a small portion of my beef stew, ignoring most of the tender pieces of meat in favor of the potatoes and cooked carrots. Still, her intake was miniscule, not enough. Strange to me was that her weight on our home scales remained consistently at around 87.2 pounds (without clothes or shoes). I did not get it.

The day was also marked with more confusion than usual, a frailty and worry about misstepping at every turn. Joan repeatedly called on me to help her to the bathroom and even to help her stand again after sitting on the toilet. Somehow we managed a short walk in the afternoon, but she was tired almost immediately and relieved to get back home to rest. The morning had been taken up with a visit from our granddaughter, Nora, who recently returned from a four-month hike throughout Central America with a friend and would soon head back to Sitka for the fishing season, serving as a deckhand on her dad's gillnetter, the Sunfish. As we talked, Joan was unable to follow the conversation, often interrupting to say, "I don't understand what you're saying." She had equal difficulty viewing photos Nora had taken on her trip (and posted on Facebook) via my laptop. The only thing Joan mentioned after Nora's departure was that Nora had been sitting in her chair (at the dining room table) without her permission which she obviously did not like one bit.

Yesterday's observations led me to think that it might be time to return the phone call to the Hospice director who sometime ago had urged me to let him make a home visit and assessment. That I was beginning to feel the impact of my caregiver responsibilities on my own health added to my decision. I needed some relief—or more relief—since I had been getting some respite with neighbors stopping by to take Joan for a walk four mornings a week for an hour or so. Of course, I was still able to work at the museum three mornings a week—but only with frequent phone contact with Joan. I could see that this arrangement might soon be impossible. I really disliked the idea of outsiders in our house, but did I have a choice?

March 26, 2011

Joan awoke this morning at 3:41 am with what was now a common refrain—"I don't feel well"—although she had made her way to the bathroom and back without assistance. She was happy to have me tuck her in to her warm electric blanket with the assurance that she did not have to get up yet.

Joan had walked with one of her pals yesterday morning but felt too tired and unsteady to walk with me later in the day. She spent most of the afternoon curled up on the small wicker sofa in the dining room while I started my bread (a two-day process) and mowed the backyard. Toward suppertime, she complained of her forefinger (right hand) suddenly hurting to the point where she could not as much as touch it without yelping in pain. Since there was no physical cause, I guessed it was a nerve issue of some kind, perhaps having to do with her diabetic condition. Later, during the meal, the finger just as suddenly quit hurting and her right eye began paining which continued for an hour or so until I gave her an OTC pain pill. Is there any connection between the finger pain and the eye pain? Research was called for. I tucked her into bed about 7:30 pm, got into my pajamas and bathrobe and read in the living room with one ear cocked toward the bedroom nearby for any sign of distress.

There was none and at 9:30 pm I crawled into the adjacent twin bed, ready to call it a day, totally done in and forcing myself to acknowledge my own limitations in caring for Joan. I really did need to pull in other help soon. The tiredness I felt was hitting me right in the pit of the stomach. No amount of breathing exercises or physical exercise seemed able to eradicate it for long.

March 27, 2011

A first occurred this morning (Saturday). Joan not only did not want to get up, she did not, preferring to stay in bed. She felt that bad—"achy," extremely "tired" and without appetite. Even when I told her that our son, John, was stopping by for breakfast and that Nora and her boyfriend, Jaycen, were joining us as well, she was not inclined to budge and stayed in bed as I prepared breakfast, set the table and welcomed everybody.

It was not until we were halfway through the meal that Joan called for me. She told me she had to get to the bathroom. The only way to get there from our new downstairs bedroom was to pass by the dining room which she reluctantly did. Once she had toileted and slipped into her bathrobe, she joined us at the dining room table and proceeded to eat and enjoy the company.

By 11:30 am the party was over. While I did the dishes, Joan curled up on the wicker sofa and remained there or in bed most of the day. She ate a small lunch and ate virtually nothing for supper except a slice of my fresh whole wheat bread and butter and a small dish of ice cream. At one point, I wanted to run to the grocery store for more ice cream but she did not want me to leave for fear something might happen to me and so I stayed put, doing inside chores (washing clothes, emptying waste baskets, etc.) and writing at my laptop in the dining room. I also got in a blissful hour of deep sleep which was rejuvenating, easing the knot in my stomach. I encouraged Joan to sit by me to watch a performance of "Celtic Thunder-Heritage" on public television which she seemed to enjoy but she soon tired of the following program on "Doo Wop" music. I did not blame her. By 7:30 pm she was back in bed, ready to call it a day. I followed within the hour after some reading. Except for the morning run and workout at the fitness center, I had been housebound the entire day. I had wanted to finish mowing the lawn, but felt reluctant to do even that, for fear Joan might need me for something. Further proof of the need for outside help.

March 28, 2011

Yesterday (Sunday) was a test and Joan passed with flying colors. She got up on schedule, ate breakfast and even agreed to take a shower with my help. She did not remember a thing about staying in bed most of the day yesterday nor would she believe that she had not showered for a week. She thought she still showered every morning. She had even more trouble believing that I often had to cajole her into showering. The reason for her reluctance had nothing to do with hygiene and everything to do with feeling tired and unsure of her footing. Suddenly, for her, the pleasure of a hot shower was replaced by the fear of falling and just not feeling up to it. Joan weighed herself on the bathroom scale at my urging. She was down one pound from 87.2 lbs to 86.2 lbs.

We managed to get in two walks, short ones, but Joan was feeling desperately tired midway through each. Later in the afternoon she wanted to take another walk, completely forgetting she had already walked twice. By supper time she had returned to her normal complaint of not feeling well, ate little of the main dish (a spinach ricotta tart) but ate all of her fresh pear salad and a piece of my fresh whole wheat bread and butter. I noted that her blood sugar levels were much higher than usual, hitting 330 mg after lunch and 217 mg at supper. She was ready for bed at 6:00 pm but stretched out on the leather sofa with plenty of pillows and a blanket to watch a segment of Cleopatra with Liz Taylor and Richard Burton. By 8:00 pm I had tucked Joan into bed and soon followed. Except for the sermon that was streamed live from the First Community Church early Sunday morning, it had been another fallow day for me, getting little done inside or outside the house, but I was thankful—joyful even—that we had gotten through it and that Joan had made some kind of modest recovery from the previous day.

March 29, 2011

Signs of decline are becoming more frequent. Another first occurred yesterday afternoon. After lunch we decided to take our usual afternoon walk, a short one down 3rd Street to Washington Street, down to 2nd Street and then north across Morris Street to State Street and then back on 1st Street through the main commercial area. We got as far as the candy store on 1st Street and Joan was too tired to proceed. I left her resting on a bench and hustled back for our car, picked her up and got her home and settled on the sofa.

She seemed totally out of energy, depleted and grateful to be home and resting. She got a lot of rest these days. I came home from the museum to check on her at about 10:00 am yesterday and found her sleeping soundly on the wicker sofa. We had tea which I saw as an opportunity to talk to her about the need to bring in some outside help, explaining my worry about leaving her alone for any length of time. Combined with her own feelings of being lonely and bored, it seemed imperative to bring in extra help. As I explained, I was feeling uncomfortable now about even going outside to mow the yard for fear I would fail to hear her if she suddenly needed me. And I can only rely on her use of the telephone to a point. If she were to fall, I pointed out, and no phone within reach, what then?

I mentioned "falling," of course, since it struck me as a much more likely possibility now than even a few months ago. Joan seemed to agree with what I was saying but I had little hope she would remember any of it. Today, anyway, I intended to make the initial contact with Hospice and set up a visit and assessment, something I had dreaded doing because of what it implied about her deteriorating condition. But I must face it and get on to the next phase, a new phase of having others around the house. Could Joan, could I, deal with the change? We had to. There was no alternative if we wanted to stay in our own house (which we had vowed to do). I felt now a sense of urgency I had not felt before. It was just the prod I needed to transcend all other considerations, financial or otherwise, to make sure Joan was properly cared for, a final act in a long play of married love and fidelity.

Whistling In the Dark

I sometimes hear my neighbor before I see him.
In the dark of early morning I hear him
whistling his way to work
Often I call out a friendly greeting
in the direction of the sound, just as often
getting a matching response.

Sometimes our paths cross and we stop to talk.
Why does he whistle?
Fear of the dark? In our little town?
Hardly.
For company against sadness?
No.
Why then?
Because there are songs in my head, he says,
music that needs expressing.

With a song in our head, or heart,
where some might locate it,
can we help but whistle?
Sadness we are able to hide for a while
at least, but happiness, joy's song?
Irrepressible it seems.
We have to whistle.

Most of us do our whistling through
puckered lips, blowing into thin air.
But others press their lips to horn
or reed, whistling brassy tunes.

Some whistle with their fingers,
tapping keyboards, plucking strings,
chiseling stone, daubing canvas,
creating sonnets and sonatas
and new worlds of form and color,
daring us to reconsider what
we think we know.

Yet others whistle with their toes,
dancing us into lively choreographies,
compelling us by sheer beauty and grace,
to try once more, however awkwardly,
to step together and, when required,
to step apart, in time.

April 4, 2011

A social worker with Hospice met with us last week to determine whether Joan qualified for Hospice at this time. Initially, I had the impression that she thought probably not. Joan seemed cheerful and responsive but as the conversation wore on, Joan was unable to remain seated at the table, excused herself to lie on the nearby sofa, trying to follow our conversation but not able to hear and, though covered with a blanket, frequently experiencing those short convulsive shakes that I found so worrisome. It seemed to me that Joan met the Hospice criteria of "debility," i.e., "the failure to thrive."

Whether the social worker agreed remained to be seen. We agreed on the one essential point: Joan's condition was way beyond the reach of a cure. My job (and Hospice's objective) continued to be palliative, to provide comfort, to make Joan's day to day existence as easy and painless as possible. Even if Hospice agreed to take us on, however, I would still need to find people to stay with her while I was at work or getting groceries or taking a break. The social worker provided some resources to explore, including COPES, a service provided by the state's DSHS. She also suggested "Remeron" as a drug that helped to stimulate appetite and elevate mood. Upon leaving, the social worker stated, with some pride and pleasure at the prospect, that she would be the case manager if Hospice decided to take us on. I hope it did. She would be first-rate: pleasant, smart, able and caring.

I awoke last night to a lot of shuffling and commotion. When I turned on the bedside lamp, there was Joan wrapped in the electric blanket, but unable to walk to the bathroom because the electric cord was tethered to the bed. I noted the time (12:11 am) as I jumped out of bed to help her. I relieved her of the blanket and helped her into her bathrobe and, while she stood helplessly by, I remade the bed and then realized she needed me to walk her to the bathroom. Her midnight confusion seemed to follow from the day's lapses. Often, over the course of Sunday morning and afternoon, she had asked where "Dad" was and whether her mother was joining us for lunch and staying overnight. Several times during the day I had to remind her that her brothers had all died. I considered it a breakthrough of some kind when she responded to my bad news with "I guess I knew that." At one point, she asked where I grew up and was pleased to hear we had both been at Ohio State University at the same time. At another point she said I could sleep in the twin bed next to hers. Her physical condition seemed no better than her mental. She wanted so much to take a walk yesterday afternoon but she got only as far as donning her jacket when she had to sit down, stating that she was "too shaky" to walk. By late afternoon she decided the only place she felt comfortable was in bed so by 4:30 pm that was where she was. I did get her up to eat a bit of salmon and potato with me at 6:00 pm, but then she went right back to bed. Not even the Lorazepam seemed to help much. I seemed to spend a lot of time these days in the kitchen preparing meals that were hardly touched. Last night I did not even bother to light the dinner candles.

April 7, 2011

Joan's Tuesday walking pal phoned me at work saying Joan was too tired to finish their walk so her husband drove down to 1st Street, picked them up and brought Joan home. She stayed a little longer at the house to see that Joan was okay. I conferred with Joan, too, via the phone and agreed that she seemed fine. A little later, around 10:30 am, another friend arrived to provide some additional coverage in my absence.

I had concluded that it was time to begin increasing home care.

My former colleague at the museum and good friend spent Monday morning from 10:30 am to early afternoon with Joan as well as Tuesday. I intended to start paying her for her hours, particularly when I was at work, but at other times as well to give me a break. Meanwhile the volunteers are a great help when they're available (one on Thursdays at 9:00 am and another on Wednesdays at 9:00 am). I may have my friend from the museum extend her Friday hours or perhaps better, cover for me on Thursday mornings when I was normally at home. A lot depended on her tutoring schedule at a public school which began the following week.

Late Tuesday afternoon, Joan felt so poorly we discussed making another trip to the Emergency Room at Island Hospital. The doctors at the La Conner Clinic were too busy to see her on the spur of the moment, but I was able to make an appointment for the next morning. Eventually she decided against the ER and soon began to feel somewhat better after I massaged her back and legs. It reminded me that physical touch can often do wonders, restoring connection with each other and with the elemental nature of being (which is the only way I can think to put it). I will make it a point now to spend time each day massaging Joan's body, particularly her back and legs, but spent a little time as well yesterday caressing her head as she rested on the sofa. I was happy to note last evening at supper that she actually ate an entire salmon patty, a serving of peas and french fries, cleaning her plate! I'm not ready yet to make any particular connection between massage and appetite but I was happy to see her eat a complete meal for a change.

Nora, our granddaughter and her boyfriend, Jaycen, were coming for breakfast so I hoped that would buoy Joan's spirit. I had just finished my income tax so I was ready to celebrate with waffles and Canadian bacon.

April 8, 2011

Nora and Jaycen arrived on schedule, enjoyed breakfast and lingered around the dining room table until about noon. Our conversation ranged all over the map. Joan was not able to keep up and lay down on the wicker sofa appearing to tune out most of the time. Such nice kids, very attentive to Joan. Nora brought Joan a few colored rocks and an unusually colored shell; she brought me a black T-shirt with her own design of a raven in white on the front.

After cleaning up and a light lunch, Joan managed to walk with me to the post office to mail our income tax return, but she complained of being tired and immediately took to the sofa upon our return. I had noticed lately, if I had not mentioned it before, that Joan's pace had really slowed, her walk now becoming much more tentative, almost a shuffle at times.

After reading another chapter from Jim Lynch's entertaining book, *The Highest Tide*, I turned off the bedside lamp about 8:15 pm. At 10:45 pm Joan was fully awake, worried that her mother had given her something to drink that disagreed with her and made her stomach hurt. I had a hard time convincing her that her mother was long gone, that no one else was living in our house with us and that she must have been dreaming. She was not convinced but I realized, noting the panic in her demeanor, that I had not given her that second pill last night (Lorazepam) which I quickly did at 11:00 pm. Then I massaged her back and legs for the next 40 minutes. It worked like magic. She began to relax and eventually fell into a deep sleep. Her mother continued to be much in her thoughts these days. Her father's presence was more prominent too. And she continued to wonder about me from time to time during the day, asking me where I grew up and other questions which revealed the distance and space that her memory loss was creating. But I happily answered her questions, going over old ground, anything to keep her at least partially grounded and connected to me and our life now. Whether I liked it or not, the separation had begun, a quiet, unintended divorce. I so disliked the feeling.

April 12, 2011

Friday afternoon the sun came out, inspiring me to get the lawn mowed and pull some weeds. Joan, I was happy to see, began her project of carrying some of the firewood stacked in the side yard around to the front porch. Later that afternoon I checked my e-mail to discover that Gorham Printing had not received fourteen of the poems I had mailed earlier nor had they gotten the six-page short story. Consequently, I spent most of Saturday morning and early afternoon retrieving the poems, converting some to older Mac software, and resending. Joan was a good scout throughout, resting on the wicker sofa. When I could not find the short story on either computer, I opted to get to the Office Depot in Mount Vernon where they would scan my only hard copy and e-mail it for me. She and I had discussed for some time whether she should go with me or stay home. Convinced finally that I wanted her to go with me, she came along and sat in the car while I got the short story processed. I had wanted to do some shopping at the Food Co-op on the return home but seeing how tired she seemed, left the shopping for another time, perhaps, tomorrow morning, Sunday, after TV church. She was glad to get home, relieved as if she had been travelling for hours which was yet another indication of just how low her energy reserves really were. As expected, she ate little and was too tired to sit with me to catch up with the news. With my help, she soon had her pajamas on and by 7:30 pm I had turned off her bed lamp.

Sunday morning, Joan felt even worse than yesterday so shopping at the Co-op was again postponed and I made do with a short run to the local market. Sunday was pretty much a lost day. Joan rested on the sofa in her pajamas and bathrobe most of the time. I had urged her Saturday to take a shower and wash her hair, but she declined because, she said, she felt too shaky and was afraid she might fall. Sunday was no different. Even when I told her she had not showered since the previous Saturday, she was unconvinced and kept asking me to feel how clean her skin was. She did not need a shower. I could only shake my head and shrug my shoulders in mute disapproval and move on to other things. Monday was a little better. I made a special point of taking time from work at 9:30 am to come home and help her shower and don freshly laundered clothes. By 10:30 am my friend (and by now our official caregiver) arrived and they were able to get in a walk to the post office and back without mishap. Joan showed some interest in our scrapbooks which I had brought downstairs for the caregiver, but was for the most part unable to recognize herself, her children or her relatives. By the afternoon Joan was feeling like she always did in the afternoons now, tired, no appetite, wanting to take another walk, but at the last minute changing her mind and lying down again on the sofa. She seemed almost totally bored and unengaged, offering to help me prepare supper, but not able to help much except to put on the flatware. (The dinner plates were too heavy). Last evening I postponed supper for an hour because she was too tired and wanted to rest some more. As usual she ate very little, avoided the vegetables (asparagus) and relished a large (for her) dish of ice cream.

An Early Spring Morning at the Marina

Night gives way to day,
nudged to nothing
by April's rosy elbow,
the shadows, night's kin,
finding their places,
in all the likely spaces,
snug alongside foc'sles and hulls.
The sailboats, well-rested
after a mild winter
in their waterbeds,
now reaching their slender,
line-laced fingers skyward
to test the wind and weather,
to see whether it's time,
once more, to hoist sail.
Standing near the pier
in this magic middle time,
the water is without ripple,
solid enough to walk on,
you think,
in faith you might, when,
suddenly, a feathered diver
breaks the surface
to set things right.

April 13, 2011

"Who is it?"

"Who is it?" This morning at 3:15 am Joan was walking from the side door to the back door to the front door, turning on the porch lights as she went, asking the question, shouting the question actually, so as to be heard by whoever she thought was outside. I stayed abed listening, figuratively shaking my head. Joan said she had heard someone "banging" at the door. I told her I was already awake and preparing to get up and I had heard nothing. That gave her pause, but only for a second, and then she insisted it was probably Jack (her brother) getting back late from wherever he had been. Joan also seemed to believe the rest of her family were asleep upstairs. The previous morning at about the same time, she had heard voices outside and went to investigate, again turning on the outside lights and peering into the dark. Once satisfied, I was relieved to see, she went quietly back to bed where I tucked her in, checking to make certain her electric blanket was operating. There was not another peep out of her for the remainder of her sleep cycle. In fact, yesterday she slept much later than usual, getting up around 7:30 am only at my insistence. I had to be at work at 8:00 am or thereabouts and I had to monitor her blood sugar.

Joan had mentioned nothing about "hearing voices" yesterday morning nor did I expect her to refer to the "door banging" this morning. What I had come to expect were questions about her parents and brothers, questions which presupposed that they were all alive and living nearby if not at our house. No matter how many times I delivered the bad news that they were all dead (said in the gentlest terms possible), she was soon back to her coveted illusion of being surrounded by her family. "Where's Dad?" she had wanted to know at supper last evening. I asked what "Dad" she was referring to because she sometimes referred to me by that name. In this case it was her father, "Pappy" Williams. Earlier, in the middle of the afternoon, she had asked the same question about her mother. Seldom these days did she think of us as being the only two occupants of the house, at night time anyway. Most nights, according to Joan, one or more of our children or members of her deceased family were asleep upstairs. So we had quite a full house. Fortunately, since they were nowhere to be found during the day, we did not have to stand the cost of feeding them.

Of course, I coveted Joan's coveted illusion. How wonderful it would be to gather Pappy and Ruth and her three brothers around our dining room table for breakfast on a sunny morning, especially if her sister flew in to join us from Salina, Kansas as well. Being associated with Joan's family, even if only through marriage, had always been a great pleasure for me, a single child and with no family to speak of. I could just imagine what a wonderful conversation we would have, particularly if Patti's deceased husband, John Shaver, joined us too.

April 18, 2011

Our house was becoming crowded with Joan's deceased family, including a few of our own distant children, and occasionally a stranger, usually a young girl. Seldom did a meal go by now that Joan did not ask me where her "Dad" was or when "Mom" was returning. I repeatedly told her that they had died and retold the stories surrounding their deaths, couched in the most loving words I could muster. When I finished explaining, she would often remark "Oh, yes, I think I remember that." The same was true with her brothers, most often Bill, who she sometimes thought was staying at our house and sleeping upstairs. My response was the same as with questions about her parents, Pappy and Ruth. I retold the story of Bill's last days at the veterans' home in Fergus Falls, Minnesota and the good care he had received from his daughter, Terri Lee. Joan usually appeared more upset when talking about her brother Don because they were the closest in age. The stranger, the young girl, was the most baffling to me and apparently to Joan as well. I would say, "I didn't see any young girl." Joan would respond with, "But you must have seen her. She was just here." When I shook my head with a "no," Joan would seem upset as if beginning to wonder if she was losing her mind. In fact, on one occasion, she said just that: "I think I must be losing it." I comforted her as best I could in my own wonderment.

It was becoming clear that Joan was moving away from me, from the real world, and into a world of her own making. Sometimes she seemed content to sit quietly, preoccupied and eating (dabbling at her food was more like it), her eyes on her plate. Other times, to my relief, her attention was directed to the outdoors, to the effect of the frequent winds on the fir trees and the general commotion the wind caused, to the family up the hill or to the need to move our stack of firewood. But even these observations were repetitive and predictable and had a certain unreality about them.

One of Joan's morning concerns lately was the worry about missing school, being late for class or missing an important exam. I thought for a while she was referring to her experience of being a teacher but it seemed more the case that she saw herself as a student. She was always relieved when I told her that she did not have to worry about getting to class, that she had finished school and graduated long ago and now could just rest on her accomplishments.

April 21, 2011

"Someone's trying to kill me!" were Joan's words to me as she shook me awake at about 10:30 pm last night. There was nothing urgent about her touch. It was more tentative, like she was not sure I was going to be there in bed and if I was exactly who I was. I coaxed her back to bed, but as I tucked her in, she made me promise several times that I would never leave without her. The fear in her eyes was real; she was genuinely frightened. When I asked who wanted to kill her, she could not provide even a clue but she was convinced of the truth of it. I had to turn on the lamp on the dresser and leave it on. She watched to make certain I bedded down in the twin bed next to her. After a while her deep breathing returned. Despite lamplight flooding the room we both slept a few hours. Later, after another of Joan's trips to the bathroom I was able to convince her that it would be okay to turn off the light. The night time confusion continued, I note. She was not sure whether she was upstairs or down, how to get to the bathroom or who I was. "What's your name?" she wanted to know. This time when I replied "Bob" She did not follow it up with the usual "Oh, that's my husband's name." And when I tucked her in bed again at 4:00 am she wondered if she ought to get up in order to make it to class on time. Again I reassured her that she did not have to worry about getting to class which seemed both to relieve her and puzzle her. There was no reference to the earlier threat against her life. Although I could vividly recall how frightened she was at the time, I wondered if this morning she would even remember it.

Several times during the day yesterday Joan wondered who I was but I was becoming accustomed to the question. Moreover, it was balanced by those lovely moments when Joan not only recognized me but embraced me and declared her love. More noticeable was the ever-increasing prominence of her mother and father in our conversation, particularly in the afternoon. "Where's Dad?" she frequently asked and was increasingly anxious to talk to her mother.

April 22, 2011

Help to maintain our house arrived in the person of a professional housekeeper who was an old friend of John and Beth's, harking back to the early Alaska fishing days. Unable to help as they would have if they still lived nearby in Conway, John and Beth did the next best thing by hiring their long-time friend to assist us in some manner each week. The housekeeper and I agreed that Thursday mornings was a good time. I would be home too, and could use the time to help with the cleaning or, eventually, use the few hours to get away to do something else entirely.

Last Thursday our newest help paid us a visit. I showed her through the house to give her a sense of the layout and where she might dig in. She was impressed with the general order but saw where we could use some help, starting with the cobwebs that had accumulated on the high ceilings and the first floor windows which obviously needed a good cleaning. As the three of us sat around the dining room table, it soon became clear that Joan did not like the idea of having anyone else around even if only to clean our house. She seemed proud to point out the good job I was doing keeping the house clean and in order—with little thought that I might like some relief to do other things.

Not only was I falling behind with inside cleaning, I seemed to have little time to complete any of my outside projects. All the advantages the housekeeper and I could cite, however, including the fact that John and Beth were paying for her services, fell on deaf ears. Joan would have none of it. The housekeeper and I agreed privately to keep Thursday mornings in mind against the time when the need for more help would become more obvious to Joan. If Joan and I could find something else to do which took us out of the house on a Thursday, she would be amenable to coming over from her home in Anacortes (a neighboring town) to get some cleaning done. So the arrangement was not terminated, just postponed.

Surprisingly, Joan has mentioned nothing about her parents for the past several days. She appeared puzzled when I told her Susan and John were not staying with us or staying nearby. When I told her they live in Santa Fe and Sitka respectively, she seemed to remember that that was where they would likely be.

Joan has continued to move the dry firewood from the rack in the side yard to the front porch, carrying one or two pieces at a time. A slow method, but she obviously took immense pleasure in having her own project and several times a day now would point with pride to the growing stack on the porch. In the interest of fire protection and pest control, I had not wanted the firewood stacked anywhere near the house but seeing Joan's delight in moving the wood under cover changed all that. When I realized this was Joan's only sustained interest these days, principles were out the window and fire and bugs took a back seat.

Perhaps the most astonishing thing to report occurred the other night just after midnight. When Joan returned from the bathroom, she pulled the covers back on my twin bed and crawled in beside me. Never did I recall her ever taking the initiative like that. I had always done the crawling. But here she was, snuggling up against me and caressing my chest and stomach with her free hand. I was, of course, pleased and responded in turn and before it was over we had a merry old time, like old times, tangled in the covers, passionate and laughing before it was over and then the pleasure of lying quietly in each other's arms. True peace.

As expressive (and passionate) as Joan was, she had written very little about our relationship. Here is the one poem I know of:

To My Lover

Your touch makes my body feel like a cathedral,
With towering spires,
And vaulted arches,
And secret, sacred niches,
That draw you in.

April 26, 2011

Easter morning. What was the greeting and response? The sequence I remember was "The Lord is risen." "The Lord is risen, indeed." Joan and I celebrated with a big breakfast of Belgian waffles and regular Green Mountain coffee and viewed a live broadcast from our home church, the First Community Church, in Columbus, Ohio.

It was a quiet Easter day as Joan rested on the wicker couch beside the dining room table as I edited my way through the proof of my new book entitled *Blue Cow*. Some copy was a mess. On 30 pages the end-note designation which I had so carefully added was missing and had to be re-added. Two pages were missing from the proof altogether, much of the problem directly related to the electronic transfer process and my own inexperience. Anyway, those tasks had been completed. The book had also been proofed (with over 100 errors!) and would be sent off to the printers today and, with it, a sense of relief.

Even under the pressure of getting the proofing completed, Joan and I managed to get our walks in and, at one point, on Easter Day had another one of those "break-through" conversations where she recognized something was wrong, that she was having memory problems. The self-revelation was prompted by her wondering who the "young girl" was who had been visiting us. When I told her there was no young girl and had not been the other times she mentioned it, Joan paused, troubled that this could be happening, that she was only imagining it. I reassured her as best I could but we both knew now that the prognosis was not good.

It was a quiet, sheltered life we lived as I scrambled now to anticipate the need for more help down the road. Among other things, I was in the process of reapplying for help from Veterans Affairs. The first step was to establish Joan's military credentials so that both of us were eligible for funding which, in effect, extended the income limit from $40,000 to $80,000. I had done that online last week.

I think I was in partial denial myself. I really hated thinking about us, about our growing limitations; I would much rather spend my time thinking about and writing about other things, but here I was. Here we were. My attention was required right here and now and I must deal with it. And deal I would. But it is a fight to keep focused on it.

April 27, 2011

Like the previous one, the "breakthrough" at Easter was short-lived. Last night as I was tucking Joan in bed, she asked where the "young girl" was. I told her I had not seen any young girl. She was surprised that I did not remember when the girl came by early in the afternoon. I asked for a description. Joan described her as a young teenager 12 or 13 years of age, possibly 14 or 15, with dark hair. When I stated again that I had not seen her, she expressed astonishment but stuck to her guns. The teenager had been right here in our house and that was that. Joan was less certain about our daughter's whereabouts. She insisted that Susan, too, had been at our house. When I told her that Susan could not have been here since she lived in Santa Fe and was there now, she hesitated some but did not seem convinced. Who this "young girl" was and how she fit into Joan's world I had yet to learn.

Last night was another restless night. Even with the second Lorazepam pill, Joan was fidgety, finding the few bedcovers heavy and weighing her down. Reading to her from Jim Lynch's fine book calmed her down but no sooner had I moved into the TV room to read something of my own than Joan was up and wondering when I was coming to bed. I could not keep my eyes open while reading anyway, so soon joined her for a little relaxed pillow talk about our kids across the space between the two beds. Almost immediately Joan had to get up again to use the bathroom. Usually Joan was up about every two hours to urinate. Last night it was more frequent. There was a period toward morning when there was only a five-minute lapse between trips. Another urinalysis may be in order, but I needed to see first what the frequency rate would be tonight.

I felt surprisingly good after my interrupted sleep last night and found myself thinking once again about how to increase Joan's nutritional intake at meals. I noticed last night that she ate all of her serving of a spinach-onion-egg dish I made and a good bit of the piece of whole wheat toast. I surmised she liked it not only for its taste but because it was easy to chew. I noticed now at meals that the meat tended to be ignored even when the meat was tender and I had cut it up for her. I simply had to focus more on vegetable dishes. I noted, though, that she barely touched my vegetable soups at noon which I made from scratch, but then, she seldom seemed hungry at noon no matter what I served. The dietary challenge continued: how to maintain her weight at 88-90 pounds and not increase mine.

One of my preoccupations yesterday was searching for my cell phone. I looked everywhere in the house, under beds and furniture, between magazines on the coffee table, in pockets. Eventually I extended the search to the museum's lawn which I had mowed the previous day. No dice. Unfortunately, I had shut the phone down so could not call my cell and trace the sound. Last night, after I had given up hope of finding it any time soon I found it. Or it found me. I was tucking Joan into bed and glanced at the top of the bed stand. There it was between the table radio and the lamp! I had looked there several times before. Much relieved, I asked Joan where she had found it. She could not remember. My guess was that she had put it under her bed pillow, the one place I had not thought to look. I noted that I was spending a lot more time these days searching for things, most notably her eye glasses. She never put them in the same place two days in a row. Oh, how I disliked the random searching. It was such a monumental waste of time and a true test of my patience, which I was discovering definitely had its limits.

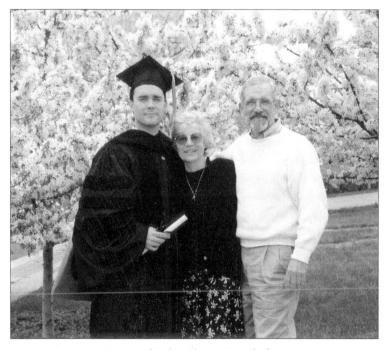

Joan and Bob with son, David after
graduation ceremony, Pittsburgh. May, 1996

Lost and Found

I looked everywhere for it, in the tool drawer,
the kitchen cupboards, behind the canned goods,

between the small stack of hand towels and under
the sink among the soap supplies. I even expanded

the search to other rooms to the dry sink, the night
stand next to her bed, even the piano bench

but no luck. I knew her strategy: hide it in plain
sight so she could find it but a thief could not.

But knowledge of her strategy did me no good. I
had already looked in all the plain places. It simply

was not to be found. To find it I resorted to the only
rational option left: I went to the Outlet Mall and

purchased a replacement. At only eight bucks or so
we're not talking about a big outlay here. The point is,

my rationale worked. Just like the strategy of washing
your car if you want it to rain. Two days after the new

purchase, I found what had been so long lost! It was
tucked under a small, raised, cheese cutting board on the

counter just to the left of the kitchen sink. Now I have
two identical items. So the moral is simple: If you lose

something just buy a replacement and you'll find it,
at least as far as favorite paring knives go.

But it wouldn't do at all, would it, if, say,
we lost something important, like our Way?

I'm told that when we lose our Way
we just have to keep on looking, searching

for whatever it is that constitutes our Holy Grail
until we find it, or in a disappointing world where

miracles still occur, the Way finds us. Now wouldn't
that be something, to be discovered?

April 29 2011

I was greatly relieved to have my cell phone by my side again. You can imagine my surprise the next morning when I went to reach for it on the bed stand where I had carefully placed it at bed time to discover it was not there. Gremlins seemed to be at work here. I asked Joan if she had seen my cell phone. "What does it look like?" she asked as if I had never shown it to her before. Joan was no help so I began my search once more starting with her bed pillow. No luck. In exasperation, I soon gave up and prepared breakfast. It was only after the dishes were done and I was helping her dress for the day that I found my side piece once again. As I was hanging up her pajamas I noticed the shirt seemed a little heavy. A quick check and there it was, stuffed in the shirt pocket with a handful of Kleenex!

Our pillow talk last night, like the rest of our daily life, seemed to be settling down to a predictable routine. Joan wanted to know where her children and other family members were, often thinking they were off to a movie or already asleep upstairs. She most always asked my name and where I lived. When I asked her where she lived last night, she referred to Portsmouth, Ohio and said, for the first time that I recalled, that she was just visiting out here with her mother. During the day she was right on target, often remarking how much she liked La Conner and our house and would not want to live anywhere else. So why this difference between night thoughts and day thoughts?

May 2, 2011

Nothing demonstrated Joan's disengagement with the world or her inability to focus and self-entertain better than what happened Saturday morning. Because several lights in the museum needed replacing and I had not been able to get to them on Friday, she accompanied me to the museum on Saturday morning. I turned on the overhead lights in the East Wing for her to look at the exhibit while I went about my job. Within a few minutes, she became restless and started following me around as I opened display cases, retrieved bulbs and moved the step ladder. It was obvious that she was bored and was anxious to return home so I cut my work short and we did just that. I found myself amazed all over again that she could find nothing in the entire museum to interest her, nothing to hold her attention, not even for a few minutes. I was impressed as well about how quickly she tired. Even the short walk down the hill seemed to exhaust her. We did not try to walk again until later in the day.

A Place to Rendezvous

Quiet, dim, with soft places, dark corners
and mute witnesses peering, behind glass,

from a turn-of-the-century parlor, as
visitors pass, the history museum a perfect

place to rendezvous, at least for two.
Frizzy blond hair, big brown eyes, a

small tattoo on her slim right wrist with
white teeth and a Bluetooth for

company to add a little twist, *Today*
enters the lobby, there to meet *Yesterday*.

He is shocked at first but likes her
inquisitive face and easy, straight-backed

grace. And *Today* likes *Yesterday's* looks.
Solid, feet firmly planted, neither too tall

nor too short, and in spite of logging boots
and a farmer's straw, a natural elegance

with experienced eyes to match his worn
blue shirt, they greet each other. Their

hands stay clasped as they walk and talk
and, eventually, in the midst of *Yesterday's*

familiar surroundings, they stop, and
embrace, their hands reaching for each other,

groping and grasping, as they search for
clues to *Tomorrow's* shape.

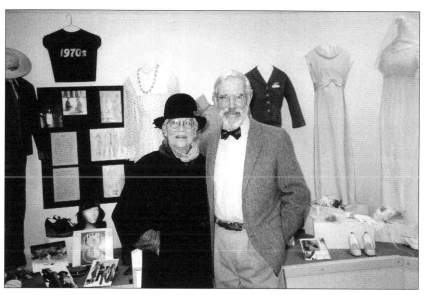

Joan and Bob dressed in 1970's clothes for a museum exhibit. LaConner, 2004

Joan made no reference to the "young girl" over the weekend interestingly, but she asked plenty of questions about her family's whereabouts, most often those of her dad and mom. Occasionally she wanted to know where our children were as well and I would repeat the names and locales. She expressed surprise that I could remember something that seemed so complex to her.

Joan watched the Sunday service at First Community Church with me on my laptop and seemed to derive some enjoyment from the chancel choir, even singing a few bars of the music at one point. She also seemed interested in my conversation about Brother Lawrence and his little book I had been rereading entitled *The Practice of the Presence of God*.

May 6, 2011

I found myself getting used to having Joan's parents around as well as our kids. I did not even mind explaining the situation—the fact that, sadly, none of our parents were here for us to talk with—and recited repeatedly where each of our children was and who they were married to, etc. Nor was I bothered overmuch any longer during those times when Joan did not recognize me and wanted to know my name and where I lived. I saw and understood that the abnormal was becoming normal and sensed the need to resist being drawn into it.

But now a couple of recent things made me worry a little more. I came down from the study early yesterday morning to find two tea bag pouches ripped open and the tea scattered on the kitchen counter. I asked Joan about it at several different times yesterday but she had no recollection of wanting something hot to drink in the middle of the night. Was this night action a prelude to other night activities that might well be harmful or dangerous—such as getting into the medicines or going outside?

The other incident occurred last night after midnight. I was awakened in the dark downstairs bedroom by a rustling movement. I turned on the bed lamp to find Joan by the dry sink, where she now stores some of her clothing accessories, with a handful of winter hats and gloves in her hands. Never, never had I seen Joan so utterly lost as at that moment. I tried gently to explain she did not need these things for a trip to the bathroom but she clung to them for dear life. I then lead her by the hand to the bathroom and tried again to relieve her of all the paraphernalia but she said "No" and this time added a sharp, "Just leave me alone!" and closed the bathroom door. I waited until she was through, accompanied her back to the front bedroom and tucked her in without any comment from her except to thank me for covering her with the warm electric blanket.

The recounting of it now so saddened me but was quickly followed by my renewed resolve to keep healthy and fit and above the fray, i.e. , not get sucked into Joan's world of illusion and fear (but remaining patient and strong enough to help her). It was also becoming abundantly clear that I would need a lot of help down the line. That I could not possibly do this alone was not an admission of my weakness (as I may have thought earlier) but recognition of reality's strength. I would bear all I could. I had no doubt that I would find the strength to bear more. But did love demand I bear all? My answer: No. There were many ways to respond in love. The first was self love, a respect for my own limitations; the second, an acceptance of the love and concern others could and would bring to bear.

May 10, 2011

Again last night about 1:00 am, Joan was up, very confused and unable to find her way to the bathroom. She seemed to think that the pillow with the oversized pillow case (which she uses between her knees to sleep with) was something to wear and was trying to get her arm through the pillow case's open end. I walked her to the bathroom, turning on the kitchen light as we went. She seemed okay after that and soon was fast asleep once more. I thought I was going to have to come up with a new name to fit this late night/early morning behavior such as "Moonup Syndrome," but then I read a syndicated column by Dr. Peter H. Gott (Skagit Valley Herald, 5/4/11) which indicated that "Sundowner's Syndrome" can apply to early morning antics as well as late evening.

By whatever name, Joan's nocturnal behavior was recognized as part and parcel of dementia. "Sundowning," he stated, "is confusion that generally occurs late in the day, although it has been known to occur during early morning hours as well." Dr. Gott went on to describe the symptoms: "As the day progresses a patient becomes fatigued and less able to deal with stress...the patient who was stimulated earlier in the day has nothing to occupy his or her mind and appears increasingly forgetful and agitated. Memory loss seems greater. Blood pressure readings may be lower. Patients may see things that aren't there or perceive things to be other than what they actually are. These visions can be extremely frightening."

All the symptoms fit Joan to a "T." The doctor's remedies, such as they were, were ones I have employed out of necessity: a mild sleep-aid was one which, when combined with the Lorazepam, was sometimes effective and might be worth trying more consistently; a strategically-placed nightlight or two was another (once in a while I had left the bedside lamp turned on to lessen the fear); being in the room with the patient during the night was also recommended. Of all the remedies, this night company seemed most important. I could not imagine Joan getting through the night, any night, without me in the room with her to reassure and guide her. Beyond these three remedies, Dr. Gott had no cure all, no magic bullet to offer. If he did, he would be a quack and not worth listening to. As it was, Dr. Gott recognized the complexity and challenge associated with dementia and ended his article on just the right sympathetic note: "Most of all, remember that anyone with sundowner's is unaware of the havoc that he or she may impose on family members and caregivers."

These nights I was still reading Jim Lynch's book to Joan after she was tucked in bed, but I had had the feeling she was less interested in the story and more interested, more comforted, in simply hearing my voice. Several times lately she had commented on my voice and how well I read. The other evening, though, she asked me to lower it. Why? Because she was afraid my voice was too loud and might awaken her mother who was asleep upstairs! When I explained to her that her mother was not upstairs, that no one else was in the house but the two of us, Joan seemed puzzled, but did not pursue the issue. Nor did I. I was discovering that the less said, the better, i.e., saying no more than was required in the way of a response seemed to result in a lot less agitation.

May 12, 2011

I needed to take Dr. Gott's advice and give Joan a mild sleep-aid at her bedtime. Last night was another reminder. After an early dinner, Joan retired about 6:15 pm. I read to her for an additional half hour. After watching the end of the Mariners game against Baltimore and checking the news, I followed suit and hit the sack at 8:00 pm. I was tired and happy enough to retire earlier than usual, doubly so when Joan woke up hungry at 10:30 pm. Although she did not want me to get up to fix something, there was little alternative. So I cooked her a bowl of instant oatmeal (she cannot seem to handle the regular variety) and toast which allowed me at the same time to clean the stove top and finish putting away the pots and pans from supper. Joan ate every bite and was soon back in bed and asleep. I no sooner began to get drowsy than she was up again to go to the bathroom. Her pattern of getting up every hour continued through the night. Each time she got up, I turned on the light and waited for her return so that she was tucked in properly against the cold. I made a point of tucking her in for two reasons: she seemed incapable of getting back in bed herself without making a tangled mess of the covers and I was concerned that she stay warm. With so little fat to protect her, she became easily chilled. Even when I was placing the warm electric blanket around her after one of her bathroom trips, she would often experience a deep shudder, from feeling cold she said. The shudder was enough like a convulsion to scare me.

Why the hunger? That was the big question. Last night I prepared Swiss steak, the meat so tender you could cut it with a fork. The mildly seasoned tomato sauce, noodles and peas made a tempting meal. Joan ate little of it, preferring instead a buttered slice of whole wheat bread and raspberry jam. And, of course, she was always ready for a small bowl of vanilla ice cream. I had already concluded that Joan was not big on meat any longer, but out of concern that she get enough protein, I kept trying. However, if she did not eat it anyway, what had I, what had she, gained? Not a thing. I simply had to work harder at finding and developing more interesting vegetable recipes and at the same time keep the carbohydrates to a minimum. Lately, Joan's blood glucose numbers were running a little higher than I liked but her weight was up to 91.2 pounds which was good news. I vowed to spend, had to spend, more time looking for just the right recipes for her. There were so few that I had reviewed that she would find at all appealing, but I still felt I must try them. Who knew, I might be surprised. After all, she liked the spinach souffle dish I had concocted and she was definitely not a spinach person.

May 13, 2011

Last night when Joan awoke to make one of her trips to the bathroom, I remembered finally to give her my version of a mild sleep-aid, an antihistamine used to treat allergies. One small pink pill (25 mg) did the trick. She slept soundly, as did I, from 10:30 pm to 2:30 am! That little pink pill will definitely become a regular part of her evening dosage, a welcome companion to the Lorazepam.

The evening meal was a success as well, with Joan eating an entire serving of a new dish I tried—an onion-bacon pie with a cornmeal crust. It had not hurt that she liked onions. She kept insisting I had invited someone to supper—it was a woman, she recalled—and that I should telephone her to remind her of our dinner date. I told Joan I would be happy to phone if she could tell me who to call. In the same conversation she paused to wonder where her mother was and if she might join us, if not for supper, then at some point during the evening. With just the two of us sitting down to supper these days, I was beginning to feel anti-social.

Joan and I had become acutely aware lately how much we missed having any of our (real) children around to drop in, to invite over for a meal, or to help out with some small project or another. Land lines and e-mails were important, essential even, but they were no substitute for the kind of more or less continuous face-to-face conversations we used to enjoy over a cup of coffee or a meal. Perhaps Joan's constant reference to Susan's illusory presence (and to one or more of our other children almost as frequently) was but a projection of this very wish: to have our children nearby.

May 15, 2011

Our conversation yesterday took a new twist. Since it was Saturday I walked with Joan in the morning, taking the usual route down to the post office, then along First Street to Commercial and back home. That afternoon, after lunch, Joan wanted to walk again and I was happy enough to oblige, this time walking south down the hill by the Catholic church and then cutting across the paved walk to the public parking lot back to Commercial and home. Upon our return I revved up the new lawn mower and cut the front lawn and proceeded to trim the yard as well, experimenting with a new trimmer. At several points, Joan came outside to watch me from the porch. Once the machines were stored, I sat down for a minute to begin thinking about dinner.

Within a short time Joan wanted to take another walk. I explained my feeling that we already had two walks under our belt and on the second one she had complained of being tired. I thought it might be too much to take a third one. Joan disagreed and became agitated because, she insisted, she had not yet walked anywhere.

My efforts to point out the various reference points on our walks (getting the mail, talking to a neighbor who was trying out his new bicycle, passing by the pocket wetlands with the long dry plants) only made her angrier. Usually she has accepted the fact that she has not been able to remember. This time, a first, she disputed my recollection. She had not taken one single walk all day, let alone two, and that was that!

Furthermore, Joan did not like the idea of me taking a walk by myself that afternoon and leaving her at the house. When I denied that and asked exactly when this supposedly took place, she said it was during the time I was using the trimmer on the front yard. But, I asked, didn't she see me with the yellow/black trimmer in hand?

Didn't she remember talking to me at the time? No. She did not. At that juncture, the conversation stopped and she said, "I don't want to talk about it anymore," the hurt and anger still very much in evidence. (All that hurt and anger could have been avoided if I could have just remembered not to ask the most useless of questions: "Didn't you remember?" Of course she did not remember. She was unable to remember even the obvious and recent experience of me wielding a grass trimmer. I had been just too surprised to think it through first. It seemed that I had my own memory problem).

Joan admitted a little later, the previous conversation completely forgotten by then, that she was not feeling well and, as had been the custom lately, spent a lot of Saturday resting on the wicker sofa in the dining room. As a matter of fact, Joan had complained of not feeling well most of the last six weeks. When I tried to get her to pinpoint the problem, she would mention her stomach but only in a vague way indicating the feeling was much more general. Efforts to persuade her to undergo GI tests to see if there was a problem had been unsuccessful. At one point, the doctor had set up an appointment at Island Hospital for tests but Joan later had me cancel it. She weighed in at 90.4 pounds yesterday so her weight was pretty stable but that was about all. Otherwise, she seemed to me to be less stable. I noticed yesterday while helping her with her morning shower, that she was very shaky and for the first time finding it more difficult to get in and out of our old-fashioned clawfoot tub. I could see trouble down the road just keeping her clean. The next move would most certainly be replacing the tub with a shower stall or redesigning the downstairs bathroom which sports a jet tub.

Reckoning

To forget what you want desperately to remember
and remember all too vividly what you long to forget
often leads to live reckoning.

Dead reckoning is something else again, more
rational and less serious. To be lost at sea
is bad enough.

To be lost and at sea on land is a lot worse
and is what turns some of us
to writing verse.

May 16, 2011

I tucked Joan in bed around 7:00 pm which was late for her but our whole day, a wet, rainy Sunday, had seemed to run late. Joan said she did not feel well and was quite content to curl up on the wicker couch most of the day resting and sleeping while I sat nearby working at my laptop. She did listen to and view the worship service from First Community Church and was, as I, thrilled by the music from the Chancel Choir.

Joan's closing words to me at bedtime were becoming routine now and no longer startled me. "What's your name?" she asks. I tell her, "Bob." Last night, she held out her hand which I shook, as if to say, "Nice to meet you." As a courtesy, I always ask her name. "Joan," she replies, "spelled like Joan but pronounced like JoAnn." With that familiar exchange, I turned off the lamp and settled down in the next room to watch the rest of *60 Minutes*. Every few minutes for the next twenty, she got up to tell me that the twin bed next to her was probably free if I wanted to sleep there. I always thank her for this offer and tell her I will probably take her up on it. Sometimes I joke with her about it. "Is there a rental fee?" I ask. Other times I want to know what to do if there is somebody already sleeping in the bed. Most often she senses that I am pulling her leg and will smile her sweetest smile.

After watching a first-rate nature program on KCTS, I piled into bed about 9:15 pm (Nobody else was in it.) and was soon lulled to sleep by Joan's even breathing. At 10:00 pm I was aroused by something and waited for her to return from the bathroom. When she did not, I got up to investigate. It was then that I heard her faint cries. I ran through the kitchen to the bathroom. The bathroom was empty. I listened again and ran for the upstairs, flipping on the lights as I went. There on the floor in her former bedroom was

Joan. Had she fallen? "No," she said, "I was just tired and decided to sit down." Relief washed over me, followed by a new concern. I had not thought of her climbing the stairs in the dark under any circumstances. Her night time confusion was obviously increasing. Later, in the early morning, she was unable again to find her way to the bathroom and was busy at one point trying to get out the door to the side yard.

I would try first providing more light to guide her at night but I had to be prepared before long to take her by the hand and walk her to bathroom. Making sure she took her sleep-aid every night became doubly important now for both of us.

May 19, 2011

Joan's former hairstylist came to our house at my request to cut Joan's hair yesterday morning. Joan was pleased with the result. So was I. Joan's hair had become much too long and uncontrollable. This was the best part of an otherwise unsettling day... and night. Not feeling well in the morning now was continuing to carry over into the afternoon and still no clues from Joan about where the problem was. She described her "feeling bad" in terms mostly of being tired and lacking in energy. She was still spending more of her time lying down on the couch in the afternoon. And in the evening she appeared more confused than ever. Talking about her mother's presence—either upstairs sleeping or out on the town and due home soon—was more or less continuous now no matter how many times I repeated the fact that her mother had died before we moved to La Conner. I kept thinking if I described in detail her mother's last days in Salina, Kansas that Joan would remember, but it had not worked.

Last night Joan worried about her brothers being able to get in the house. She thought they were in a bar some place and would not be home until late. Most confusing though, was her increased inability to recognize me as her husband. For a large part of last evening she had no idea who I was. Several times during the night she asked, "What's your name?" Also to be noted: even with more light in the kitchen, she could not seem to find her way to the bathroom. I was surprised that the extra light did not seem to make any difference. Once she leaves our bedroom now she veers right to the side door and attempts to unlock it. I get up most times during the night now and lead her in the right direction.

A catastrophe occurred last night apparently, but I was never able to determine exactly what it was. Joan awoke at 1:00 am, alarmed at what had occurred and wanted desperately to telephone her mother and father to let them know she was all right. I asked what had happened but she could only stammer something about "a pear" or "pair" or "pare-nt." Never, after repeated attempts, could she give me a coherent answer or even an incoherent one. Rather than tell her the sad news one more time which might upset her and keep her up the rest of the night, I opted to play along, suggesting that we wait until morning." Mom will be up and worrying," Joan contended. "Yes," I agreed, "maybe so. It may also be the case that she has gone back to bed by now. Do you really want to disturb her again?" Finally, she bought my argument and we both managed to sleep until her next bathroom run at 3:30 am. Tonight she was able to steer herself to the bathroom without guidance. No mention was made of the catastrophe. I would ask her about it at breakfast but my guess was that she would have no memory of it.

This morning Joan had an appointment with her doctor. I wanted to work out a way to deal with the slight rise in her average blood glucose level which has moved from the high 100's to the middle

200's. Part of it was her diet, but then it had not changed all that much over the last months. It also needed to be noted that her endurance had diminished, was diminishing. She was doing a lot more sleeping and resting on the sofa during the day.

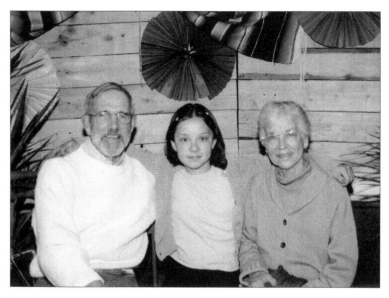

Bob and Joan with granddaughter, Nora.
Conway Elementary School. May, 1999.

Morning Song

It's May, early morning. I open the door and without
warning, music galore, surround sound.

Nearby, unseen, the song bird's short, piercing trills,
cut happily through the air, reminding me
of the day's lyric potential.

High above, my gaze directed there by hundreds of
Canada geese honking their way north, I see, etched
faintly against the changing sky, a flying road sign,
its arrowhead directing the way home,
the vee to vie for tundra food.

Down the road I hear the resident turkeys, their gobbles
more frequent and louder by the moment as they
descend from their favorite roosting to forage, once
again, on the town's good will.

Low overhead, two blue herons, on silent wings,
their gravelly voices signaling their swift presence,
heading for the shore or someone's fish pond,
ever the elegant and patient thieves.

Lyrical trills, determined honks, insistent gobbles,
gravelly caws, if not the songs and sounds
of paradise, are very close, at least on this early
May morning in La Conner.

May 24, 2011

I was groggy this morning due to interrupted sleep (so what else was new?). Joan woke up at the usual approximate two-hour interval at 10:30 pm and then again at 1:00 am she went to the bathroom, and again at 1:35 am, 1:53 am and 2:36 am. The last time she returned from the bathroom with a towel and roll of toilet paper in her hand, but seemed to have no idea why. When I asked her to get in bed so I could cover her up, she did not know how to do it. I had to tell her to sit down on the bed and then put her head on the pillow. Within a short time of covering her up and increasing the blanket temperature (she complained of being cold) she wanted to get up again because she had to get dressed. Without turning on the lamp, I urged her to stay in bed until daylight when everyone else was getting up. My argument was not persuasive and before long she was sitting up again, ready to throw back the covers. I marshaled other arguments and she stayed quiet until 4:30 am at which time she had to get to the bathroom. I waited for her return and when she did not, I got up to investigate. I met her just coming out of the bathroom carrying the small white trash receptacle in her hand full of disposed toilet paper and Kleenex. She reached in the container to show me the paper. I told her she had plenty of that under her pillow so she let me return the container and waited there in the cold kitchen until I could lead her back to bed and warmth where I again tucked her in and made her promise not to get up until I came back downstairs to fix breakfast. She promised. So far, so good. It is 5:05 am and no noise has been detected by my monitor which picked up the slightest sound.

I had now to rethink my own early morning routine. Obviously I had to stay at the house so for the time being I would intensify my floor exercises and make use of the Health Rider right here in my study. Perhaps I could find time later in the day to work out at the fitness center or take a run, but probably not until I found someone to spell me. Adjustment on my part was the order of the day.

I was forewarned about the morning restlessness two mornings ago when I was writing away upstairs and surprisingly heard Joan's plaintive voice calling my name. I jumped up to go to her but she was already half way up the stairs. She said she had been walking around downstairs for some time (around 5:15 am) and was surprised that no one was up yet. Apparently she expected our children or her parents to be here at the house which, of course, by now was not new. She continued to ask where her mother was during the course of the day as well as other family members, especially her brother Bill.

Suddenly, unexpectedly, I heard Joan coughing downstairs below me in the kitchen. I ran downstairs to find her sitting at the dining room table huddled over a cup of hot water. She did not know where I was and decided to fix herself a cup of coffee but could not find the coffee container. There had been a time when she would have remembered that it was in the door of the refrigerator. I immediately set about getting her a proper breakfast, first some toast and coffee and, a little later, some fresh muffins. Why had my fail-proof monitor failed me? I checked it out to discover that I had inadvertently turned down the volume control. That fixed, I sat down with Joan to read the morning paper and eat something myself. As was typical these last few weeks, she complained of feeling terrible and was not going to school. I told her not to fret. She did not have to attend school. She had already graduated. This knowledge, I knew, would not sink in, and tomorrow morning she would express the same anxiety about missing school. Now, at 8:15 am, against her objections, I had monitored her blood glucose (too high at 290 mg) and injected her in the stomach with both the long-term Levemir (5 i.u.) and short-term Novolog (4 i.u.) and she had gone back to bed. I had come back upstairs to finish this section, making sure the monitor was turned to the proper volume!

Not having showered or worked out and having slept only fitfully, I felt terrible, too. I hated beginning the day this way. But I had better get used to it and change my routine accordingly. It seemed just that quick, in the course of a few days, to be a new ball game.

At the appointment with the doctor, it was noted that Joan had gained about 10 lbs. since last September. I think the doctor was as surprised as I, given the little Joan ate. She did like her ice cream though, two small bowls a day and also continued to enjoy a little wine at the supper hour. I was not worried so much now by Joan's wine consumption since I had began diluting her wine glass with an equal amount of sparkling water. She had taken no notice of the change to this date and, in fact, I thought it actually improved the taste of the inexpensive Australian wine we drank.

The only important change in strategy was to up Joan's long-term insulin from 4 mg to 5 mg to see if that would help offset the slight increase in her blood glucose level from the high 100's to the middle 200's. The doctor thought that the 5 mg was about the max for her small body type. I concurred. I would still like to find a way to get her to consume more vegetables, but might have to settle for less. Her liking of canned peaches and pears was some help, too much sugar, but easy for her to chew. I did not know how else to explain her recent style of eating just tidbits of food from the end of her fork or spoon, often examining the bit before consuming. I could not stand to watch her eat most of the time and would often read aloud to her during meals in the style of some monastic orders. In fact, I was beginning to feel I was living in a monastic retreat of some kind, more prayerful inwardly and less conversant with the outside world in spite of myself. And surprisingly, I sensed now and then a spiritual presence I could not shake, a presence that was somehow on this spiraling journey too. God riding shotgun. It was probably just my imagination working overtime, the result of reading too much of Brother Lawrence.

May 27, 2011

Most endearing was our little conversation yesterday afternoon as we sat in the twin swivel chairs holding hands. Joan and I had just gotten back from one of our frequent walks and I had turned on the television to watch some of the early matches of the French Open. Until this year, she had enjoyed watching tennis. Not now. Like most other television, she could not seem to make sense of it. After a few minutes I turned the television off. Then Joan spoke to me like I was an old friend whom she had been visiting. "I've got to go home now. I'm worried about mom being alone and I feel I should be there to help." I asked her if she was thinking of her home in Portsmouth. "Yes," she said, "I think so." I then had to tell her, as I had so many times before, that her mother had died a long time ago when we still lived in Vermont and carefully went through the history of her mother's move to Salina, Kansas and the wonderful life she had had there with Patti, Don and Bill all nearby. She nodded her head as I recounted the story, seeming to remember.

How wonderful, I told Joan, that she was concerned about her mother and wanted to help her. "Endearing" is the term I thought of to describe Joan's tone and attitude at that moment and so complimented her. We were quiet a few minutes as we thought about our mothers. "Did we have the same mother?" she wanted to know. Undaunted, I went on then to describe my mother's life, her husbands and her life in Fort Lauderdale. At the end of my description I thought there might have been a mini-break through. I was wrong, still in denial myself about the extent of Joan's memory loss. It was not long before Joan decided she had better phone her mother! She just was not sure where to find the telephone number.

The active night life continued. Last night Joan was up at hourly intervals beginning at 9:00 pm through 2:00 am or so. Several times it was a nightmarish dream of some sort that awakened her. Once she sat up in bed, crying "Mom!" Another time she cried out "Oh, no. There's water all around me!" I was quickly out of bed to reassure her, forcing her to put her feet on the floor to show her there was no water. Several of the other times I walked her to the bathroom. On one occasion she was certain the toilet was not functioning and was reluctant to sit down. Judging by the way she tested the toilet seat—first, lifting the lid and then pressing her hand against it—she was apparently afraid it might collapse. I wondered if the fear exhibited here had anything to do with her experience as a child being forced to go outside to the privy and her fear of falling through the hole to the suffocating mess below.

May 30, 2011

With the introduction of Melatonex to Joan's intake before bed, her night life had calmed down, with much longer stretches between bathroom breaks. The OTC product, a derivative of melatonin, contained some Vitamin B and a time-release feature. One pill (3 mg), the recommended dosage, seemed to do it for two nights running now. One immediate effect was that I felt more rested. It was less clear what aftereffect the pill had on Joan. Yesterday morning she was really dragging. She usually started out the morning stating that she did not feel well but yesterday morning she curled up on the wicker sofa and was not the least bit interested in food. About 9:30 am she ate one of my freshly baked muffins and a cup of coffee which I followed up later at noon with a proper breakfast of crisp bacon and a small omelet. She managed to eat about half the small helping. I would have to watch closely this morning to see how she felt. We managed to get in two short walks yesterday, but she tired quickly and did not feel up to helping me plant the flower boxes with bright Impatiens in the afternoon.

She had driven with me to Christianson's Nursery the day before and helped to pick out the colors, but mostly held my hand as I picked out plants to replenish the butterfly garden. I was holding my breath the entire time, worried that she might stumble on the uneven ground or hit her head on the low overhanging baskets as we made our way through the greenhouses. Happily, we made it without mishap and with the help of a young employee. I had not been able to find a time when she felt well enough to drive to the Food Coop and Haggen's for groceries, something she once liked to do just to be company for me if nothing else. It appeared that shopping together would soon become a thing of the past. Sad, really, although I had never minded shopping by myself.

Joan was upset when I got home from work Friday noon and asked that my former colleague at work and good friend no longer continue as her companion. Why? Because Joan felt she had to entertain her, to act the hostess and it wore her out. Was this something that was correctable? I did not know. What I had to deal with was the fact that Joan did not want my friend to be her caregiver any longer. Reluctantly, I was now looking for a replacement and would have my first interview with a person who had been working as a professional caregiver now for many years, lived close by and came highly recommended. My friend was a pleasant, adaptable, unflappable woman, and wonderful company, but had no experience working with dementia patients. The new prospect would meet with Joan and me at our house this coming Wednesday and we would see what happened.

June 1, 2011

Over the long weekend I had a chance to consider Joan's request not to continue with my friend and colleague as the caregiver. In light of the fact that Joan had no memory of her experience with my friend and, in fact, could not even recall her name, my friend and I, after talking it over, decided that the solution was to reassure Joan that she was not obligated to be the hostess, to entertain. Sure enough, on her Tuesday morning visit, my friend urged her to lie down on the sofa at one point and rest which Joan happily did, sleeping soundly for a long stretch. By the time I got home from work that day, Joan looked rested and was obviously pleased to have my friend there. So my friend continued her caregiving role on the Monday-Tuesday-Friday schedule. I talked with the professional caregiver today as a possible back-up, part of a support team which I would need, and needed now, to help me manage the care. Before long the two caregivers planned to talk to one another about Joan's condition with my complete approval.

After the second night of Melatonex, Joan awoke feeling more like herself and ate a good breakfast so I concluded that taking the sleep-aid on a regular basis was harmless, i.e., with no aftereffect. I noted that even after taking the Melatonex the second night, she still had a short spell between 12:00 am and 2:00 am where she was up frequently. It was recommended that I give her the Melatonex later in the night which seemed worth trying. The problem was that she refused to take the tablet at that time so I will go back to giving her the Melatonex along with the Lorazepam at bedtime.

Memorial Day morning Joan accompanied me to the Food

Coop to do some needed shopping and to cash in the gift card our son David had so thoughtfully given to Joan for Mother's Day. Before I was halfway through the aisles, she said she was too tired to continue and wanted to get home. I quickly grabbed a few more items and checked out, leaving the selection of a gift for another time. As I said earlier, shopping with Joan was coming to a close which was too bad because it had been one of the few things we still had been able to do together.

We had a small filet of Copper River salmon last night along with sweet potatoes and peas and onions. I was pleased to observe that Joan actually ate everything on her plate although it took her an extraordinarily long time. I also did not provide any bread with the meal which helped focus her attention on the main course. I probably should discontinue serving bread at all meals but I did not have the heart to deprive Joan of something she really enjoyed. Compromise was probably the order of the day, selective omission. I must keep in mind, too, that Joan was diabetic and the fewer carbs the better. Trying to keep her weight up and her blood glucose down remained a challenge. As was common now, she wondered why we did not set more places for supper, for her mother and father apparently. I felt I had once again to explain their deaths and the wonderful years her mother had after selling the house in Portsmouth and moving to Salina.

June 2, 2011

Joan kept wanting to have supper early. I complied with a Mexican corn tortilla dish and salad of which she ate but little. I thought it was one of my better meals and so ate her share. By 6:00 pm she was in bed, happy to call it a day. The Melatonex did not seem to have any effect in the early hours. While I did the dishes and watched the Mariners game, Joan got up several times to visit the bathroom, but later, between 10:30 pm and 3:30 am when I expected the most activity, she was quiet, sleeping soundly.

A little after that, however, she awoke totally confused. I turned on the light to find her picking at the bed covers as if looking for something. I asked what she was doing, but all I could hear was something having to do with "glue." I finally told Joan to stop messing up the bed, that I would straighten it up when she got back from the bathroom. (Did I mention that last night she had stripped the top sheet completely off the bed and spread it over her dining room chair?) She turned around and stuck her tongue out at me and proceeded to the bathroom and just as soon returned, not able to find it. At this point, I took her hand and led her through the living room and kitchen to the half bath but she was uncertain what to do next. I waited to make sure she figured it out and after she urinated, led her back to the front bedroom and tucked her in. She asked where I was going to be. She appeared so bewildered and frightened I reassured her that I would be right in the other twin bed. Normally, at this time (3:45 am) I would get up and begin my routine of showering, writing and working out, but not this morning and perhaps not for many months to come. I stayed abed listening for Joan's deep, even breathing but it never happened; there was only shallow, erratic breathing like she was having upsetting dreams of some kind. At 4:30 am she was up again and made her way directly to the bathroom without assistance.

When she returned to the bedroom I tucked her in once again and told her I was going to take a shower and do some writing but would not leave the house. She then muttered something from under the covers that made me stop and take notice. To clarify the mutterings, Joan said plainly that she no longer trusted me, that she did not believe I was going upstairs to shower and write! Why? She would not, could not, explain it or saw no reason to, but I was totally dismayed. The one thing that has kept us together, through thick and thin, had been "trust." Was this the beginning of a serious break in our relationship? If it was, it would make managing and coping down the road much more difficult for me and everyone else. Discord was distrust's daughter and bore careful attention as well as constant affection.

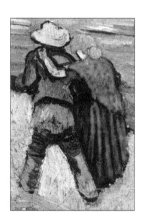

June Sounds

Cracking open June's brightly painted door
Ever so slightly, is enough for them to waft through.
Sounds familiar as the recurring solstice and
Inevitable as the shortened shadow of summer's first day.

I hear the distant sounds of Mendelssohn's *Wedding March*.
Bride and groom, their steps to an uncertain future
Outpaced by racing hearts.
Two to become one in imperfect union.

The notes of Elgar's *Pomp and Circumstance* wind earward.
Gowned students, Lock-stepping their way to a battered freedom
With diplomas in one hand and Ipods in the other and a certain
Pride, each one to become two in annual reunion.

Applause, from many a lauding lunch, sounds 'round the valley,
Random, intermittent, like reservation fireworks.
The ritual of the hand slap, which if heard all at one time in
Stride, Skagit-wide, would form a thunderous clap.
Colleagues settle, instead, for lifting up with gentle acclaim
The heroes among them who, without a word, happily
Exchange fireworks for good works and let it go at that.

Other sounds, like applause less musical, fill the void.
One is the collective sigh of grown men, begetters of the begotten,
Fathers forgotten, who by act of congress have their say

Finally, honored and anchored in June's middle days.

Fathers, once abandoned, now abdomened, in June,
Leads naturally to the best sound of all:
My mother's first breath and lusty wail.
Newborn on the fourteenth, a century ago.
Letting the world know

She was here to stay for ninety years or so
Mother's Day may be celebrated in May,
But for me, you see, it is much too soon.
I celebrate it a month later in June.

June 11, 2011

Our son, David, arrived from Slippery Rock, Thursday night and stayed through Monday. David spent a lot of time with his mother while I was at work, walking and talking with her. He treated us with two of his favorite things to do when visiting us: dining at Nell Thorn's restaurant and eating a take-out meal from the local Thai restaurant which he considered among the best. Both were enjoyable occasions for David and me but we were less certain about Joan's reaction since she seldom entered into a conversation any longer. From time to time, though, during the visit she would evidence her pleasure by embracing David and telling him how much she enjoyed having him here. At other times, she did not recognize him at all. At one point when David was helping me with the gardening. She wanted to know who the strange man was working in our front yard. David sensed, too, that there were times when his mother did not seem to know who he was and was acting instinctively, like she should know.

It was David who questioned the wisdom of going ahead with our plans to have a big 60th wedding anniversary celebration next September. His worry stemmed from the observation that Joan seemed unable to handle any noise or the usual hustle and bustle that was involved in dining out. She did okay at Nell Thorn's but when I took Joan and him to lunch on the sunny deck at La Conner Seafood, Joan was upset during most of the meal by the loud voices of the two waitresses, several times turning to them and the patrons they were talking to, telling them to quiet down. It got so tense that David finally decided to take Joan home early while I stayed behind to pay the bill.

So how would Joan react to a big party of as many as a hundred guests with all the hubbub that a potluck and dance music would create? Maybe it would be too much for her. It certainly would be the case that she would not remember any of it anyway, so why not just keep it low key? I had felt it might make some difference if she were the center of attention but who knew really? Perhaps it would prove too taxing. It was good that David could spend some time with us at this point to see for himself what our situation was and how I was coping with the changes. He clearly saw the need to get help, and liked the plan to apply for funding through Veterans Affairs. He clearly saw as well that his mother's condition had deteriorated drastically since his visit last October.

Should I go ahead with plans for our wedding anniversary? David would not be able to attend. It was unlikely that Matt would be able to attend either. But Susan and John and Beth might make it. So the question remained, to go ahead with the celebration or not. I was inclined to say "yes," full speed ahead. I would do some consulting first, however.

June 13, 2011

The main person to consult was Joan, of course, although I was no longer certain she was able to grasp the reality of what I was asking. For what it was worth, she felt we should go ahead with the original plan at the Civic Garden Club. She seemed to think it was okay as long as our friends were doing the work. A party of 100 people impressed her. She would probably prefer less but she reasoned if at any point she could not handle the noise or crowd she could simply leave. I would not want that to happen at our anniversary celebration. On the other hand, the party as planned had all the elements that made for success: friends, food and music. Whether we were present or not, our friends were going to have a good time for a few hours. So, I acted on my inclination and added an exclamation point to "Full speed ahead!" The celebration was on!

For the last few nights now, Joan's nighttime activity had calmed down. The restlessness and bewilderment had disappeared and she had slept soundly for long stretches, i.e., two or three hours at a time which, in turn, had allowed me to get more sleep. For the first time in a long time, I just stayed in bed Sunday morning, watching the morning light fill our downstairs bedroom, enjoying the luxury of a decent night's rest until 6:00 am. Yeah, I know, it's scandalous. Last night, however, we were back to the more usual routine: Joan up about every hour (starting around 10:30 pm until 3:30 am or so) to go to the bathroom, in most cases able to find her way with little direction. As we got nearer the morning, she kept insisting she had to get up to get to school. I was able to convince her to stay in bed until I started breakfast at 6:00 am or so. Actually, what convinced her to stay put was the prospect of getting up in a dark, cold house without me there baking and preparing the morning's fare.

As I noted again over this weekend, Joan's daytime activity consisted primarily of resting on the dining room sofa and going for walks. She ate—slowly—but appeared to have little interest in food except for vanilla ice cream. This Sunday, like most Sundays now, I spent an enjoyable hour viewing the worship service at First Community Church on my MacBook. Initially, Joan had shown some interest in the services but not this morning. She slept through most of it and, near the end of the hour, had no sense of my engagement in the excellent music and sermon, wanting only to take a walk. She did not remember that we had already walked but I soon joined her, knowing that exercise was a good thing for both of us as was the camaraderie, so off we went at her ever-slowing pace.

June 14, 2011

Veterans Affairs asked for additional information in connection with my request for funds to help with the cost of home care. For Joan to qualify, she needed to submit a separate application for medical benefits which I completed recently. With a few exceptions, my application and hers were identical. Most important, I also completed the Durable Power of Attorney (effective immediately) form. The manager at the Bank of America in La Conner notarized it and two friends witnessed Joan's signature at Town Hall. Joan had had no difficulty signing the application at that time several days ago but yesterday afternoon she could barely scrawl her name on the second form, appearing greatly confused and tired throughout the process. Joan's two signatures bear no resemblance to one another. I wonder what Veterans Affairs will make of that? To me it signified that obtaining legal power to make decisions for both of us had come none too soon. Parenthetically, it was a good thing Veterans Affairs required the Durable Power of Attorney document. I thought I already had completed such a form but what I had filled out was the Durable Power of Attorney form for Medical Decisions which was important too, of course, but quite different.

My monitor told me Joan was up and walking around downstairs. This was a new pattern I may have mentioned earlier. Usually she would still be sleeping at this hour (5:30 am) but not now. The other new twist was that she had awakened at 8:30 pm or so last night (just when I was thinking of getting ready for bed) thinking it was morning and wanting something to eat. I fixed her hot chocolate and an English muffin which she ate without uttering a word, sitting at the dining room table looking at a magazine. This must all be connected to the fact that Joan was retiring much earlier these days, usually around 6:15 pm or so. But why so early? Part of the Sundown Syndrome, I suspect. Lately, in the afternoon, Joan seemed both tired and restless. I tried yesterday to convince her to get some rest while I dashed to the post office and grocery store. As worn out as she seemed, she wanted to go with me and would have seen my refusal as a sign that I did not want her company. So, naturally, she accompanied me and seemed no worse for wear. To tell you the truth, though, I worried most every step of the way, afraid that Joan would stumble and fall, so unsteady was she on her feet these days. Against my own habit, I slowed down, holding her hand most of the time and pushing the cart with my other as we made our way through the grocery aisles.

June 25, 2011

"Who is coming to dinner and when?" Joan asked me this question again and again last Wednesday afternoon prior to the arrival of her nephew, Randy Williams, and his wife, Lucie. We always got together with them a couple of times a year to keep in touch, usually over the holidays. They were always kind enough to drive from their home in Coupeville to meet with us. They arranged to visit us this time because they were aware of Joan's deteriorating condition and wanted to offer what support they could by bringing the food and good conversation. "Just who is coming to dinner?" Nothing wore me out more than answering the same question with the same answer over and over again. It was no exaggeration to say that I responded to Joan's incessant question during the afternoon at least a couple of dozen times.

An older woman who worked at the local drug store told me she cared for her father around the clock for the last four years of his life and the thing she most needed to get her through it was patience. I had no trouble believing that. Patience was a crowning

virtue, essential to my care for Joan and—I was surprised to learn—
I was in woefully short supply of it. I was not nearly as patient as
I needed to be and so was quickly learning to ease up, to establish
broader priorities and to throw the clock away.

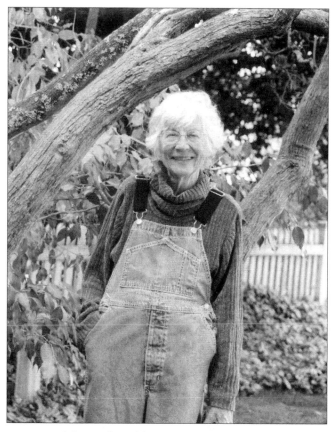

Joan in bib overalls and her winning smile. LaConner, 2006

Patience

The Seattle Times headline reads:
"Drug Prices Plummet as Patents Expire."

The remarkable Mrs. Skeele reads:
"Drug Prices Plummet as Patients Expire"

Whether "patents" or "patients"
the fact seems to hold. In either case,

drug prices will fall, and then some,
if there are no patients left at all.

Has the good wife stumbled on a
stubborn truth? Do we prefer, too often,

a patent on patience, keeping the price
high, enjoying our impatience too much

to go generic, to make virtue cheap and
such? How else do we explain our

giddy pleasure at lording it over the
slow and plain, eager to show

the less quick the way to go? Still,
we shouldn't feel too guilty for

patience, like the other virtues, can
never be reached with complete ease.

Virtues, after all, are part of God's
wish list and the Devil's proper tease.

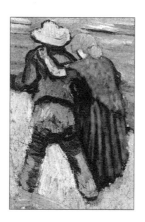

Randy and Lucie arrived on schedule at 5:30 pm, bringing with them steaming containers of food from the local Thai restaurant and a hot guitar. Later, after a delicious dessert of a little bit of vanilla ice cream stirred into a small glass of chocolate wine (Yes, there was such a thing. It was put out by the Dutch and marketed as Chocovine), Randy entertained us on the guitar and harmonica with a number of his latest songs, all of which impressed me with their originality and lyrical quality. Joan seemed to enjoy the music as well. I invited Randy to perform at our 60th wedding anniversary party September 10 and he seemed pleased to do it. Randy is an architect and building contractor and Lucie is a medical doctor (OB/GYN). That they took time from their busy schedules to be with us was a wonderful gift. They want to visit again soon. Lucie even offered to stop by on her way to hospital duties at St. Joseph's in Bellingham to cover for me for a few hours. Randy and Lucie soon departed for the hour's drive home. Only with prompting later that evening did Joan have any recollection of the visit or who the visitors were. The next day she had no memory of our meal together whatsoever. It was a sad and devastating state for her to be in and a challenging one for me as I tried to remember for both of us.

June 28, 2011

Does memory loss occur by degrees? It appeared so. Just when I did not think the loss was going to get any worse, it seemed to. Returning from our walk along First Street after lunch, Joan wanted to know where our house was. After walking the same route for months, she suddenly could not recognize the adjoining street (Benton St.) or our prominent yellow house when we turned the corner onto Fourth St. Once inside, and for the remainder of the afternoon, she kept asking when we were going home. Nothing inside seemed familiar to her. When I asked where our home was, she could not tell me. For the last few weeks, she had told me she would soon have to return home to Portsmouth (Ohio). I asked if she was thinking of her family home. She looked at me as if to say, "How dumb can you get?" Of course, she was not thinking of Portsmouth. "Well, where then?" I asked. She was not able to answer and could only shake her head in bewilderment.

This episode bothered me almost as much as the previous night. Quite often lately in the early morning hours, I have had to show Joan where the bathroom was, sometimes taking her hand and leading her there. This time I had to lead her back from the bathroom as well to her bed and tell her how to lie down on it, curled up on her left side! The whole process seemed foreign and strange to her, her body almost catatonic. I tried not to show my alarm but I was quite stunned. Changes, bad changes, were happening too fast for me. Much to my relief, last night was more normal. It helped that I went to bed when she did, reading to her and staying in the bed next to her after turning off the bed lamp at 8:00 pm. (Normally at such an early hour in June I would not need the lamp. The sun would still be up and shining right through the curtains on our west windows but yesterday was gray and overcast for most of the time.)

July 4, 2011

If I were to try to compose a piece of music based on Joan's night behavior, I would entitle it Sundown Variations in B Minor. The last two nights were different yet from what I had observed and experienced before. The night before last, Joan's routine started out as usual, getting up every couple of hours to urinate, usually finding her way to the bathroom by herself, sometimes with my help. At a little after 1:00 am, however, she began getting up about every ten minutes without any articulated reason except that she thought she should. Each time I would coax her back to bed, reminding her of the hour, and that I would be sure to let her know when to get up. I was, after all, the breakfast cook. No amount of cajoling seemed to work. Then Joan said something about how good it felt to be rubbing her own foot. Yes, of course! Immediately I hopped out of bed and with my right hand braced on her headboard, I leaned over her and, without removing the bed covers, began rubbing her back and hip with my left hand. Within five minutes she was breathing easily and before long was into a deep sleep.

Why could I not seem to remember this simple remedy? It occurred to me that possibly Joan's restlessness would never get out of hand if we were sleeping together in our queen size bed. I would automatically reach over and make physical contact as I had done most of our married life and that would settle her down. Perhaps I should reconsider and move the big bed downstairs. It would be an easy remedy if I could just exchange spaces, placing the twin beds where the queen size bed was. The problem was the twin beds don't quite fit the vacated space.

Last night was more of a challenge. To my surprise, Joan slept more or less through the noise of the fireworks from 10:00 pm to after 11:00 pm but at 11:45 pm woke up and, against my protests, very calmly put on her running shoes and bathrobe and prepared to walk to her "friend's" house where there was a lot of "care" and "concern" for her. What friends, she could not say nor could she tell me where they lived. She might have made it to the side door if I had not told her she really was not properly dressed, pointing out that she was in her sleepwear not her day clothes. She opened her robe, looked at her flannel pajamas and decided not to walk. She then began looking for "Bob," going toward the bathroom, calling out Bob's name. Not finding him, she came back to our bedroom, took off her shoes and robe and climbed back into bed. A lot of the time these days, Joan did not seem to recognize me as "Bob," her husband of 60 years, often asking me where he might be. So I was not surprised that she went looking elsewhere for him last night. Thus the "B minor" in the title of the *Sundown Variations*. The real "Bob" was disappearing. The mythological "Bob" was taking over.

July Colors

In July, the fourth day holds sway.
Its door, history-lighted
And like any door, two sided,
One festooned in red, white and blue
The other draped in a darker hue.

When I push open July's door
Celebration is the first to greet me.
Town folk gathered along the shore
All eyes turned upward to see
The night's colorful offering.

Amid appreciative murmurs and outright glee
The flares thrust straight up in a sizzling white
Then noisily burst forth in a dazzle of color
Painting the upturned faces, however briefly,
Making clowns of us all.

Clowns, especially those who, knowing the dark
Make a virtue of light and mirth,
See something more in the night's pulsing glare,
A sadness running through the joys of earth.
Dire works in the fireworks.

Between the skyward shots and arching sprays
Of gold and green, white and red

Is that black, silent interlude
When the embers, amber and dead,
Float down through the swirling smoke
To capture by the water's ebb.

For the document we celebrate this bright night
Declares Independence from the British Crown a must
But no matter how necessary and just
Separation did what separation tends
Pitting friends against friends.

Neighbor with neighbor contends
The fiercely loyal against liberty's sons,
Strident division, with cannon and guns,
Tears at civility's core,
Creating America's first civil war.

July 6, 2011

Sometimes, the earlier you go to bed, the less sleep you get. Last night was a case in point, yet another "variation," but before the sun actually went down. Joan, as usual, was ready for bed shortly after supper at 7:00 pm or so. I said I would like to catch the news on television and see how the Mariners did, at least in the early innings against Oakland. Joan was quite happy to join me for fifteen minutes or so, but then begged off to get ready for bed. I helped her get into her pajamas and returned to the television for a little while longer, but soon realized I was tired too and joined her, reading to her from John Vaillant's book on the Amur Tiger until I began to lose the sense of what I was reading. I was suddenly ready to sleep. The problem was Joan could not sleep and kept asking me to turn off the light so she could. I carefully explained that this was one light I could not turn off. The sun, still above the horizon, was shining through the curtains and lighting the entire room. After I had finished my explanation, she would ask me again if I would please turn off the light and pointed toward the overhead ceiling fan insisting that was the source of the problem. Many years ago I had replaced the lighting fixture with the ceiling fan but my explanation fell on deaf ears. My repeated explanation of the light's solar source were as useless.

By this time I was wide awake and so returned to the adjoining room to watch the later innings. At about 9:40 pm or so, just when I was beginning to feel relaxed enough to return to bed, Joan appeared, ready for breakfast. In spite of my best arguments, she found it hard to believe it was still evening and began to rummage around the kitchen to find something to eat. I ended up making her a bowl of oatmeal and some toast and, in the process, I had again become wide awake. By now the sun was down, the front bedroom was darkening, and I saw that she was tucked in. She appeared content and was soon breathing deeply. I, on the other hand, could only wonder—at 10:30 pm—when sleep would return. But it did, finally. It was not until 2:30 am that I was awakened by her visit to the bathroom, but I was thankful to get four hours of uninterrupted rest. At her next bathroom trip, on schedule at 4: 30 am, I got up, dressed, showered and was at my iMac writing these words and ready to seize the day. Oatmeal and toast were not on the breakfast menu.

July 15, 2011

Nine days have gone by without any major dramatic event to record but Joan continued to get my attention. For the first time, she had not been as enthusiastic about going for the early morning walks with her friends, cancelling out three days in a row now. Lately her complaint about not feeling well was accentuated by her lack of appetite. At breakfast she used to eat two or more of my warm muffins along with a cup of coffee, often exclaiming over the muffins. Now, she eats one muffin, drinks only a half cup of coffee and offers no expression of enjoyment. She pleads exhaustion and returns to bed or the sofa to sleep for an hour or so. She was still unable to point to any specific part of her body as the source of discomfort.

I have been checking Joan's blood sugar at regular intervals and giving her insulin injections as required. The blood sugar was under control with no severe highs or lows. Her desire to set the table with extra plates for her parents or our children has diminished. Every once in a while during the day, she would still ask me where Susan was or inquire about her brother Bill or other deceased family member. Depression most certainly was part of the problem here; I wanted to try to counteract that by getting her to the Senior Center for lunch on Tuesdays. So far my friend and caregiver had not been able to persuade her to stay and partake. I also would try to get her into a daycare facility one day a week. I had heard particularly good things about one place called Gentry House in Anacortes. They operated in small groups of adult dementia patients with good staff and good results. Getting Joan to participate was the challenge. I knew I would like the respite. Right now, I am helping to set up a new exhibit at the museum so I am able to get out of the house for short periods, thanks to our wholly reliable caregiver. Currently, she is contracted to come to the house every Tuesday from 9 to 3. She is available for more days as needed.

July 19, 2011

As before, I did not have to guess who was coming to dinner, only now Joan did not try to set extra places. Her expectations, however, remained high. Soon after beginning to eat, she would ask me where this or that family member was. Last night she asked about her mom. I told her she was not here. "Does she have a car?" Joan wanted to know. "No," I said. "I wish I had known that. I would have picked her up," she replied. She did not follow up her question nor did I offer further comment. I had begun to follow a modern military policy. When it comes to responding to questions about absent family members, I practiced "Don't ask, don't tell." It seemed simpler, less confusing to Joan that way.

Sometimes, of course, an extended answer was called for. Last night at supper, for example, when Joan learned her mother would not be present for dinner, she went on to ask about Susan's whereabouts. In that case I reminded her (again) that Susan lived in Santa Fe now. Joan was surprised (again) that she lived there, and even more surprised at how long she had been residing there. But, then again, Joan was surprised at how long we had lived in La Conner. She had guessed six or seven years. When I told her it had been 25 years, she could not, would not, believe it. The same was true with our marriage. When I told her we had been married 60 years this coming September, she shook her head in denial as if it was totally impossible. Even when I did the numbers, subtracting the year of our marriage from the current year, she was unconvinced. All this reminded me of just how extensive her memory loss was. Along with the loss of memory was the loss of time—which should be obvious. But it was not obvious when you were the caregiver and you were not ready to acknowledge your beloved's wholesale forgetfulness. It was because memory loss was a loss of rationality that I no longer expended my time on explanation. Repeated explanation was a waste of time and sapped my energy like nothing else. Constant repetition wore me down.

I observed what appeared to be another subtle change in the Sundowner's Syndrome from early evening to early morning: the latter was apt to be a much more confusing time. Last night before midnight, for example, Joan was perfectly able to make her way through the living room and kitchen to the bathroom with ease. By 3:30 am however, I had to guide her every step of the way, even pointing out how to use the toilet. After she urinated I then showed her how to flush the toilet and walked her back to the bedroom. She figured out how to position herself in bed, asking my opinion, as I placed a soft pillow between her knees and a smaller one to hold against her chest, and then tucked the blanket around her body. At 4:30 am I heard her on my monitor upstairs and went down to investigate. She was intent upon getting up to fix breakfast for a number of people who were soon due to arrive. I coaxed her into returning to bed and waiting for me to tell her when to get up. She seemed relieved that she did not have to decide that. Upon leaving to return to my computer upstairs, Joan asked, "What's your name?" "Bob," I replied.

July 23, 2011

"Pitch battles" were becoming more frequent these days as I found that sometimes I simply had to say, "No, we cannot do that." Yesterday was a good example. Several days ago I had taken our VW camper to my auto repair shop in Mount Vernon to check out the electrical system. At lunch time I received a call from the shop saying the car was ready to pick up. I explained to Joan that I would hitch a ride with someone who was heading to Mount Vernon and then drive the camper back home. She could not see why we did not just drive over in our Saab. I could drive the camper back and she would drive the Saab. I tried to avoid the issue for a time, explaining that it was just as easy for me to find a ride which would save her the trouble. (Every time she was in the car, she had to put up with a certain amount of pain. Her frailty was at the point where the slightest bump or jar would bother her back or neck and make her feel nauseous. I was always surprised when she wanted to accompany me anywhere in the car. But she did, and after each trip she wished she had not. Now, of course, she had little if any memory of the pain.) Finally, she confronted me directly. "You don't want me to drive, do you? After all my years of experience, you don't think I am capable of driving my Saab, do you?" I agreed, I did not. And I gave her the biggest reason: her eyesight. Most every time she was in the car with me she was quick to let me know that she saw double, that there was not one but two cars ahead of us, not one but two lanes, etc. My argument quieted her down some. I backed it up declaring the responsibility I felt for her safety and that I would be totally remiss to allow her to drive. I then returned to my original argument and proceeded to find a ride to Mount Vernon with a friend who was heading to Mount Vernon momentarily. What I did not mention to Joan, and would not mention, was her susceptibility to disorientation and confusion. I was absolutely convinced that she could not find her way home from Mount Vernon and that the traffic she would encounter would be a nightmare for her. I had no doubt this battle would occur again. I had to watch now that Joan did not decide at some point to grab the keys and drive off. Had I reached the time when I had to hide the keys or lock them up? So far, I had felt that Joan, subconsciously, did not really trust herself to drive a car without my approval—she was depending on me increasingly to make decisions for her—but was I correct? And for how much longer did I dare leave the car keys within easy reach? I hated deception. But here I was, of necessity, playing the game.

July 28, 2011

Another daily "pitch battle" had to do with Joan's diabetes. After every meal I monitored the amount of glucose in her blood by pricking her finger and injecting her in the stomach with insulin using a flexpen, the amount of insulin determined by the glucose level. The higher the blood sugar, the more insulin I injected. She had grown to hate the entire procedure. I could not blame her, but the alternative was much worse. At least one of the three times each day, Joan fought the procedure, wanting to know why she had to submit to such torture. As often, I explained. For some reason, I told her, her pancreas was no longer producing insulin which was what controlled the amount of sugar in the blood. Therefore, I had to supply the insulin by injection. In effect, I was acting like her pancreas.

Working in conjunction with her doctor, I had tried using just long-term insulin (Levemir) which meant only one shot a day but that had not been sufficient to keep the glucose at 150 mg. The only solution seemed to be a combination of Levemir with short-term insulin (Novolog) which meant two injections every morning and one injection after lunch and supper. The battle continued, of course, because Joan could not remember from one moment to the next what I had already told her hundreds of times. She could not remember the consequences of not taking insulin either, which under normal circumstances would be enough motivation. When all other arguments failed, I explained to her that most diabetics self-medicate and that she should, too. Since she could not tolerate the idea of pricking her own finger and injecting herself in the stomach, I would win and she would comply...until the next meal. "Patience," I kept repeating to myself, "Patience." As the caregiver, I did not want to, must not, allow my weariness to slop over into exasperation, but I knew there were times when I was right on the edge.

In fact, last night, I did slip over the edge. Like most nights from midnight on, Joan was restless. Last night it took the form of increasing numbers of trips to the bathroom, sometimes as often as every half hour or so. Each time, I turned on the bed lamp and awaited her return so I could tuck her back in bed. She needed the light to find her way back and if I did not tuck her in, her bed would soon be a mess and I would end up having to remake it. It was also the case that she was chilled on even the warmest nights so it had become important to my mind to snug the electric blanket up against her back. At 2:45 am or so I tucked her in and turned off the lamp, as usual, hoping to get another hour's sleep when she said, "I have to do something with my bridge. I can't sleep with it in my mouth." Since I had seen her put the bridge in her white plastic container in the bathroom before bedtime, I told her she had obviously just put it in her mouth on her last trip to the bathroom. "Why," I asked, "don't you just leave it in your mouth until morning?" Many times she had preferred to sleep with her bridge in her mouth, thus the suggestion. "No, I can't stand it in my mouth," she responded.

At this point, I got up once again, irritated, totally disgusted, and swearing to myself like the sailor I once was. I took Joan's bridge and stomped (Can you really "stomp" in bare feet?) back to the bathroom only to discover that Joan was trailing behind me. She wanted to see where I was putting the bridge. I showed her and we returned to the front bedroom one more time. No sooner had I tucked her in and turned off the lamp than she was up again! She felt she might have to urinate. By then, I was too wide awake to care and after she came back to bed, I called it a night, made my bed, turned off the bed lamp and headed upstairs to shower and write. It was 3:00 am on the nose. I made a mental note to get a urine sample to the medical center at first chance. I would try again, as well, to get Joan to take a second Melatonex.

At 5:15 am, as I was preparing to dress for my morning run, guess who was climbing the stairs looking for me? Joan agreed it was too early to get up and was quite happy to go back to bed while I jogged. I walked her back downstairs, tucked her in bed, turned off the kitchen and dining room lights and proceeded with my routine.

August 1, 2011

A third "pitch battle" appeared to be brewing. For the last several weeks now, Joan had begun to resist even more my efforts to get her to shower and wash her hair. Usually after some wrangling I succeeded, but not yesterday. Even when I told her that she had not showered for a week, she would not believe me, but even if it were true, she argued, she had not been sweaty or gotten dirty so what was the problem. This from a woman who had always bathed every day and prided herself on her personal hygiene. Part of the resistance seemed to have nothing to do with substance and a lot to do with control. She did not like being told what to do (Who does?) which was why I tried to get her to see the logic of my request or desire. But as I pointed out before, and should know better by now, logic holds little sway in her irrational world. Only when I convinced her that I had her best interest at heart was I going to succeed, but that, too, was difficult because she was always suspicious of others' motives, including mine. So the battles continued. Who knows, this morning Joan might want to shower and offer no resistance whatsoever.

Last night was relatively calm; Joan was up only three times to make her way, unescorted, to the bathroom. The only variation was her alarmed voice saying out of the dark that someone had knocked on our front door. I said, "No, there was no knock. I was awake. You must have been dreaming." Joan said, "I wasn't dreaming. I was awake too." "If someone was at the front door," I said, "they will knock again." In the face of my indisputable logic, Joan jumped out of bed, turned on the hall light and the porch light, calling out "Who's there?" and peering through the window next to my bed but, of course, she heard and saw nothing and soon returned to bed. I tucked her in once more, turned out the lights she had left on, and slid into my own bed…again.

The previous two nights had been absolutely horrible, overactive, puzzling and exhausting. The first of the two nights began strangely. Joan had retired to bed early and woke when it was still light (around 9:00 pm I would guess), walked into the living room where I was watching the Mariners lose again, carrying her plastic water bottle with its blue cap and plastic straw. I noticed she had a scowl on her face. She was obviously mad about something. In response to my inquiry, she waved me away, and pointed to her water bottle. It was then I realized she was treating the water bottle like a telephone, listening and talking into the plastic straw. She did not like what she was hearing but would not tell me anything about it after she put down the "phone."

At that point, I turned off the television, tucked Joan back in bed, changed into my pajamas and read to her from *The Tiger*. She was soon asleep. I had realized slowly that she enjoyed having me read to her at night more for the sound of my voice than the content of my words. My soothing voice this night did not soothe for long, however, for soon she was up to make her usual trip to the bathroom, followed by more trips every half hour or so through the night until about 3:00 am, many of the trips requiring my guidance. A long rubdown with me standing over the bed and reaching her back and legs, seemed finally to calm her enough to relax and stay put. I awoke much later than usual and was not able to get in any writing or exercise before breakfast preparations.

The next night was more wearing and frightening. This time there were few bathroom trips but Joan was often awake complaining of feeling terrible and experiencing what I could only describe as pre-convulsions. Uncertain whether the convulsive episodes were diabetically related, I took a blood sample which read 123 mg—well within the normal range. What was puzzling, though, was that her glucose reading immediately after supper was only 136 mg. Since I had not given her any insulin, and her food (sugar and carbs) had entered her blood stream by then, why was her glucose reading so low? Perhaps it was just the long-acting insulin (Levemir) kicking in, but it had me wondering. After doing all I could to make her comfortable, including another long rubdown through the bed covers, she finally got some rest as did I. I awoke the next morning at 6:45 am! Never had I slept so late in the last 20 years. Again, I had no time to exercise or write before breakfast which I did not wish to see continued for long. I understood, on the other hand, that some adaptation was going to be necessary as Joan and I moved through these next hilly months together.

August 2, 2011

I am happy to report that I won the recent "pitch battle" over the issue of showering. Joan slept in yesterday morning, not joining me at the breakfast table until about 9:30 am. As usual, she said she did not feel well and her slow shuffling walk in slippers and bathrobe and her pale, somber face confirmed it. She perked up a little bit with hot coffee and one of my fresh muffins, as she usually did, but seemed totally self-absorbed, hardly glancing at the paper—or at me, for that matter. Eventually, however, she consented to take a shower partly because I told her it would revive her some, make her feel a little better. Once I had helped her to shower and helped her dress in fresh clothes, she admitted she did, in fact, feel better. I noted in passing that the process of showering itself puts a big strain on Joan and it helped me to understand her reluctance. She was so frail and shaky and seemed to have so little strength for the task. Once in the shower, though, she seemed content to soap down and wash her hair without my assistance. Getting her to shower again in a few days would involve the same battle because she would not remember how good it felt.

I am also happy to report that Joan slept comparatively well last night with only three trips to the bathroom. The first time, I had to help her find her way through the kitchen but that was due to not turning on the night lights before retiring for the night. The next two times she handled on her own. Turning on the bedside lamp as she made her way to the bathroom made me feel like a lighthouse keeper as the light guided her back to bed. Tucking her in bed and rubbing her back for a few minutes exceeded my role but it seemed to reassure her so I had made it part of my lighthouse duty.

As if to make up for the relatively tranquil night, the daylight hours yesterday seemed zanier than usual. During the course of the day Joan kept remarking about David (our son) working at the museum up the street. As often as I would correct her, telling her that David was in Slippery Rock with his wife Nora and the two children, Joan was surprised to hear he was married and living elsewhere. Ten minutes later, she would again wonder when David was getting off work at the museum. Also, much of the day she could not figure out my identity. Frequently she asked where "Bob" was. I would tell her, "I'm Bob," and then she would say something like, "Oh, yes," and smile. At one point, I told her we were married and she would not believe it, even when I pointed to a picture of the First Community Church where the crime took place. Her mother was much on her mind yesterday, too. Frequently, she asked about her mother's whereabouts as if she were out shopping and was expected to return at any minute.

Last night in bed, Joan asked again about her mother. Again I explained that her mother had died when we still lived in Vermont and that she, Joan, had, in fact, flown to Salina, Kansas one weekend just to spend time at her bedside at the Presbyterian Home where she was being cared for. A week later she died. Joan seemed to absorb what I said, obviously pleased that she had made the trip. Five minutes later, however, in the midst of the darkened bedroom, she wondered why her mother had not made an effort to come out here to La Conner and then answered her own query: It's too far for her to travel. Lately, Joan's been referring to our house here in La Conner as "her" house. Yesterday, I corrected her. She said she was quite surprised to hear that our house was jointly owned (and probably did not believe it for a minute). I would be interested to see what she said about home ownership today.

August Picnic

Hinges well-oiled, the sturdy door of August,
Its patina worn smooth with wear and care
Opens the first Thursday wet or fair
To a convivial scene sedately robust.

Under the protective firs, snug against the hill
Between the new bandstand and old shelter
Gather some young and many an elder
To celebrate and honor in common will

The adventuresome who with gilt-edged dreams
Headed northwest, daring hardship to invest
In a future fraught with peril and promise, to wrest
A living from the rich earth and broad streams.

Now, after a century and a half of lives that mattered
The pioneering struggle oft told in book and song
How it went, the things done, right and wrong
Prompts a knowing nod from the proudly gathered.

For life, any life, is a struggle, and continues still.
The fields cleared, the big river mostly tame
The diked delta yielding ample seed and grain
The Valley, a modern Eden it seems, has more grist to mill…

August 8, 2011

All that I described in the previous entry had continued over the past week, Joan's mother and sometimes her daughter, Susan, taking center stage with David, our youngest son, identified with the museum up the hill. Joan's nights had settled down to a pattern of awaking about every hour and a half to use the bathroom, only occasionally losing her way. The only break in the routine came three nights ago when she slept straight through from 9:30 pm to 2:30 am. Oh, what a treat that was! Five hours of uninterrupted sleep. I felt like the lighthouse keeper (my alter ego) would feel with a whole night off.

I was struck again last evening by the progress the dementia had made over the weeks. After supper, Joan drove with me up the hill to deposit our week's worth of recyclables in the museum's recyclable bin for pick up the next morning by Waste Management. While there, I wanted to remove used paint supplies from the museum's East Wing and haul them next door to the Library for storage. My thinking was that Joan could look at the new exhibit, Native Journey, while I loaded our camper. To my surprise, she showed zero interest in the remarkable display of native artifacts and instead watched me haul paint cans and trays and other items, offering every so often to help (but could not because it was all much too heavy for her back). The longer I worked, the more anxious she became to return home. She needed to get to her bathroom. At my urging, she reluctantly let me take her to the women's restroom in the North Wing. She was spooked by the two stalls and chose the one with the open door indicating to me that she did not think she could urinate in such a strange place. When I turned to leave, she wanted me to stay right there in the restroom and wait. To ease her fear that she would not be able to find her way back to the lobby (which was just a few feet away), I waited and led her back to familiar ground. At this point, I drove her home and returned to the museum to finish the job of loading the camper which took maybe another 30 minutes. Rather than stopping next door at the Library to unload the pile of supplies, I drove straight home. I was glad I did because Joan was standing there at the front door anxiously waiting for my return. We embraced as if we had been parted for days. She then told me she had been looking all over the house for me and had even gone up to the museum but could not find me. This latter statement I seriously doubted. She could not have missed seeing me, nor I her. The camper was parked right in front of the museum entrance. But there you were. Our particular evening at the museum which had nothing at all to do with the wonderful display of native artifacts had a lot to do with other, sobering, facts, so very sad and frightening.

August 12, 2011

There seemed to be no end to the variations of the Sundowner's Syndrome. Just when I thought the pattern of Joan's getting up at regular intervals of one to two hours to urinate every night was going to be the standard, she surprised me two nights ago by sleeping soundly from 9:30 pm to 2:30 am and again, after urinating, from 2:30 am to 5:30 am. Since she slept over longer intervals, so did I, and as a result I felt refreshed in a way I had not for some time. I expected that Joan would feel better too, but apparently not, for she came shuffling to the breakfast table complaining about how bad she felt. During the course of the morning she rallied as usual and seemed much better.

The next two nights Joan reverted to standard except for one 45 minute stretch from about 1:30 am to 2:15 am where she kept going to the bathroom, returning to bed, and then, a few minutes later, getting up again to go to the bathroom once more. I finally figured out what was happening. Joan often (at night) thought she must save a urine sample (and once in awhile a feces sample) for the laboratory and that was what she seemed to be doing now: holding her urine. I eventually walked with her to the bathroom, and while she sat on the toilet, I urged her repeatedly to let go, not hold the urine and explained that was what toilets were designed to do, capture the urine (and feces) and transport it through the town pipe lines to the treatment plant. Finally, Joan convinced herself it was probably okay and urinated.

In the process of our bathroom conversation, I discovered something that had long been a mystery: why the excessive amount of toilet paper in the small waste basket next to the toilet? It seemed I was emptying the waste basket every other day so rapid was the accumulation. To my amazement, I watched her take the toilet paper from the roll, fold it carefully, wipe herself and then, instead of releasing the paper into the toilet, she retained it, examining the paper, and then tossing it into the basket. I explained to her that this paper was designed to disintegrate in the toilet water and tried to convince her to just let the paper drop into the bowl. She could not bring herself to do it. After that 45 minutes, I was worn out, and slept then, as did Joan, until 6:00 am, almost as late as the record time of last week!

Consequently, I had no time for writing or for my usual exercise routines. I was finding more and more frequently that I was unable to get to my writing until much later in the day, which I did not like, but there seemed to be little I could do about it. I was waking up later each morning but did not feel all that rested even then. Just as serious, my exercise routine was too sporadic. I needed to keep to my alternate day workout program at the fitness center or I would begin to lose the strength level I had attained over the years. Ditto the walking/running routine to help keep my metabolism up and my caloric count down. Perhaps I would find a new way to make it all work, but I must say I missed the early morning routine I had worked out over the years. But the new reality required a different approach and I had not found it yet. And I must make certain that I did.

August 18, 2011

A former neighbor, who had moved to Prague with her husband and three children two years ago, was back for a visit, staying at her mother's house on Maple Avenue across the street from the barbershop. Wanting a chance to visit with us before her return to Prague, she invited us to her mother's on a recent afternoon. Joan was happy enough to incorporate the visit into our walk, but was ill at ease once we arrived and gathered in their living room. The mother and daughter were hospitable as always, offering Joan sparkling water and a comfortable chair to sit on, but the four dogs underfoot and the general hubbub with children coming and going soon proved too much for Joan. Within five minutes of conversation, she said she could not stay any longer and we were soon back on our walk. The two hosts were sympathetic and well understood Joan's condition. The next morning I delivered a blueberry coffee cake, fresh out of the oven, as a way of thanking them for including Joan and me in their visit and to wish our former neighbor and the kids *bon voyage* as they departed for Prague that afternoon.

Joan's growing intolerance for noise and fast movement around her made me think it was probably wise that I canceled our big plans for our 60th wedding anniversary.

I was not particularly surprised to see some intolerance for Joan's behavior occurring as well. One neighbor who had been faithfully walking with Joan every Tuesday and Thursday morning for months now, had decided she "no longer has the strength to walk with her twice or even once a week." It was not that Joan's walking pal was not sympathetic, far from it, but she wrote that she was "wearing out walking and, I regret to say, anticipating walking with Joan." Although the neighbor did not point out any specific issue, I readily understood her feeling. My walks with Joan were becoming less pleasant (as I have mentioned before). She did things like yelling at drivers to slow down when they were not driving fast to begin with and becoming easily annoyed at pedestrians who hogged the sidewalks, sometimes making unnecessary remarks in passing. Because of a hearing problem (which she continued to deny) Joan became especially annoyed at people who slammed their car doors as she was walking by or at motorcyclists with their loud engines—noises which did not even faze me. I would not say that annoyance and antagonism defined our walks entirely; there were still those times when she held my arm tightly and told me of her love for me. There were other cuddly moments as well, warm and delightful, when we sang one of our few songs in harmony. But the negative aspects of our walks were there and seemed to be growing.

I always listened to this neighbor. She was a perceptive person. I listened to her now as she wrote, "Joan can be a sweetheart and I know you love her. I will also tell you … that Joan is past the point where most people I have known with dementia entered assisted living." If I wanted to keep Joan at home, she urged me to get sufficient help so that I have some respite and did not fall ill. Yes. She was absolutely correct. I had the right person as helper, I believed, in our caregiver who covered for me every Tuesday from 9 am to 3 pm, and, starting today, every Thursday from 9 am to 12 Noon. This arrangement should work well for the time being.

Our neighbor concluded her note, "I wish you the best with this. I admire you both and am sorry to see you struggling. I hope I have been a help to you." My response to her thoughtful note could only be overwhelmingly positive! She had been a great help! I would miss seeing her and I knew Joan would miss her too. Now it was time to move on to the next page in the big book.

August 19, 2011

Yesterday I mentioned our neighbor's concerns to our caregiver. When I referred to Joan's unsocial behavior during walks, the caregiver smiled as if remembering her own experiences with Joan and said that she had dealt with it by avoiding places where there were more than a few people. With regard to Joan being in an assisted living complex somewhere, her only remark was a question: that was where Joan was now, wasn't it? I guess she was right. Joan's in assisted living at home. That she got plenty of assistance these days was clear. Our neighbor's concern, of course, was for my health and survival. The day and a half away from the house should be enough for me for the present but bore watching, particularly the impact of disrupted sleep on my health and my performance during the day.

For two nights in a row now, by way of example, Joan had awakened at around midnight, restless and confused, only to settle down again an hour later with my help. The first time she awoke saying, "I don't know what to do." She would shake her head and repeat it time and again: "I don't know what to do." I could get no clues from her about her statement and so proceeded to address the immediate reality. She, in fact, did know what to do which was to get back in bed and get a good night's rest. First things first. We could deal with her question in the light of day over a cup of steaming coffee and one of my freshly-baked muffins. After helping her back to bed, I spent some time rubbing her back and legs through the bed covers which I was learning seemed to do more to relax her than anything else. It was like my hands provided reassurance, confirmation, maybe, that she was alive and loved.

The same was true last night. A little after midnight Joan sat up in bed and started talking about the "game" she had to get to or play in, none of which I could make sense of, nor could Joan. She could not name the "game" or where it might be played or why she had to get up in the middle of the night to get ready for it. Here again I talked her back to bed. Night time was for sleeping. Since she had eaten so little for supper last night, I thought she might be hungry, but if she was, she would usually mention it and she did not. So, as before, I let my hands do the talking. My small, arthritic hands, the fingers gnarly and distorted, still useful, bringing warmth and reassurance to my loved one after all these years.

Getting Joan to sleep again, I felt, was a major accomplishment, her deep breathing, the sound of victory. In some respects though, it was a hollow victory since the effort had left me wide awake. After an hour I was able to get back into my sleep cycle, but last night I failed completely, spending a good hour and a half worrying about how best to celebrate our upcoming 60th wedding anniversary. I had already scotched plans for a big gala at the Civic Garden Club with a hundred invitees complete with a Deejay and an organized potluck, concluding that it would be too much for Joan. Even going to a restaurant with a few family members and friends might be more than Joan could handle or enjoy. In fact, at this point, I was not sure she could "enjoy" any social event. Susan was coming to visit and help us celebrate; Randy, Joan's nephew, and his wife, Lucie, were aboard for the evening. Should I include others? And should we eat out or should I cook something myself at home? With these questions I finally fell asleep to be awakened by Joan who was getting up at 3:40 am for her usual trip to the bathroom. I resisted the temptation to roll over and, instead, got up, showered, did my usual floor exercises and started writing. I will now drive down to the fitness center for a short workout if I determine that Joan will remain asleep or, if she wakes up, will stay abed until my return.

August 22, 2011

In some respects, yesterday, Sunday, represented a point in our journey where all that had been happening was summarized, heralding what the days would likely look like down the road, followed by a night that revealed its own terrible future. For one thing, it became abundantly clear that Joan was unable to find anything to engage her mind, the only notable exception being the *Poetry* magazine which she would become absorbed in for short periods. Reading the Sunday paper together at the dining room table over a second cup of coffee (or in my case, tea) had always been a favorite time. Not any longer. Joan may look at the headline or reread aloud to me a few lines of something on the front page, but that was it. The television news made no sense to her and watching tennis, particularly women's tennis, held no interest now. She wanted to get outside so I urged her to help me with watering the plants, but she said she could not hold the hose. Observing her walking across the lawn was painful for me as she made her way slowly and tentatively. It looked like she might fall at any moment. She used to like to keep the rose bushes trimmed, but said she could not use the small shears any longer. This Sunday she reclined on the sofa waiting none too patiently for me to finish reading the paper so we could take one of our two or three short walks during the day. Walking seemed about the only interest remaining but even the walks, as short as they were, seemed to tire her too quickly to be enjoyable.

Perhaps most noticeable was Joan's confusion and anger. Several times during the day, she asked where various family members were, thinking David and Susan were nearby, and was surprised to learn they were living elsewhere. The same with her deceased brothers. Each time she asked about them I explained that they had died and what the circumstances surrounding each were. Often Joan was shocked all over again that she had not been informed. None of this was particularly new except the frequency of the questions. The issue of her children and her family's whereabouts seems to have taken center stage, much more of a preoccupation than ever before. Of all the preoccupations, it was her mother's presence that was closest and most constant. Most of the time her mother, Ruth, was sleeping upstairs or shopping somewhere nearby, and would soon return. Occasionally she had her mother living in the family home in Portsmouth, Ohio and thought she must remember to telephone her at first chance (but never did).

The first angry episode occurred yesterday afternoon over lunch when Joan asked, again, where "Dad" was. Instead of asking, as I usually did, what "Dad" she was referring to, I assumed she meant her father, "Pappy," and explained that he had died long ago when we were living in Alexandria, Minnesota. Joan was incensed, nostrils-flaring angry, at my answer. As if she did not know about her own father! In the process of trying to explain myself, I said something like his having died "long before your mother" which made Joan even angrier. According to Joan, I had made the reference to her mother just to make her feel bad, to make her see that I was the kingpin here and in charge. One of her normal characteristics had always been to question the motives of others which was part of what made her a good lawyer. Now, though, she tended to impugn my motives as well as those of others. I, we, were all out to make her look bad and ourselves better.

That irritableness came out again later that night (actually early morning) when she awoke (one of her many times to go to the bathroom) and was trying to take the cover off one of her bed pillows. Since I had seen her do this before on several occasions and did not want to struggle—in the middle of the night—getting the pillow case back on, I piped up with "No, no, Honey, just leave the pillow alone. I want it here when I tuck you back in bed." Joan's retort was an angry, "I know all about that!" and stomped off to the bathroom.

Joan's anger appeared to stem from the same thing in both cases: rebellion against my authoritarian manner. I had no interest whatsoever in a being a dictator, but I guess I was. I knew of no other way to deal with her irrational and suspicious nature at this point. She needed a lot of direction. Giving her choices did not help much if at all and usually just ended in more frustration for both of us. In most cases she literally could not make up her mind and, in fact, was relying more and more on my opinion, while at the same time resenting it.

Last night became even more of a concern for me. It was not getting up every hour to turn on the lamp while Joan traveled to the bathroom that bothered me, though that was tiring enough, nor was it her wanting to get up every five minutes for a period of twenty minutes (just after 1:00 am) because she had something she had to do which she never defined. I told her not to worry about the time, that I would remind her when it was time to get up. She got up one more time. When I reminded her of our agreement she said she thought I had forgotten to wake her up. Finally, then, she slept until about 4:00 am. when she got up to make another trip to the bathroom. As usual, I turned on the bed lamp while she wended her way east and then waited ... and waited ... for her return. After five minutes or so, I investigated and found her standing in the middle of the little bathroom, a roll of toilet paper in hand, unable to figure out what to do next. She said she did not want sit on the toilet seat since it had no bottom. I explained to her that that was the point, that was the way toilets were designed, so we could conveniently eliminate the waste from our body. Thomas Crapper (1835-1910), who was one of the first to promote the use of the inside toilet, would have been proud of my explanation. Only reluctantly did she finally drop her pajama pants and try to urinate, at last succeeding. This was the second incident where Joan could not recognize or operate the toilet. Would I soon have to accompany her on each of her trips to the bathroom? How much more personal or intimate would the operation become and could I handle it? I was not sure I would be able to but, like everything else that was happening in my caregiving role, I would probably slowly work myself into it.

Talking with Joan about what happened last night was a surprise to her. She did not remember any of it and felt bad that she kept me from getting my rest. It became obvious, too, that she had no problem operating the commode during the day.

August 28, 2011

These last few days we seem to have reached a plateau of sorts, the Sundown Syndrome becoming as predictable as the Sunup Syndrome. Joan continued to get up frequently at night with the times varying from one to two hours with a certain amount of disorientation and confusion some of the time, often later in the sleep cycle. It was imperative as a caregiver that I slept in the same room with Joan. I could not imagine how she could function otherwise. Last night, for example, after she had urinated and returned to bed at 2:15 am, she wanted to get up and begin the day. What would she have done if I had not been there to persuade her to stay in bed until I started breakfast? She might well have started to dress and begun rifling through the kitchen cupboards to prepare her own breakfast as she began to do one time before, even turning on the gas stove to heat the water! So the number one strategy at this point was clear. There were no alternatives. I must sleep close by my wife or find another friend or professional caregiver to do that for me. I could not right now see the latter ever happening, but then again, it was early in the game.

Joan's Sunup Day usually began with the words "I don't feel well" as she dragged herself to the breakfast table. She was also usually cold even in July and would not have thought to grab her bathrobe or have known where to find it anyway. So I would fetch the bathrobe and a certain cushion from her bed that she liked to sit on at meal times and get her settled with hot coffee, fresh muffins (or whatever I'm baking that morning) and the Seattle Times. Occasionally, she would read me an item from the paper, often the same item numerous times, but most of the time there was little conversation since I was trying to catch up on the news as well. Following breakfast the first fight would begin—involving persuading her to let me draw blood and inject her with insulin. She would finally yield when I talked of the consequences of not doing it. As I mentioned earlier, my arguments were pretty practiced by now.

Eventually, Joan would perk up enough to want to get dressed and take her morning walk. I would walk with her to the bedroom and lay out her clothes, normally these days just simple attire: sweatpants, a hoodie and running shoes with fresh underpants every day. Once she decided among three baseball caps and whether or not to wear gloves (she had worn gloves most mornings through the summer), found her sunglasses and keys (which could sometimes take several minutes), we would take a short walk, hand in hand, to the post office and thence home via First Street, sometimes stopping at Town Hall to greet the staff. I noted that Joan's walking pace was getting ever slower, now more of a stroll, and she tired easily. Once home she would lie down on the dining room sofa and rest and sometimes sleep while I would read the mail, do some writing on my laptop or tend to some chores if the weather was right. It was not long before I would be thinking about lunch, meals most days continuing to be a real challenge since she had never developed an appetite and even if on rare occasions she might be hungry, she would eat little, hardly enough to meet her nutritional needs. As I had grown well aware of by this time, vegetables and meat were not among her favorites. At supper it was the bread, butter and jam she always went after first. That she had maintained a consistent weight of 90.2 pounds over these last months continued to astound me. I could only chalk it up to the carbs and the small dish of ice cream I served her daily at lunch and supper.

Following lunch. once again Joan would typically resist my entreaties to let me monitor her glucose level and give her insulin, compelling me to repeat all my arguments. In the end, though, she would always relent, and the insulin, if needed, was administered with only an occasional howl of protest.

August 31, 2011

"Sunup Time" for Joan had become as unusual as "Sundown Time." Her afternoons were most always chock full of illusory friends and guests among moments of clarity. After our early afternoon walk, she and I would return to the house, she to rest on the sofa, me to read or take on one household task or another. Squeezed in between these activities, Joan would ask a lot of familiar questions regarding the whereabouts of family. "Where's Dad?" was one. Her mother was sometimes upstairs resting or out shopping. Her brother Bill was visiting and should soon be here for supper, etc. In each case I would explain as patiently and thoroughly as the situation required that the person in question had died sometime ago or, in the case of our children, lived elsewhere now. She was amazed each time to hear the news, of course, since she could not remember what I had told her many times before.

The most puzzling thing that occurred frequently now, still was the appearance of a young girl or young woman who sometimes slept with Joan at night and visited during the day when I was home. "How could you possibly have missed her? She was right here talking to me a few minutes ago." When I repeated that I had never seen her, an expression of what I wanted to call alarm passed over Joan's face, a worry that she was losing her connection to reality, but I might have been reading into it. It was worrisome though, somehow much worse than her sitting at the dining room table and looking out into the side yard and seeing figures moving beyond the trees.

Elsewhere

Elsewhere is the most beautiful place,
everyone's dream from time to time, at least,
in this we all agree:
Elsewhere is always where we want to be,
the place most sought,
when where we are is not
where we want to be.

When Here proves unbearably difficult,
some kind of final assault
on our sense of what is fair and humane,
and our tolerance is severely tested
and strained.
Oh, how then we long to be Elsewhere,
any where but Here.

For there in Elsewhere, we like to think,
we're in the land of opposites,
where motives are pure and water
is safe to drink,
and there's a lot less pain.
Here's hell somehow countered,
if even for a moment,
by heaven's gentle reign.

But we know, in our skeptical mood,
that Elsewhere is not really out there
somewhere,
but are we willing to consider the alternative,
that Elsewhere might be close by,
just out of easy reach,
beneath and within
Here's harsh bravado
and war-warmed speech?

Could it be that Elsewhere does exist,
that we might find Elsewhere
where we least expect
any secret to unfurl,
not outside but inside,
in the stillness at the center
of our deadly, daily swirl?

September 1, 2011

Having just described, before the poem, what was a more or less typical day, guess what? Yesterday morning and afternoon passed without a single reference to Joan's deceased family, the young girl or our children…until the middle of a late supper. Joan was in the midst of eating some substantial food for a change—in this case a halibut fish cake and an ear of corn—when she suddenly blurted out "Patti!" When I asked about what brought that on, she seemed surprised at my question because Patti (her sister), was here, had been visiting here for some time, apparently. When I told Joan that Patti was not here but at her home in Salina, Kansas, she did not dispute it. In fact, an expression akin to self-doubt seemed to have crept in. Joan, in quick succession, asked after her brother Bill and brother Don. She was miffed that she had not been told of their deaths. I said that we both had been told at the time, and again explained the nature of their deaths and who informed us. She appeared satisfied and we soon went on to other things as I, once again, cajoled her into letting me monitor her blood to see if she would need any insulin for the night. The monitor registered a glucose level of 195, so I injected her with 2 i.u. of the stuff with the handy flex pen.

Sunday had been a bad day. Yesterday, the last day of August, was worse. With my revamped exercise routine in place, the morning had started well, but it was downhill from that point on. I was looking forward to baking some scones for two expectant neighbors from a recipe I had tried before, but for reasons I could not altogether determine, the scones did not turn out well. So I tried again, using a second, more familiar, recipe with equally unsatisfactory results. This was not the way a baker liked to start his day.

In the midst of my frustration, Joan came into the kitchen saying she did not feel well, and it was obvious she could not eat or drink anything—not even a cup of hot coffee—and she soon returned to bed. I baked some fresh muffins for her which coaxed her out of bed and to the breakfast table at 9:30 am or so, but she ate little. She wanted to walk, so after helping her dress, we took our usual route to the post office and back to "her" house (For some reason lately, Joan always referred to our house as "her" house as if I had no stake in the ownership.). The little excursion seemed to wear her out so she retired to the sofa to rest and she actually slept awhile.

Lunch was later than usual but, again, Joan ate little, barely touching her soup or sandwich. She did eat a small dish of ice cream. By 2:30 pm, I had cleaned up the kitchen and begun to think about the supper menu, and realized I had to get to the neighborhood store. Since I needed only a few items and did not need any help making selections, I suggested that Joan stay home and rest. She seemed to agree but, at the last minute, unknown to me, decided she wanted to go. Unfortunately, I did not hear her shouts over the noise of the engine as I drove off, leaving her in the dust. When I returned, Joan was angry that I had not waited for her and accused me of deliberately driving off without her, and that I really did not want her to accompany me to begin with. I vehemently denied the charge and expressed my particular dislike of having my motives impugned all the time. I told her that the next time I went grocery shopping, she was going with me whether she wanted to or not! It became a genuine brouhaha, a shouting match, for a few minutes and then we quieted down.

It was not too much later before Joan came up behind me as I was at the kitchen counter preparing supper (and still irked), embraced me and said how much she loved me. Just like that, Joan seemed to have forgotten all about our stormy conversation! The problem was it was not as easy for me to move on as if nothing had happened.

I helped her get ready for bed. She needed help identifying her pajamas and finding her toothbrush and toothpaste. She asked me to come to bed with her and since it was later, about 8:30 pm, I happily agreed. It had been a long day. I carefully climbed into her twin bed. She nestled her head in my shoulder and rested her right leg across my hips. In a bigger bed, I would have had room to maneuver so I could use my hands to soothe and massage. Not tonight. I was pinned on my back so depended on Joan to use her hands. She did for a few minutes, running her right hand over my chest and then, the movement stopped and I soon heard her soft breathing. Quietly I slipped out from under her leg and the covers, and, as quietly, collapsed into the other twin bed hoping against hope, tomorrow would turn out to be a little better.

September 3, 2011

A first! After many months of interrupted sleep, last night Joan slept through the night which meant I slept through the night. She had awakened a little after 11:00 pm to go to the bathroom. Since she had not taken her second Lorazepam earlier, I gave her one then, thinking it might reduce the restlessness or anxiety she had been dealing with the last several nights (expressed as her need to get up, dress and go somewhere without being able to specify where). Such periods usually lasted about an hour, just long enough to make it difficult for me to get back into my sleep cycle. What was the cause and effect of her good night? Did the Lorazepam allow her to sleep through the night or was it some other factor? She had already taken her two Lorazepam pills for the day so I would not give her one tonight. But I might tomorrow night if she reverted to the previous pattern.

I felt wonderful after the uninterrupted sleep and I thought Joan would too. But she did not. Just the opposite. She complained of not feeling well at breakfast, ate only one of my fresh muffins, drank some hot coffee and went back to bed, sleeping most of the morning while I watched Ohio State play its opening football game at home, my home, in Columbus.

Joan was not hungry at lunch time but I made her a small tuna fish sandwich anyway along with a thick chocolate milkshake. She ate about half of each. Feeling somewhat better, Joan got into her sweats and we took a walk to the drug store and grocery to pick up a prescription and a few other items. All during the walk Joan wondered why we had not driven. At one point I asked her if she wanted to wait at a convenient point in the shade while I fetched the car to give her a ride home. She declined the offer, insisting on soldiering on. It was slow going. Her pace seemed noticeably slower these last weeks. With so little nutrition, I did not know how she managed at all. And yet, she had this spirit, this determination, to keep going when, in fact, she was noticeably tired, wearing out.

Shortly after we got home from the walk and I was doing some preparation for supper (a neighbor had given us some smoked salmon and I was beginning to cut up vegetables for a chowder soup), Joan asked, as tired as she was, if she could help. "What can I do?" she often asked from a reclining position on the sofa and so she asked today. When I told her everything was under control and she did not have to help, she was relieved. "Oh, good," she said. I told her again what I had told her many times, that she did not have to "do" anything. All she had to do now was to "be." Over the decades she had done her share, "doing" for the kids and for me. Now, I told her, she could rest on her laurels and just "be," if not the Queen of the Nile at least the Queen of Esary House, basking in my admiration and taking her ease. I did ask her to help in the kitchen once in a great while but most things she did not feel up to.

September 5, 2011 (Labor Day)

I had not pursued the strategy of giving Joan a third pill (Lorazepam) at night because she seemed to have broken the pattern on her own. The last several nights she had slept for longer stretches. Last night, for example, she went to the bathroom at 10:30 pm and did not get up again until 3:30 am. at which time I got up and started my day. At 4:30 am I could hear her stirring around on my upstairs monitor. I went downstairs to find she was in bed with the bed lamp on, ready to get up for breakfast. Usually she was relieved when she learned she could sleep awhile longer, but this morning she was disappointed, and groaned when I told her she had two more hours of downtime.

Now, as I sit at the computer writing these words a half hour later, I can hear the reassuring sound of Joan's deep breathing over the monitor, relieved that all is well for the moment and that I can keep writing and maybe get in my morning walk/run (and fitness center workout) which I usually begin at around 5:30 am.

I still wanted to work bicycling back into my routine. I had Joan's mountain bike, a Bridgestone, reconditioned at Skagit Cycle. It had been resting and rusting on our side porch, its back wheel locked into a trainer, so Joan could use it as part of her exercise program, but she had not used it for several years. With new tires and a new chain, the bike handled well and the multi-gears got me up and down the hill with relative ease. Joan had not noticed the bike's disappearance from the side porch, nor had she recognized it as the bike I was now riding. Nor was she apt to. Her other two bikes which had been stored in the shed I had sold to Skagit Cycle, the money from the sale about covering the cost of the reconditioned Bridgestone. I had secreted the bikes out of the shed and off the side porch without Joan's knowledge. I did not feel entirely comfortable operating behind her back, but I knew that otherwise I could never put the Bridgestone to good use or remove the other two from the shed. One of my projects this year was to clean out the shed and make it useable as a workshop once again. Getting the bikes and other unused tools, etc. out of there was the first step.

September 16, 2011

Our big day, our 60th wedding anniversary on the ninth had come and gone, the decisions about how and where to celebrate it, blessedly over with. I found myself immensely relieved that the celebration had turned out so well.

Its success was helped along by our daughter, Susan, who had arrived early from Santa Fe and by the museum staff who had invited us and Susan to the Research Library at 10:00 am on Friday, our wedding date, to honor the occasion. They put on a beautiful spread, complete with freshly smoked salmon, cream cheese and bagels, sweet rolls, coffee, tea and, since the weather was still hot, a pitcher of lemonade. Two large bouquets of flowers added color and cheer to the already friendly gathering. That two members of the Board of Trustees were present was a surprise to me but a welcome one. It was a wonderful occasion. Joan seemed to enjoy herself and Susan was impressed with the spirit of the staff. I had a chance to regale them with stories of our courtship which everyone seemed to enjoy.

The highlight of the hour was our anniversary gift of a beautiful Pendleton blanket, which I was told, our good friend and Joan's principal caregiver helped select. The prominent colors were soft browns and white, one side more or less the reverse of the other, except for two dark blue stripes. The dominant symbol was a cross, the design with its four arms of equal length, repeated throughout (I now had it spread out on the Lincoln bed in the upstairs bedroom to glimpse at from time to time). Two of the staff helped us by carrying the vases of flowers home, the flowers becoming a focal point for our anniversary party the next night. As I told the staff and Board members, the museum meant a lot to me, never more than now, as I wound up my part-time career as its facilities manager. In a way, this anniversary celebration had the feeling of a retirement party as well, a perfect ending to my tenure (with a few breaks) of nineteen years. A little while later, over a late lunch, I asked Joan how she liked the party at the museum. She could not remember it.

As mentioned earlier, I had abandoned the idea of a big gala with music and dancing and a potluck in favor of something smaller by way of an anniversary celebration. Finally, I decided that, instead of going to a restaurant, I would have the restaurant come to us. This way I could have the party at our house, but I would not have to do all the cooking. To this end, I consulted with Casey, the chef and owner (with his wife, Susan) of Nell Thorn's. After a number of suggestions, he came up with the perfect menu, something that was both of local origin and easy to serve: roast pork shoulder (pulled pork) from the nearby organic farm (we could see the pig pen from our dining room window at one point as the farmer moved the pen around his closest field), roasted vegetables and potatoes and a side dish of faro. I would bake rolls, corn bread and a chocolate, gluten-free cake topped off with chocolate sauce and ice cream.

Did it work out? Was it successful? I thought so, but not without a lot of help from Susan who had washed windows, vacuumed, dusted and helped me shift furniture around to accommodate the five guests. Never had I appreciated the energy and strength of the young more than when watching Susan's whirlwind attack on our innocent little house. Given the warm weather, putting the wicker furniture (from the dining room) on the back deck had been a good idea because after we opened the wine the guests brought, we ended up sitting on the deck, sipping it and talking. As I had at the museum, I spent some time talking about our courtship and wedding, deferring to Joan from time to time. Only when we were hungry and ready to eat did we go inside, uncover the dishes and turn to. Winding down outside and then moving inside and having such excellent fare was a winning combination—another wonderful, deeply satisfying celebration of our 60th. I could not have been happier at the way it all worked out. Most importantly, Joan seemed to enjoy it too, although she had no recollection of it the next morning. This year I saw our celebration as a two-stage affair, low key and quiet but varied and unharried. Who could ask for more?

Who could? I could. I could ask for one more impossible thing to make the anniversary celebration perfect. If only Joan could have remembered that Susan was her daughter! As it was, Joan did not recognize Susan at any time during the four days, did not see her as a family member, and several times asked me to follow "the young woman" upstairs to be sure she did not steal anything. I was concerned naturally, about how Susan would take her mother's inability. On the surface, at least, Susan seemed to understand and accept it objectively as part of dementia. But how could you really accept such a notion? It hurt. It was painful—more disconcerting, I thought, than Joan's inability to recognize me most of time.

September 24, 2011

The pattern of not being able to remember haunted our relationship every day and seemed to me to be worsening. Amazingly, I had adapted to it without blinking an eye. Even the recent afternoon I spent trying to convince Joan that we were married—and had been for a long time—did not upset me. My first defense was to recall the wedding itself, showing her pictures of the First Community Church where it all took place. When this rang no bells, wedding or otherwise, I turned to the wedding pictures themselves. These too were unpersuasive because now we looked nothing like ourselves back then. Finally after much discussion, I asked Joan if a copy of our marriage license would suffice as proof. I had to ask because in today's culture even bona fide birth certificates were coming under question as did President Obama's claim to be an American citizen born in Hawaii. Joan, at least, was not a "birther" and would be quite happy to accept the fact of our marriage upon my show of proof. Delighted to be able to convince her with a single sheet of paper when all other arguments had failed, I ran upstairs, unlocked my fireproof file and rummaged through our valuable papers. The marriage certificate had to be among the papers, but guess what? Last will and testaments, insurance policies, birth certificates but no marriage certificate! As of this date, Joan continued to think we were not married. But given her non-existent recall, would seeing our marriage certificate make any difference anyway? Probably not, in the long run. She saw me mainly as a good friend and confidante, someone who looked after her and cared for her and who also frequently angered her with insistence that she let me draw blood or inject her with insulin or take a shower.

Once in awhile, she saw me as her lover and invited me to bed. The desire to be comforted and held was there, just beneath the surface, as the reality of the loss of her brothers and parents became gradually more apparent. Not a single day went by that I did not have to mention that all, except her sister Patti, were deceased. Last night, when I told her once again that none of her family was alive anymore, Joan shook her head and said "Why can't I remember they're all gone?" That, right there, was the beginning of a break through, a glimmer of recognition of her incognition. The pain I felt for Joan as she was going through this process of diminishing self-awareness (if this was what it was) was intense, making me shudder at the extent of her loneliness and isolation, compelling me in quiet moments here and there (like now) to shake my fist and cry out against such a fate. I did not want Joan, I did not want anybody, to suffer this way. There had to be better ending to a decently lived life.

Saturday Visitors

On Saturday mornings, every now and
then, comes a knock at the door.

Two young men, neatly dressed in dark
suits, black shoes and proper ties,

Bibles and pamphlets in hand, greet us,
standing there, earnest and scripture-wise.

One of the two, the younger, smiling
and genial, had visited before.

We had had a good conversation,
leisurely, around our dining room table.

He recalled it, too, my insistence that he
keep his curiosity alive to enable,

in good faith, truth to shine through.
This time I asked, jokingly, if he was

staying out of trouble. "Yes, of course,"
he replied, as if to say, "After all,

I am a Christian." Is it the mark of a
follower to be trouble-free? Saint Paul

spent a lot of time in jail, I recall,
and Jesus, though not a Christian,

was he not, in his short career, the biggest
troublemaker of them all?

No one, I see, was saved on this Saturday
morning, at least not me.

September 26, 2011

One of the little aggravations that kept cropping up and tested the level of my patience was the constant misplacement of things. We were always looking for Joan's eye glasses, either pair. For the last week now, we had not been able to find the bridge to her lower teeth. You would think the problem would be easily solved by always putting items back in the same place, but that was not the way it worked because Joan had no memory of what that "same" place was. Most of the time Joan could remember where to put her bridge if I gave her a series of clues (the back room, in the white plastic container, on the rim of the tub), but this time she did not do that, placing the bridge somewhere else, presumably in a container of some sort. I had looked high and low with no luck. Joan tried to help in the search but she could not remember what she was looking for and the first thing I knew she was picking up some other object such as a book or the remote to the radio, and asking if this was it, if this was what we were looking for.

I had noticed too, that her ability to identify objects essential to her daily routine was disappearing entirely. For the last several weeks now, I had had to remind her to brush her teeth and then go with her to the tub room to point out the toothbrush and the toothpaste tube. The same applied as well to dressing and undressing with no ability to distinguish her pajamas from other articles of clothing, for example, but that had been going on for a while. How much worse was this going to get? I believe I already mentioned that once or twice now I had had to instruct Joan on how to use the toilet. And I still could not convince her to deposit the used toilet paper in the toilet and not in the small waste receptacle nearby. As a result, I had to remember to discard the bathroom waste frequently or it soon became too difficult to avoid handling in spite of plastic liners. Caregiving, I was discovering, involved taking care of myriad details all day long. Easy to see why it had become a full-time profession in its own right. I now foresaw needing more help—probably a lot more help—down the road.

September 28, 2011

I must keep reminding myself that between all the odd, perturbing moments that make up life with Joan these days, there still were those times when Joan would come up to me to tell me how much she loved me and would kiss me and want me to hold her which I did gladly. Sometimes, though, the exchanges just before the affectionate overture were so severe I could not make the transition. In a short time, Joan would have forgotten her outburst already. I would not have. And even though I realized these angry reactions were part of the dementia, they still affected me and I had to feign my response to them. In fact, it was getting worse than that. Now, I noticed that there were increasingly long periods of time when I did not want Joan to even touch me and would try to avoid her embraces. What was going on here was not clear except that our relationship seemed less and less real. Was it perhaps the inevitable outcome when your lover was moving into another world? Probably. But I did not like the feeling. I did not want her to feel isolated or lonely. I did not want that for myself either, but that was what was happening. Silently, against my desire, a divorce was taking place and I was unable to do a thing about it.

For the last two days now I had engaged Joan in conversation to see just where she was in terms of her perception of me. As I had already mentioned, she did not believe we were married and so far I had not found any official document to verify it. Now Joan was unable to believe we had had any children together. I was totally astonished yesterday when she denied having given birth to her daughter and could see no connection with the name "Susan," though at other times she had asked about "Susan" in a familiar way and wondered if she was not upstairs sleeping or would not soon join us for supper. Add to the mix Joan's perception last evening. As I was tucking her in bed at around 7:00 pm she wanted to know who the "boy" was that had been in the kitchen. I said I had been the only one in the kitchen before and after supper. "Well," she said, "if you were there you would certainly have seen him." There were, for a change, no questions about her deceased mother's whereabouts, none of the feeling she had yesterday morning when she was not feeling well and wanted her mother to come and pick her up and drive her home. I kissed her goodnight, too tired to read to her and, an hour later, after cleaning up the kitchen and washing a load of clothes, I called it a day too.

To my relief, Joan did not wake up again until midnight which meant I had gotten four hours of uninterrupted sleep. After trips to the bathroom, we both slept for another three hours. When she arose at 3:00 am though, she reverted to behavior I had not seen for awhile. She began picking up and pulling apart her bedcovers as if searching for something. I asked her what she was doing, what she was looking for. She told me it was none of my business, to just leave her alone. I then asked her to stop it, it was just messing up the bed which meant I would have to remake it and I did not like making a bed at three o'clock in the morning. Totally irritated now, she grabbed the two small velveteen pillows she used when sleeping and marched off to the bathroom. I straightened up the bed covers and, when she returned, I tucked her in again (after having retrieved her two pillows), gave her a quick kiss and turned off the light for another hour's sleep.

September 29, 2011

I went to bed last night worried anew about Joan's poor appetite. She ate so little yesterday that it was beginning, once again, to frighten me. For breakfast I fixed her oatmeal but she ate little of it. She did eat one and most of a second of my freshly baked muffins and a cup of coffee but that was hardly packed with nutrition. At lunch I heated up a slice of turkey-broccoli quiche—which was excellent to my taste—with some small strips of ham and a piece of toast, but she hardly touched it. Nor was the supper any more successful. Thinking maybe she would enjoy some tender, slow-cooked Swiss steak this time around, I presented her with an attractive plate of it along with a little broccoli with shredded cheese and fresh cornbread. All she did was cut up the food and spread it around the plate. She ate a small dish of ice cream at lunch and a small bowl of chocolate pudding at supper (both with gusto) but that was it for the day!

I thought maybe she might wake up in the course of the night wanting something to eat as she sometimes did, in which case I usually fixed her hot chocolate or oatmeal. She woke up all right but was not hungry. The first time, at 11:30 pm, she sat up on the edge of the bed and tried to explain, in a garbled way, what was bothering her. I heard the word "process" and she pointed to her drinking glass full of water and finally I figured out she wanted to urinate but would not or could not, disturbed in some way by the fact that she would soon have to get up again and repeat the process.

I tried to explain that sometimes people sleep through the night because their bladders were big enough to hold the waste water but most of us, especially when we got older, had to get up more frequently, our bladders telling us when. Finally, taking Joan by the hand, I led her, singing happy anniversary to the tune of happy birthday, to the bathroom. There she stood while we had another conversation about urinating and how the toilet functioned for our benefit. Finally she consented to sit and try to urinate and finally she did, coaxed along by my running water from the faucet. I then led her back to bed where she was content to have me cover her up—but turning off the light seemed to terrify her. She consented to let me use a small nightlight which shed a little glow throughout the room. It was a little after midnight.

At 2:13 am Joan sat up in bed again, saying she had to get up now, she had an appointment to keep and had to get ready. I tried to reassure her that there was nothing pending on her schedule and that, in fact, she could stay in bed and sleep as long as she wanted. I urged her to go back to sleep because no one else was up and she would not want to wander around alone in a cold, dark house. She lay back down only to get up five minutes later to see if it was time now to dress for the day. I assured her it was not time and to go to sleep. Another five minutes, the same thing etc. Finally, I stood at her bedside and rubbed her back and legs for a spell and that finally did it. By this time it was 3:30 am so I went upstairs to shower and write. Now, at 5:45 am Joan came upstairs looking for me, worried that she was the only one in the house. I walked her back downstairs carefully, tucked her in bed once again. At this point, she seemed quite her normal self, content to sleep a little more, knowing I would be down soon to begin breakfast. It was scones today.

October 1, 2011

Rain was forecast for tomorrow so I tried to get some gardening done, replenishing the soil and transplanting a few large sedums. At one point, when I was lifting a bigger plant into place, Joan, who had been watching from the porch, suggested I wait and get some help from "Bob" when he got home from the museum.

When I told her I was "Bob" and gave her my last name as well, she would not believe it. I stopped what I was doing, got out my driver's license, which she took and studied carefully. She finally agreed, my name was Bob Skeele but I was not her "Bob Skeele" and continued to ask me questions about my background which indicated that she had no idea who I was and was totally bewildered when I told her I was her husband and had been for 60 years. On the other hand, she felt perfectly comfortable about inviting me in the house and showing me where the kitchen sink was where I could get a drink of water. When I told her I owned the house she was content to think she and the other Bob were simply renters. It was a funny afternoon, strange but funny. I found myself laughing with Joan over my inability to convince her we were husband and wife and had been for so long a period.

The identity issue did not subside any when I was in the kitchen preparing supper. Joan kept wondering where "Bob" was and why he was not home by now. Meanwhile, she began as usual to set the table. I put our two dinner plates in place but she was convinced others would join us, her mother or one or more of our children and so got another plate and set the table for three. I had told Joan many times that I did not mind at all if she set a third place—there was a long-standing tradition in some cultures of always setting an extra place in case a stranger arrived unexpectedly—but of course no one, family member or nomad, ever joined us.

There was a new wrinkle in the nocturnal routine last night. About 9:45 pm Joan awoke more restless and anxious than ever. Usually the Lorazepam and Melatonex kept that to a minimum but not tonight. She just kept tossing and rolling, complaining the bed covers were too heavy and tossing them off even though they were no different than any other time. After we talked for a few minutes, she was able to identify what was bothering her: fear. She was afraid—but of what? Finally after a lot of questions she was able to tell me. She was afraid of falling and found herself holding onto the edge of the mattress. As I was thinking of possible solutions, she popped up with one that had just crossed my mind: moving upstairs into a larger bed. A second's thought, however, quickly changed my mind. She had a hard time getting used to new spaces and the thought that she might wander and tumble down the steep stairs clinched the argument. I settled instead for rubbing her back and legs to see if the old magic would work. It did, although it took longer. After 15 minutes leaning over her bed, I finally got on my knees and reached under the covers and rubbed gently and thoroughly until I heard her breathing deeply. It was 10:30. A half hour on my knees and I did not think I could get up and make it the two feet to my bed but I managed, relieved that she slept, which she did until 3:09 am, a wonderful rest break for both of us. By 4:22 am she was ready to get up and begin her day. This time it was not so hard to convince her to stay abed until I started breakfast after six o'clock or so. It was now 6:30 am and no sounds from below. It was time to bake blueberry muffins.

October 7, 2011

The most worrisome of all of Joan's nighttime behavior occurred the night before last (Wednesday night, Thursday morning). It began with Joan saying she was hungry. I could see why. She had eaten little for supper per usual so I got up and prepared a dish of hot oatmeal, most of which she ate. My hope was this would settle her down for a good night's sleep. No such luck. Instead, it was not long before she began saying, "I don't feel very good," repeating it at short intervals almost in the form of a moan. She could not pinpoint the problem except to say she felt cold, accompanied every so often by involuntary shaking. I turned up the heat on the electric blanket to double the usual. Her body was warm to the touch, even hot, but still she felt cold. The only remedy was my only medicine: my hands. So, once again, I began massaging her back and legs ever so softly which would help for awhile, but soon she would be feeling cold again. Except for the occasional shaking, which lasted only a second or two, there was no other sign of a problem. In this manner, we got through the night.

In the morning Joan looked and felt normal. She did not remember saying she did not feel good and corrected her own grammar with a shake of the head. "Well, it is, not good…I don't feel well." She also did not remember feeling bad or cold. I, on the other hand, was groggy. I worried that I would fade during the day, but it never happened. My work at the museum was unencumbered as I clambered up the tall stepladder to change light bulbs. I recalled asking the doctor about Joan's feeling of being cold after the first time she experienced it some months ago, but he dismissed it. I was not so sure. I was told that if there was a loss of heat in the body's core, there would be constant shaking.

Last night, by contrast, was peaceful with little disruption of the sleep cycle for either of us. I got to bed after I watched the Detroit Tigers win the AL division against the NY Yankees around 9:00 pm and Joan only got up once after that until 4:15 am. Blessed rest! I had no idea why she would sleep so well one night and not the next. I, on the other hand, had no trouble explaining my own sound sleep: no sleep the night before and Detroit's victory.

October 8, 2011

Given the way it started, I was not at all sure how the day was going to turn out. For some reason, Joan elected to sleep in and did not slip on her bathrobe until after 9:00 am which was fine with me since it allowed me the time to read the morning paper and sip tea at my leisure. Before joining me at the breakfast table, she headed for the bathroom and almost immediately called out for me to help her. I ran to the next room to find her standing in front of the bathroom door. "What do I do now?" she asked. It turns out she suddenly (to her) had no idea how to use the toilet. Calmly (I had had some practice on this issue), I went through the process with her, step by step, ending with explaining the toilet's flushing mechanism. I left her, closing the bathroom door behind me and hoping for the best. Soon she joined me and I heated her muffins and the water for instant coffee as if all were normal.

The rest of the day, to my relief, did not follow the morning's start. Joan seemed fine and even had enough energy to accompany me to the supermarket later in the morning without becoming too tired midway through my shopping list. It had rained most of the morning, but the afternoon cleared enough to walk to the post office to pick up the mail and was pleasant enough. We only got into a couple of old, recurring arguments, the oldest being that I always take the other person's side in any discussion and never support her. My rejoinder was just as old: I would support her view any time I thought it was the right view. Why would I want to uphold her view if I did not agree with it? That was carrying marital loyalty too far. The other conflict, more recent, was Joan's hearing impairment. As mentioned earlier, almost every time we walked, there were moments when Joan had to stop, put her hands over her ears to muffle what, for her, were intolerable sounds. She was unwilling to acknowledge or ask herself why no one else was bothered. It was so frustrating to observe her pain and discomfort, knowing that in the case of sensitive ears, there was a solution.

As I wrote, it was approaching 6:00 am. Joan was up. I pointed out that it was a little early for her to be up. Did she want me to start breakfast or did she want to go back to bed for a little while? She would go back to bed, she said. So I came downstairs to our relocated bedroom to tuck her in to find the bed totally dismantled, the sheet, bedspread and electric blanket in distinct piles in the middle of the mattress. As I expressed my puzzlement, she became angry at my questioning and implied criticism; shut-up-and-make-the-bed was her fervent wish. I made the bed and tucked her in it, but she was not a happy camper. She would get up in due course and probably not remember a thing about the messed up bed or her irritation with me. I should forget, too.

October 15, 2011

The last tether that gave me a modicum of freedom with minimum risk had been severed. I was surprised to discover yesterday that Joan could no longer figure out how to phone my cell number using the land phone. Even with my cell phone number printed on the face of the land phone, she was unable to punch the right sequence of buttons. I noticed too that she had a difficult time reading the numbers so maybe it was more a problem of poor eyesight. I intended now to make an appointment with the eye doctor . Examining Joan's eyes properly had been a problem the last ten years because she seemed to have an allergy to the saline solution the doctors routinely used to dilate the eyes. The last doctor who discounted such a notion had to quickly change her opinion when she tried to dilate Joan's eyes and got an immediate positive reaction with swelling, etc. Perhaps now my doctor would have an alternative. It would be worth a shot. It might also be the case that Joan's saline allergy no longer existed, but how to determine that without risk?

I was pleased that Joan was able to survive and even enjoy a dinner party at a neighbor's house last Saturday night. It was a 60th wedding anniversary party for good friends of mine so we were invited. It ended up being a re-celebration of our 60th as well—altogether a splendid evening with wonderful food and conversation. I was proud that Joan was able to make her own way with little fuss until she tired at about 8:00 pm or so. As usual, she remembered none of it. Afterward, I wrote a poem entitled "If We Were Artists" to commemorate the occasion for Joan to read which she did, but with no connection to her experience of it that night.

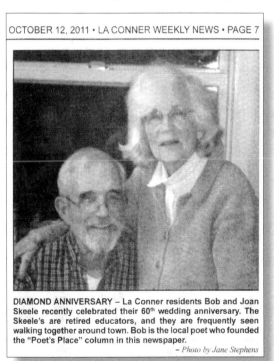

OCTOBER 12, 2011 • LA CONNER WEEKLY NEWS • PAGE 7

DIAMOND ANNIVERSARY – La Conner residents Bob and Joan Skeele recently celebrated their 60th wedding anniversary. The Skeele's are retired educators, and they are frequently seen walking together around town. Bob is the local poet who founded the "Poet's Place" column in this newspaper.

– *Photo by Jane Stephens*

Bob and Joan pose after celebrating their 60th Wedding Anniversary. LaConner, 2011

If We Were Artists

If Joan and I were artists we would paint you,
Ed and Miki Sundin, just like Carl Newman did.
If we were artists
your portrait would be like his wife
Helene's, the two of you, seated just so,
would gleam of color and beauty.
If we were artists
your portrait a life full of
serene's kin, humor and warmth.
But though artists
we're not, that's how you
come across, as you hit 60 years
of wedded bliss
and knowledge of
who's boss.
Color and beauty are there.
So, too, are warmth and
humor and the prospect of
another kiss.

If we were artists and doubled the size
of the frame and stretched the canvas taut,
could we capture your 60th celebration?
Probably not.
If we were artists, we could depict
the place all right, our hosts'
well-appointed tree house,
the elegant table set for eight,
the glass ware and service ware

fairly gleaming with an invitation
to sit and sate.
If we were artists, really good,
I suppose we could even convey
the celebrants' merry faces
as they sipped champagne
and reflect on yesterday's traces.
But if we were artists, however skilled,
could we do justice to what is heard
and felt in the room so filled
with music, in the background
the the big band sound,
and to the fore the music
of long-standing relationships,
the soft lyrics of family and friends,
the conversation at once tender
and new, but solid to the core,
with you, the celebrants
at the center of it?

I guess I just had to settle for the fact that we at least did something of a social nature together which got us out of the house and
which I remembered even if Joan was unable to. During the course
of the evening, the hostess of the party took a picture of us and
submitted it to the local paper. I had often seen pictures of couples
in the paper who had celebrated their 60th wedding anniversary. It
had never occurred to me to submit a picture of our own. I thought
it a good picture. Joan was not so sure. I was surprised she even
recognized us in it. Maybe she did not.

October 17, 2011

I truly dislike the kind of night we had heading into yesterday (Sunday) morning. Joan woke up at about 1:30 am and started to get up, putting on her bathrobe. I explained to her, as usual, that it was too early in the morning, that this was the time of the night that everyone stays in bed to rest for the day ahead. "Well, that may be so," she said, "but I'm hungry." This had happened occasionally before, and after Joan had wandered around a cold kitchen for a few minutes, she would return, happy to get back in her warm bed. But this time I waited … and waited … but no Joan. There was nothing to do but shake off my deep sleep and see what she was up to. She had turned on every light in the kitchen, the dining room and the porch and was busy trying to piece together breakfast. A carton of eggs was on the dining room table, as was an open box of cookies, some broken pieces of which were in a cereal bowl. She had a single egg in her hand but obviously was not quite sure what to do next.

I had no alternative but to pick up Joan's start and poach the egg and make some toast and tea while shaking myself awake and resenting every minute of it. Her poor appetite was becoming increasingly a problem of late. She seemed to have even less of an appetite these days, if that was possible, and must therefore eat more frequently. She had eaten little for supper Saturday night and went to bed almost immediately afterwards. It was no wonder she would be hungry seven hours later. To make sure she ate enough, I fixed her a bowl of hot oatmeal. For someone who was hungry, she did not eat much, consuming only part of the egg yolk, a half piece of toast and maybe three spoonfuls of the cereal. While she was eating, I prepared the makings for buckwheat pancakes for the next morning and ate a piece of her toast and remaining oatmeal. By 2:30 am she was tucked back in bed and was soon breathing deeply. I, on the other hand, could not get back to sleep at all and had to settle for trying to rest my body as well as I could, occupying my mind with approaches to my next writing project. I awoke late for me (about 7:00 am) feeling like I knew I would, totally unrested and groggy (the term "punch-drunk" came to mind) and with it not as much patience as I needed to care for Joan.

I was happy to see she enjoyed the buckwheat pancakes for breakfast. She ate three small ones which was her normal limit. After some resistance, I won the next two morning battles. As usual I had to repeat all my arguments as to the importance of letting me prick her finger to obtain a blood sample. Only then would I know how much insulin she would need. "Who said I need insulin, anyway?" she asked. "How does the doctor know?"…"Why not just ignore the whole procedure and let me be?" Finally, I got her blood sample and the reading showed a lower glucose level than usual. As it turned out, the readings following lunch and supper were equally low, requiring no insulin at all. So maybe Joan's wish was coming true but at what price? Why was her glucose level down? It must have to do with eating less.

In fact, one of my more frustrating moments of the entire day came at lunch. It was the first time I had ever seen Joan actually refuse to eat. When I placed before her a succulent dish of vegetable stew over a bed of brown rice she took one bite and that was it. She would not eat it. Why? The brown rice was too hard to chew, she insisted (it was just normal brown rice, thoroughly cooked) and she did not like the hunks of beef in it (the beef was extremely tender, easily cut with a fork). I removed the stew dish and soon had a small omelet and fresh toast for her to eat. She ate maybe two bites of the omelet and a half slice of the toast with jam. She did not do much better at supper, barely touching her roasted vegetables. On the other hand, she had no trouble, thank goodness, eating a small dish of ice cream for dessert at both meals.

The second battle I had lost the day before but won Sunday morning: Joan reluctantly consented to take a shower. As usual, she could not believe she had last taken a shower the previous Saturday but belief, we knew, often had an element of incredulity about it and did not change the picture. It had been a week. A shower was in order but I had to proceed with care. The previous day I had gotten her to climb the stairs to the bathroom but she was so exhausted by the 18-step climb (she was literally shaking from the effort) that she did not feel she could continue and so we turned around and after a minute's rest returned to the first floor. This, her Sunday climb, was less tiring for her for some reason, and we proceeded with the morning toilet. So far Joan was still able to climb into the tub, carefully holding on to the strategically placed safety bars, and bath herself but I continued to wonder how long before I would need to remove the old claw-foot tub and replace it with a shower stall? By the time she had showered I was back with fresh underwear and clothes and could help her dry herself, step from the tub and dry her hair. Her weight today, without clothes, was 90.8 pounds. How she maintained that weight constantly amazed me. I was pleased to hear her say later that she was glad she had made the effort to shower. She felt better for it.

As I was roasting vegetables for Sunday evening's fare, I heard someone ring our little handbell on the front door. Who would be calling at this hour, late Sunday afternoon? I opened the door to find one of my dearest neighborhood couples standing there, she holding a paper bag with an array of pink blossoms poking out the top which she presented to us as their way of congratulating us on our 60th wedding anniversary and also as a means of thanking us for remembering her birthday several weeks ago with one of my freshly-baked coffee cakes. I could not have been more pleased to see them and quickly invited them in for a glass of wine.

The potted flower, it turned out, was not your normal plant but an orchid! We had never purchased an orchid before let alone received one as a gift. Upon closer inspection I could see why the orchid drew such special attention. It was absolutely beautiful, five delicately arranged blossoms, the five light pink petals of each peppered with minute, darker pink dots and light purple centers. I was worried about our ability to care for it properly but they assured us that it would thrive with only minimum attention. After a delightful half hour sipping wine and talking, the couple departed to get home to their own supper. After Joan and I finished ours and I had cleaned up the kitchen, I spent a good bit of time admiring the orchid once more. It now stood on the pass-through counter at eye level for our constant enjoyment. I continued to be deeply touched by the young couple's thoughtfulness.

Leaves and Departures

Walking up Washington Street hill
on the new cement sidewalk
enjoying a beautiful fall day,
the air fresh with a slight southerly
and the sun, having just broken through
the morning's fog, taking away
any lingering chill, I pursue
one of my favorite fall rituals,
kicking the brown leaves,
western maples mostly,
as I make my way home.

And then I notice something
I'm sure others have noticed too:
Many of the leaves
plastered to the new cement
by the night's soft rain,
leave an imprint of
themselves,
the five points and veined
patterns clearly stained
on the hard surface,
as if an intimation of immortality,
at least for awhile,

until the next rains
wash the stains away.

I'm left to ask myself:
Is our immortality
any more certain?
We leave an impression,
our acts and words
too easily rinsed clean by
memory's indelible lapse.

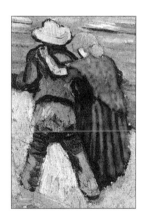

October 19, 2011

Sunday night was a pleasant change. Joan retired early, about 7:00 am and slept until I came to bed at 9:00 am after watching Masterpiece Theater. I enjoyed the Inspector Lewis series on PBS. A quick trip to the bathroom and Joan returned to bed where I tucked her in against the warmth of her electric blanket. The next thing I knew it was 4:15 am. We had both slept seven hours straight! I could hardly believe our good fortune. But alas. The next night made up for it due mainly to my own forgetfulness.

Joan retired as usual around 6:15 pm or so but seemed restless and could not get to sleep, turning and tossing and complaining about the bed covers being too heavy. With the complaint about the covers I remembered I had not given Joan her anti-anxiety pill, Lorazepam, that afternoon, a major error on my part. I had given her a second Lorazepam along with the Melatonex on schedule at bedtime but it was too early for them to have taken effect so I now had one nervous, agitated bed partner to try to calm down.

I tried physical contact as the first approach, actually climbing in bed beside her but that lasted about 2 minutes. It made her feel too uncomfortable. She did not know where to put her arm. She did not like her head snuggled against my shoulder. The only strategy that worked immediately was for me to read to her. So I read, and read, and read the short but compelling descriptions of the adventures of a young mother with three children as they explored the northwest coast aboard their 25 ft. cabin cruiser (*The Curve of Time*, Blanchet). Finally, the Lorazepam and Melitonex began to kick in, and Joan slept, with frequent trips to the bathroom, the trip at 3:30 am or so being another one of those disconcerting times that Joan underwent every now and then. She could not remember how to use the toilet. By the time I took her through the process and tucked her back in bed, I was wide awake. Thoughts of sleep were replaced with the pressures of the new day. It was 4:00 am and time for me to get up anyway and start baking.

I had planned some time ago for a luncheon, inviting my friend down from Bellingham on a day that our caregiver was there with Joan. The two of them had worked together at the museum for a time. My menu included peach cobbler and homemade whole wheat bread and corn meal muffins to go with the main dish, a New Orleans-inspired concoction called "Jambalaya" (KCTS 2010 cookbook) so I had my morning cut out for me. In addition I wanted to bake muffins for Joan's breakfast and for delivery to my Tuesday customers. I enjoyed the quiet time between 4:00 am and 6:00 am to bake and write and this morning was no exception. With our friend and caregiver keeping Joan busy through the forenoon, I was able get everything done on schedule. By noon time the four of us were sitting down to lunch in the sunlit dining room to some good wholesome food and conversation.

Joan as usual did not eat much and she felt left out of the conversation, often breaking into it with comments like "I don't understand a word you're saying" when in fact we were all talking in a normal tone. Each of us kept reassuring her that we were not neglecting her and wanted her to be part of the conversation but Joan seemed unconvinced. I noticed at the end of the meal that Joan enjoyed entertaining our guests with our singing of "Honey," "Let Me Call You Sweetheart" and "Around the Corner" which we kept practicing on our walks every day. I wanted us to learn a half dozen songs or so that we could sing together at the drop of a hat. It did us both good to have something we could do together that other people enjoyed too. Music. Singing. Who could ever have too much of that?

October 20, 2011

Yesterday morning (Wednesday) was a slow starter. Earlier in the morning while still in bed, Joan complained about her stomach hurting. When I asked if she could locate the pain, she patted her left side. I left the bed lamp on for awhile trying to decide what to do about it. Cold pack? Hot pack? Pain killer? Joan wanted none of those and before long she was again asleep. I turned off the light and slept until about 5:00 am or so and began my usual routine, showering, doing floor exercises and writing. Before I knew it, it was 7:00 am and much too late to get in even a short walk. I hurried down to begin baking. At one point Joan put on her bathrobe and came to the breakfast table but said she did not feel well and wanted to go back to bed which she did until after 9:00 am, eventually joining me for coffee and muffins.

Because Joan did not feel well, she wanted me to forego testing her blood. I told her I could not do that. I had to take a blood sample at regular intervals, especially mornings, no matter how she felt. Then ensued one of those long arguments, yet again, about why she had to undergo the blood testing and insulin injections. Finally, Joan consented, as she always did, with my clinching argument: fear of the future. If she did not comply, she would soon have a serious health problem from which there was no recovery. And that was absolutely the case. Lack of insulin management would soon lead to serious complications and in Joan's case, earlier than later.

No sooner had I completed the blood testing (Her glucose was high—252 mg) and had given her the appropriate injections (long term and short term), then Joan was ready to take her morning walk. When I suggested she come into the front room with me to change clothes, she resisted. "What's wrong with the clothes I have on?" she wanted to know. "You've got your pajamas on," I pointed out. "So who cares?" she asked. Taking another tack, I said "The pajamas are not warm enough. It's cold out today." She felt her pajama pants with her thumb and forefinger. "Maybe you're right," she said, and before long I was helping her to identify her running pants and hooded sweat shirt.

The morning walk was pleasant enough with some sun and blue skies to enjoy before the rain moved in tomorrow. We picked up another load of mail at the post office. I always wanted to get rid of a lot of our mail at the post office by throwing it in the recycle bin but Joan always wanted to bring it home (only to have me throw it away later). By this time it was almost noon so upon on our return I fixed lunch, warming up the Jambalaya soup and cornbread muffins. Joan ate a lot of the cornbread and jam but little of the nutritious soup and was soon ready to take another walk. She had, of course, completely forgotten that we had already walked.

Since walking was a good thing, we took a second one, this time along the main drag, Morris Street. As we sauntered along, hand in hand, a younger couple crossed the street and stopped us to say how wonderful it was to see an older couple holding hands. Then she apologized for using the term "older" for fear of insulting us, I reassured her that we were not insulted, that we were old. "How old?" he wanted to know. I told him my age and he would not believe it. Joan volunteered her age (after asking me how old she was). On impulse, Joan and I serenaded them right there on the sidewalk with our rendition of "Oh Honey." The couple was so delighted they embraced both of us before moving on to their destination. Music. Singing. It touched people. It touched us. We should become troubadours.

Oh, Honey

Oh, Honey, Honey,
Bless your heart,
You're the honey I love so well.
I'll be true, sweetheart to you,
Cause you're the honey
I love so well

October 23, 2011

Joan's wake-up/get-up time varied from morning to morning as had been noted. Once in a while she would arise like the sun, slowly brightening. This morning, Friday, was like that, starting out with a flare but then, after eating, just as quickly she wanted to go back to bed. I shrugged and said "Why not? There was nothing we had to do this morning. "Go back to bed, I'll clean up the kitchen and do some writing." "No," Joan said, "It would be too lonely to go back to bed by myself. You come with me." "Sure, why not? The kitchen can wait," I replied. I was ready, happy to comply with my lover's wish. Occasionally Joan wanted me to come to bed with her when she retired in the early evening. I usually declined because I was just too tired and with too many little chores left to do. This morning, though, I was rested. I encouraged her to join me in my twin bed because I used a tempur-pedic mattress which distributed our weight more evenly. Aware of Joan's fragile frame, I slipped into bed gingerly. She quickly pulled her body alongside mine as I began ever so gently to massage her back and legs. Within seconds, it seemed, Joan was beginning to breathe rapidly and like two eager teenagers we were soon tearing off our clothes to get at each other, fragility no issue now. Where did Joan's strength come from so suddenly? I tried to keep pace with her crying, moaning urgency, completely taken in by her warmth and moisture, until the primal music and motion, compelling and overwhelming, slowly subsided and Joan's measured breathing struck a cadence equal to my returning heartbeat. The difference was that she slept and I was wide awake.

I soon slipped out of bed and into my running clothes, still shaking from the frustration of an unsatisfied yearning and drive. My medications (Avodart and Simvastatin) do it every time, robbing me of the chance to be more in synch with my lover's deep and abiding satisfaction. Oh, to relax and sleep as I once did, the sleep of a spent lover. Still, in the light of day, there was much to marvel at and enjoy. Who would ever think that Joan and I, at our age, were capable of such youthful frolic? I was surprised too, and pleased, frustration and all, that occasionally we could derive such immense joy from each other in this intimate, frolicking way.

October 25, 2011

With all of Joan's deceased relatives moving in and out of our house and our children hovering around, often close by, it was a wonder Joan was not more self-conscious when it came to the more personal activity of going back to bed. But she did not seem to be. No matter how often I explain the circumstances of her parents' deaths and those of her brothers, they were, in Joan's mind, never far away. Her mother was often upstairs sleeping or out shopping. She frequently wondered why her mother had not joined us for supper. Same with our own children. Joan fully expected one or more of our kids to show up at supper time. There was also the intermittent presence of the mystery girl or woman Joan kept referring to who was just here and to whom she had been talking and was totally unbelieving when I told her I saw no such person.

Nor did she seem to experience any confusion regarding my identity when in bed together. At most other times, though, who Joan thought I was, was up for grabs. Right in the middle of lunch the other day she asked, "Are you married?" This time I did not play it straight. Instead I replied, "Yes, I'm married to a beautiful woman just your age." "Do you have any children?" she wanted to know. "Yes," I said, "We have four wonderful kids, all grown and married." "Where did you grow up?" "In Columbus." "I grew up in Portsmouth, Ohio," Joan said, and then went on to tell me about her upbringing. This in the middle of the day, part of Joan's continuing problem of identifying me. Last night, the same thing. After helping her get undressed and into her pajamas and in bed, she looked up at me and asked, "What's your name?" This time I play it straight. "Bob," I said. She seemed content with that. I gave her a final kiss and turned off the bed lamp.

I kept bringing up the identity issue because it had become such a part of our daily routine. While I did not understand completely what was happening, I saw it partly as Joan's struggle to keep her world intact. It was my job as her lover and caregiver to reassure her, to let her know in whatever ways I could, that she was loved unconditionally by me no matter what my name was or how she saw me from one moment to the next. I must be, I would be, that steady presence as we walked this strange, bittersweet journey together, helping her to keep her world safe and secure. The struggle to keep her healthy was part of the journey and where I found the most resistance. Through no fault of her own she had become her own worst enemy.

October 27, 2011

As we moved through the daily routine of eating, moving about and sleeping, I kept getting surprised by the little ways Joan's behavior changed. "Little" was the right adjective. The changes were small in themselves but I could begin to see, when taken together, where they led. What I was thinking of in this instance was the "butter and jam" episode. The other evening for supper I began setting the table. I put on the two dinner plates and Joan put out the eating utensils, often now, uncertain what a table setting consists of, so I was no longer astonished to see several forks and knives at her place or mine.

This particular evening I also placed a plastic tub of faux-butter on the table (I was trying a new product called "Earth Balance" and I wanted Joan to read the information on the container). The next time I looked around, Joan had taken one of her teaspoons and dug out a half cup of the stuff and put it on her plate. While she was doing something else I scooped the butter back up, placed it in the container and removed it from the table. Joan took no notice of my subterfuge. To avoid a reoccurrence, I took two small butter dishes, placed a dab of faux-butter on each along with a dab of jam, and placed them on the table (to go with the rolls I had in the oven). After working at the stove, I returned to the table to discover Joan had taken her spoon and eaten all the butter and jam on her plate! So much for my strategy. When I asked her if she had liked the taste she had no memory of having eaten it. Was this behavior due simply to being hungry and just eating what's immediately available? Perhaps.

Since Joan generally consumed very little at lunch, I compensated by having a snack available for her in the middle of the afternoon. She, however, most often refused because she did not want to spoil her appetite for supper. This in turn forced me to start the evening meal much earlier in the afternoon than I normally would. So, yes, it could be, in part, that Joan was just hungry. But here was the thing: always in the past she had waited for supper, waited for a side of toast, or a warm roll, to appear on which to spread the butter and jam. Why the sudden change?

I was beginning to see this minor "butter and jam" episode as part of a general breakdown in habit or routine. The way we learn over time to do things without having to spend time thinking about them was no longer automatic in Joan's world. When memory went so went all the learned responses. From how to use the toilet to table manners, mother-taught in most cases, all began to disintegrate slowly, requiring more and more dependency on me, her lover and caregiver, to the point where I may not be able to handle it. This had certainly been the case with my friends who had gone through what I was now in the throes of experiencing. I must force myself to anticipate future need and prepare for it with great love and care for Joan and for myself as well.

October 28, 2011

As I had wanted Joan to have an ear exam, so had I wanted her to have her eyes examined but I was still unable to convince her to do either. With respect to the ears I had mailed away for a set of ear amplifiers that look exactly like the ear phones some cell phone users plugged into their ears. My thinking was if once she heard what it sounded like to hear voices and sounds easily, she might be persuaded to undergo an exam. It was a long shot, admittedly.

In the general area of future need, I had again begun to piece together a plan for dealing with an emergency scenario where suddenly something happened to me and Joan was left unattended. So far three people were prepared to respond initially to such an emergency: my friends who lived just up the street would be contacted first. As the first responders, they would notify Joan's primary caregiver and then would notify our children from a list of names and phone numbers I had provided. The caregiver would come to the house immediately to care for Joan with the support of the first responders. The next step was to get in place an agency or individual who would provide long-term coverage, if necessary. The professional caregiver who lived below us on Whatcom St. came to mind. I must remember to have the caregiver practice taking a blood sample from Joan and injecting insulin if she was willing and if not, finding someone who could do it three times a day. Diabetes was a complication in any number of ways.

Yesterday, Friday, began early and ended late. I came downstairs at 6:00 am after writing, ready to take a run down to the fitness center, but Joan was already up, robed and ready to eat. I expected she would have to wait at least a half hour for me to get the muffins mixed and baked and then I remembered that I had frozen two waffles from last Sunday. I quickly had those in the oven and within minutes Joan was sitting down to an instant breakfast. While using frozen waffles in our small household was unusual, it was apparently fairly commonplace in most American homes. I recalled reading some time ago now of the panic that was created nationwide when Kellogg's had to shut down its Eggo production plant for a period of time.

It was an overcast, blustery morning and Joan did not want to take our usual morning walk so we relaxed, reading the morning paper, having second cups of tea and coffee. Soon I opened up my laptop and began writing a poem regarding hunters whose guns I kept hearing in the distance. From time to time Joan would stand by me as I wrote.

Note to All Hunters

Duck hunting season has begun.
I didn't have to read about it,
I could hear it in the breaking light,
the hunters' shotguns
blasting away
single shots, Pow, pow,
pump action, bam-bam-bam
echoing across the wind-tossed bay
hitting my ears as a sort of
soft, intermittent stutter
even as my eyes catch the
swaying limbs and the
wild flutter
of the swirling leaves.
I'm not worried about the ducks
in such raucous weather.
It's the hunters nearby
and in all seasons
that concern me rather.
This from a San Francisco newspaper:
To all you hunters who kill
animals for food, shame on
you. *You ought to go to the*
store and buy the meat that was
made there, where no animals

were harmed.
Do you see what I mean?
With subscribers like the latter
above, is any hunter safe?
Is the country, for that matter?

At one point Joan stopped next to me and I began to rub her legs and hips thinking to ease her stiffness. Before long my hands had wandered between her legs moving gently back and forth, the frequency of the movement increasing with Joan's slight, responsive swaying. "Do you want me to stop?" I asked. "Yes," Joan replied, then "No, don't. It feels too good to stop." "Should we go back to bed?" I asked. It was about 10:30 am and we both hesitated for a moment. Quickly Joan headed for the bedroom, asking me to be sure the doors were locked. "What do I do now?" Joan asked, her question surprising me. I told her to take off her clothes as I peeled mine. We piled in my twin bed, pulled up the soft covers and for the next half hour were in an ecstatic wonderland with all kinds of pleasurable sensations, sometimes intense and at other times relaxed, until we felt sated and ready once more to dress and continue our day. I was left with the same vague feeling I had had before, not quite satisfied but happy for the experience of intimacy with my partner of so many years.

Eventually we got in our morning walk but it was cold and windy. We were only too glad to stay in our warm house for the rest of the day. Joan's questions about her family prevailed. I cannot believe the number of times now I had had to explain that her mother had died many years ago before we left Vermont. Each time she was incredulous. After supper I settled down to watch the final World Series game at St. Louis with Joan at my side but her interest quickly flagged and I helped her get ready for bed and then turned to the supper dishes and the usual kitchen clean up. With the Cardinals ahead 5 to 2 in the late innings, I gave up and headed upstairs to get into my pajamas and brush my teeth, stopping just long enough to make one little correction in my "Hunter" poem.

Coming back down stairs I was shocked to find Joan just entering the side door from the outside! She had put on her nylon jacket and running shoes and was carrying her slippers inside one of her knitted hats and had wandered outside in the dark. For how long? Probably just a few minutes, her inability to see in the dark the only thing that kept her from walking the streets. Where Joan was headed, I could never determine beyond some vague reference to "offices" downtown where "they" were waiting for her. Whatever the place was, it was obvious that she saw it as a welcoming place, a comfortable, safe place to be. It took me sometime to calm Joan, to talk the issue through, but it was clear that she was seeing our house as a prison, some place that she had to escape from.

A few hours later Joan was up again, this time bent on going "home." She shook her head impatiently when I asked if she meant "Portsmouth," her family home in Ohio. She said her "home" was where her mother was now, just down the block from here. When I said her home was not down the block but right here where she was now, Joan shook her head vehemently denying any connection to the house we had lived in for the past 24 years. That the bed she had been sleeping in tonight was where she had been sleeping for many months was also denied. She had slept in the bed only the one night, she insisted, and had to get back home to her mother right now. After talking along these lines for some time, my every defense of ownership countered by Joan's denial, she began to tire and said she was hungry. Here was something I could help with, so right away I fired up the gas stove and soon had hot oatmeal and toast ready for both of us. A little after midnight I tucked Joan in bed one more time, her last words before sleep a series of questions, asking me again what my name was and asking me to promise to protect her and keep her safe. Yes, of course, I responded. I, Bob, would protect her, stating that caring for her was now my full time job, a sacred calling really, the most important of all undertakings.

I was up again at 4:30 am intent upon entering these recent oc-
currences in this journal. Joan's venture outside by herself at night
represented a pivotal moment in her lonely, frightening journey,
one I expected at some point. What I had not expected was the
motivation: Joan wanted to escape our house and get home to her
mother. Joan's mother, Ruth, had a habit of escaping her home in
Salina, Kansas at night and wandering the streets when she was
Joan's age. I wondered what her motivation was? Was she, too, looking for her mother?

October, 31, 2011

The next night was just the same except Joan awakened two hours
later at 1:00 am., hungry and ready to get up. I had no other alternative but get up with her and fix her more oatmeal and toast. She was
then quite willing to return to bed as was I. We both slept later, until
after 6:00 am this time. Contrary to Joan's one o'clock foray, she was
happy to snuggle in her electric blanket and sleep some more while
I showered and prepared breakfast. Much to my regret, the routine
of going out for a run and working out at the fitness center before
breakfast seemed to be a thing of the past. Because keeping to some
kind of exercise program was essential to my health, I was beefing
up my floor exercises and working much longer and harder on Joan's
Health Rider which I found provided some aerobic benefit.

Sunday was overcast, rainy and blustery and Joan did not want to
do anything. I could not coax her into taking a shower and washing
her hair which was overdue (Joan would not believe it had been a
week since her last). In fact she stayed in her pajamas and bathrobe
all day spending most of the morning sleeping on the wicker sofa in
the dining room. I made some of my good whole wheat bread (using the Wheat Montana recipe) and read the *Sunday Seattle Times*. I

enjoyed the leisure but felt a vague unease and wished to be getting some exercise and doing some writing but was unable to focus on the latter. The day was totally uneventful and what entertainment I might have gotten from the Seahawks game against the Bengals was ruined again by their poor performance. Five dropped passes did not help. I cannot imagine how Pete Carroll could possibly last one more season as the head coach.

I was happy to see that Joan ate a little more for supper. I fixed us some fresh cod which I had cut into thin strips and coated with a Creole cornmeal mix and served with boiled potatoes, roasted onion rings and string beans and, of course, my home-made bread. I tried to convince Joan to stay up a little later but she felt tired and ready for bed by 6:00 pm. With the evening Lorazepam and a Melatonex under her belt she slept well until 3:00 am. At that time she began fidgeting, wanting to get up every few minutes. After an hour of trying to convince her to stay put, I finally got up, turned up the heat in the house (the furnace and baseboard heat in the dining room) and with Joan's promise to remain in bed, proceeded to shower, do my exercises and get these few paragraphs written before hearing Joan moving around downstairs.

November 4, 2011

Two mornings ago, Joan had a doctor's appointment at 9:00 am which spurred her finally to consent to shower and don some clean underwear and duofolds, the latter to fight the changing weather. With so little fat on her body, Joan was cold or was easily made uncomfortable by the cold so the cotton/wool long johns truly helped. Her doctor noted that Joan had been able to maintain her weight. Fully clothed, she weighed in at 94.0 pounds, a pound heavier than the previous time. He also agreed with me that it made sense to increase her Levemir dosage (insulin) from 5 mg to 6 mg each morning to see if that might bring her blood sugar down more consistently below 200 mgs.

Yesterday was Joan's 87th birthday. After trying to think through carefully how to celebrate it, I finally decided to do something at home at the noon hour and to keep it small in keeping with Joan's intolerance for hubbub. We ended up with just five of us, staunch friends and neighbors, an easy fit for our round dinner table. Her biggest gift was from our friends up the street, our first responders. They provided the complete luncheon. All we had to do was order from Nell Thorn's luncheon menu. They picked up the orders and brought them to the house, each plate set before us hot and ready to eat. The food of course was delicious as anything from Nell Thorn's always was. Joan settled on pan-fried oysters. As it turned out, we all ordered seafood. I provided the birthday cake and ice cream and fresh decaffeinated coffee for dessert. It would not have been a proper birthday had I not had candles on the cake. The minute I showed up with the lighted cake we broke into a lusty rendition of "Happy Birthday" to Joan's pleasure.

Our next door neighbor got Joan a colorful pair of hand knit wool gloves fully lined. One of Joan's walking pals had the same idea with cold weather approaching and got Joan a pair of bright blue Thinsulate gloves and two pairs of warm socks. Our friend who cared for Joan on Tuesdays and Thursday mornings normally would have attended but had emergency dental work over the noon hour. Joan seemed pleased with the event, the warm attention and respect paid her around the table over the hour and a half. I thought again how lucky Joan and I were to have landed in La Conner and to have such quality friends.

Our son, Matt and his wife, Annie, phoned to wish Joan happy birthday but surprisingly Joan did not hear from the other three children. Joan did not seem to notice. Although Joan had ordered the oysters for lunch she ate little so I served them warmed up again for an early supper along with a piece of my spinach-ricotta pie which I had baked the previous night. Both were excellent but per usual Joan ate little and was soon ready to retire. I had her tucked in bed by 6:15 pm. Shortly after I came to bed at 8:30 pm, Joan awoke and said she was hungry. When you desperately craved sleep and were hopelessly in love at the same time, which won out? My bones said "stay put, you need your rest" but I never had a chance, something within demanding, countering the weight of my body's need, and so, like any other husband whose wife was unwell and disappearing, I got up and fixed her a bowl of oatmeal and a piece of my whole wheat bread, toasted and buttered. This time she rewarded me by eating most of both and was soon back in bed.

Her snack had given me just enough time to read an article in the newest issue of the AARP magazine on the caregiver's need for companionship when the spouse had dementia and there was no longer any physical intimacy. There are ethical issues to consider but the article's conclusion seemed to be that our rules would and were changing as we lived longer and as dementia increased. Right now over 5 million Americans were affected. By 2050 the number with dementia was estimated to triple. Someday it would be acceptable, perhaps even by the church, to have an extramarital relationship when the spouse had dementia. Adultery would be redefined or an exception made in light of emerging reality. Would this knowledge have any relevance to my life down the road?

November 6, 2011

After shuffling back and forth to the bathroom on the hour most of last night, Joan stated at 4:00 am that she did not feel well. Again she was unable to pinpoint the problem except to say that she felt nauseous, that her stomach was "tight." I had repeatedly urged Joan to have her stomach scanned for possible causes but she continued to resist the notion just as she had for her faulty hearing and eyesight. Was she afraid of a bad diagnosis or what? I knew avoiding doctors ran in the family. Her father was a prime example. Joan told me of the time her father accidently sliced his cheek open and instead of seeking medical help got a needle and thread and stood in front of the bathroom mirror and sewed himself up! More recently we learned of her brother Don's waiting until the very last minute to seek medical help for what turned out to be acute anemia. He did not make it. By the time he got to the Emergency Room his organs were failing and the emergency room staff could not save him (what I did not learn until much later was that he had been diagnosed with advanced cancer six weeks earlier).

There was resistance from Joan all along the line, much of it due to dementia I would have to think. I did not have the slightest idea, for example, what started her placing her soiled toilet paper in the nearby waste basket rather than in the toilet bowl but it created a sanitation problem and I could not get her to change this odd (and recent) habit. At one point she said she did not want to put the toilet paper in the toilet bowl for fear of clogging the sewer line so I had shown her how easily the paper disintegrates or dissolves upon contact with the water. Would she remember to place the used toilet paper in the bowl if I removed the waste basket? No such luck. The first I knew, there were wads of used toilet paper on the surface of the cabinet, the water tank and along the edge of the wash bowl. I guess I was stuck with making sure I emptied the waste basket at frequent intervals.

Yes, yes. Of course. There were a lot of bigger issues to worry about so why sweat it? Joan appeared incapable of learning now.

I was the one who must keep learning and adjusting and shifting priorities to make sure Joan remained safe, healthy and comfortable. The change in my exercise routine, a big one for me, seemed to be working okay. I missed not running outdoors in the early morning and the fitness workouts but I was discovering that I could get many of the same benefits by making more use of Joan's old Health Rider, a sort of rowing machine which promoted strength training, muscle toning and cardiovascular health. The test would be to keep from being bored to tears in the process.

November 7, 2011

The title of this section might be "Why I Sometimes Have Difficulty Getting Anything Done Around the House." Yesterday, Sunday, I wanted to get started on one project I had had in mind for some time. Several days earlier I had parked our Eurovan camper in the side yard for that purpose: namely, to haul miscellaneous stuff (wood scraps, old bottles and other odds and ends I was never likely to have need for) from our small shed behind the house to the transfer station. Before I could even put the tarp down to protect the camper's interior, Joan was on the porch telling me that the camper was not made for hauling, that I should use a pickup truck for that job. I agreed with her but I did not have a pick up so I was making do. Otherwise, I had to pay someone else to do the hauling. Her next question threw me: "Have you got Bob's permission to use the camper?"

"I am Bob," I replied, none too patiently.

"You may be Bob but you're not my Bob," Joan countered. And so the conversation went much like it had at another time while I was working in the yard and showed Joan my driver's license with my picture and the name "Skeele." Joan was not convinced then and nothing I could say now would be any more convincing. See-ing Joan's growing concern and agitation, I backed off, drove the camper from the side yard to its normal parking space in front of the house and moved on to collecting wood from the woodpile for our first fire of the fall.

Later in the evening during supper, Joan brought up the subject of "this man" who tried to manipulate her into using the camper. She didn't trust him, didn't like him at all, she said, and was glad when he was gone. Having said that, Joan still was unsure who I was sitting across from her at the dining room table. In fact her confu-sion about my identity went on all day long. In the morning she had asked several times where "Dad" was. I explained I was "Dad," that is, the father to our children. And that I was also "Bob," her husband. I answered to both names. In the afternoon over lunch the question had been "Where's Bob?" I explained that I was "Bob" but she seemed uncertain, all sorts of questions in her eyes about the truth of what I was saying. Perhaps, the most surprising question came at bedtime after I had tucked her in and turned off the bed lamp. "What's your name?" she asked. I told her, not at all surprised at that question which she asks most nights. What surprised me was her implied question about gender. When I stated that my name was "Bob," she commented, "That's a strange name for a woman." I quickly explained that I was no woman, I was a guy, her husband of many years, in fact sixty years. Joan could only manage a slight laugh in response which I took to mean that she did not believe me, or did not believe the part about the sixty years.

With that, I closed her door and went back to cleaning up the kitchen and wondering how long I could keep doing this, caring for Joan, without more help. Being a companion to Joan was becoming more tiring and I was trying to decipher exactly why. It had in part to do with her inability to entertain herself. With no interest any longer in reading, writing, playing cards, doing crossword puzzles or even watching TV, she concentrated on what I was doing and did not want me out of her sight, continually pummeling me with questions to the point of distraction. It was becoming more of a fight to focus on a recipe or read a paragraph. Forget writing. The only time I was able to do any writing was when Joan was resting or before she woke up in the morning such as I was doing at this minute.

November 8, 2011

Compared to yesterday (Sunday), today was much less difficult perhaps because it was raining a lot of the day and I could not pursue any outside tasks. Even Joan's questions about the whereabouts of "Dad" and "Bob" were minimal. She did ask several times about Susan and John (our daughter and oldest son) thinking they were nearby and might be dropping in for a meal. And her questions about other family members, her brothers Don and Bill, particularly, as well as her mother, seemed always to spring up several times during the course of a day. It was left to me in each instance to tell her (again) that they have all died and to explain something of the nature of their deaths and how Joan felt at that those times. It seemed to ease her mind to know, for example, that she actually flew out to Salina, Kansas from Vermont to be by her mother's bedside just a week or so before her death. But then, only minutes later, she would refer to her mother in the present tense, wondering why she had not returned for supper or alternatively, that she should telephone her mother in Portsmouth or wherever Joan thought she was living at the present time.

I was reminded again yesterday that Joan needed constant attention. We ventured to the local drug store and grocery store in the afternoon. Joan did okay walking with me through the aisles in both places. However, at one point I asked Joan to wait by our shopping cart while I backtracked to pick up an item. When I returned, a minute later, she was not there. I quickly went to the store entrance and there she was, staring outside, looking for me. Seeing the sheer relief and delight on her face when I called her name and she turned toward me simply melted my heart. I could only hold her, all problems momentarily forgotten, so dear was she and so vulnerable and frail. I had my work cut out for me just to keep her safe, I thought to myself as I held her, and yes, what a privilege.

My prayer these days consisted of only one refrain: give me strength, never let me weary of, what it took to care fully for another. But my prayer had a caveat which I suppose may disqualify it. The caveat? Give me the wisdom to know when I could no longer handle it and needed the assistance of others.

Friendly Fire

There's always something special about
the fall's first fire, the fireplace casting its

flickering shadows against the ceiling and
walls even as its heat begins to reach out

to touch them, two old veterans of WW II,
still alive, still married, still in their own home

on this Veteran's Day with its double-ditto
date, 11-11-11, six vertical figures, standing

straight and tall like proud soldiers,
too soon to disappear in the next days

victim to the progression of time or
the conflagrations of war, take your pick,

the former leaving little to remember,
while the latter rotating in and out of hell

leaves too much to recall. Consolation
comes later to those who are left,

the worry of gun fire, sniper fire and
rocket fire replaced with an open hearth

and a fire of a more friendly kind,
embracing the old veterans, holding them

close until the flames disappear and the
embers slowly, quietly, turn to ash.

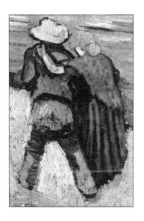

November 14, 2011

I was floored that six days had gone by without a journal entry. Enough was happening at any one time to keep me busy but much of it is repetitious which, in a way, was a prime reality of caregiving: the relentless deconstruction of what was normal. Joan continued to feel unwell, her morning complaint now followed the last several evenings with the same complaint which was new. It seemed to be the case too that her appetite, never good, was even less. She wanted fruits mostly and bread and jam, all high sugar. Along with it was her habit, mentioned before, of eating increasingly smaller bites of food, often examining each morsel of food for foreign objects. It was all I could do not to march around the table and force her to eat a normal spoonful without pre-examination. To control my own impulses, I ignored her, read a magazine, anything, to keep my eyes away from her plate. There had been occasions when in fact she did eat what for her was a reasonable amount of food but there was a lot of waiting involved. Mostly though, she simply did not eat enough. That she felt tired, rested on the sofa more than she sat up or stood, and could barely endure our short walks spoke in part to nutritional lack.

One time recently, before supper, she completely contradicted everything I just mentioned. As I usually do, I set the table, placing the diluted wine, bread and butter and a fruit salad (in this instance) on it while waiting the final minutes for the low carb pasta to cook through. The next thing I knew, Joan had drunk most of her wine, eaten all her salad and bread. The pasta and sauce? Naw. She was not hungry. And, at 5:30 pm, was ready for bed.

Over the weekend I had been installing venetian blinds on the six dining room windows. There were good reasons for having blinds, mainly as a sun blocker and for privacy. I made the installation a priority because Joan was bothered lately by the lack of the latter. Every night when I turn on the dining room lights, Joan felt exposed as if all eyes were on her and our neighbors had nothing else to think about.

November 15, 2011

No question about it though, Joan liked the new blinds and every night now asked me to turn the tilt wands to seal out the dark and any peering eyes that may be looking our way. At other times, she made comments that puzzled me. Looking out the dining room windows yesterday morning, she asked me what all those horizontal lines were! Was her eyesight failing her, a growing suspicion of mine? Was her increasing inability to distinguish one object from another solely a function of memory loss or was it, in part at least, due to failing eyesight? Joan still refused to have me schedule an eye exam but I would keep trying.

When I came home from my time away yesterday afternoon, Joan was sitting on the wicker sofa wrapped in a light blanket sipping tea under our caregiver's watchful eye. The caregiver told me that Joan complained of not feeling well. Joan did not look well either, pale face, eyes red-rimmed, puffy. She seemed to perk up some with an early supper of baked salmon and onion rings but was ready for bed by 5:30 pm. I coaxed her into watching the news on television but within a few minutes she wanted me to help her get out of her clothes and into her pajamas. She slept well through most of the night waking up at two hour intervals to walk to the bathroom. At her 3:30 am trip, I got up to shower and write but not before I tucked her in and listened again for any sign that would tell me where or in what way she was not feeling well. All she could say was that she was nauseous, too sick to attend school today. I reassured her that she did not have to worry about school and that she should just rest for now. She seemed satisfied with that. An hour and a half had passed and I heard nothing but her slow breathing on my monitor upstairs. Joan's physical health seemed to be declining slowly, feeling bad in the afternoons as well as the mornings. I felt helpless to stop it. On the other hand, was Joan telling me unconsciously, by refusing treatment, to let nature take its course?

Joan just called out something on the monitor, panic in her voice! I dashed downstairs to find Joan heading for the front door because she heard someone knocking. I turned on the porch light and reassured her that no one was there. After a quick trip to the bathroom I tucked Joan back in bed, turned up the electric blanket a notch and left her content to sleep awhile longer.

November 17, 2011

Bundled up against the frosty morning, Joan and I made our usual way to the post office. The clerks were still putting up the mail. One of the clerks said hello to us through our postal box. I asked if she would like to be serenaded which of course she did. Joan and I then proceeded to sing our song "Oh Honey" in perfect harmony into the little mail box opening. She was delighted. So were the other clerks who by now had stopped to listen, everyone applauding. Seconds later, a young couple came through the post office door so there was nothing to do but serenade them as well. They too were pleased. She exclaimed "Wow. You could make a mint standing on a street corner singing that song!"

Joan and I, in good voice, were obviously on a roll. By the time we were approaching the other end of First Street, it occurred to me that we really ought to serenade the owner of the Next Chapter Book Store. We stepped to the back of the store where the owner was making coffee and again sang our signature song, "Oh Honey, Honey..."

She could not have been more pleased. She came around the corner, hugged us both and told us how much it had meant to her to be serenaded after such a horrible start to her day. Before we turned to go she insisted on making us cups of hot cocoa to take home with us! We did just that. After arriving home, Joan and I sat down at the dining room table to sip our free drinks, shared one of my morning muffins and relished the moment. It was so sad that Joan remembered none of what had just happened, the singing and the listeners' response. No question, though, that she enjoyed the singing at the time. In fact, her harmony, her pitch, was faultless all three times.

The caregiver came at 12:15 pm to free me to attend a museum function at the El Gitano restaurant in La Conner. The entire staff was gathered there to wish me well along with two other retirees. The new director bought my lunch and they honored me with a nice card and a gift certificate for the Thai Restaurant. It was a lovely occasion as it always was to be remembered and appreciated particularly by this group, several of whom I had worked with for almost twenty years.

Our caregiver stayed with Joan a while longer so I could sneak in a haircut at the barbershop across the street from the Mexican restaurant. Joan seemed quite content with my former colleague and friend around which pleased me and reassured me for the future.

As usual, Joan began feeling a little restless in the afternoon which reminded me to give her the Lorazepam pill. We took a short walk in the dark, blustery weather but Joan tired quickly. By 4:00 pm she was ready for bed, thinking it was a lot later. She did finally eat a small supper of a ground ham patty (onion, green pepper, corn flakes mixed in) and baked French fries and a small bowl of ice cream. I got her to sit beside me for a few minutes to watch the news on television but by 5:45 pm she was heading to the bedroom, calling on me to assist her by identifying what to take off and what to put on. The anticipation of being snug and safe in her bed with me nearby to make sure the doors and windows were locked seemed to be Joan's happiest moment anymore.

She had, incidentally, mentioned a few times how much she liked the venetian blinds in the dining room and the privacy it afforded in the evenings. I liked them too, and had now ordered similar blinds for the glass walls on either side of the side door.

November 18, 2011

Joan continued to drag herself to breakfast these mornings, feeling terrible but could not define it. By the time she had her coffee and two of my fresh muffins she has perked up some and after her insulin shots was ready to walk. We had cut the length of our walks down considerably from a year ago but she had started to complain that the current route to the post office and south along First Street and back home was too far. Still, she managed two walks yesterday, one with the caregiver in the morning and with me in the afternoon.

With the change back to Pacific Standard Time, Joan was slipping into a predictable afternoon pattern where everything was pushed up. As a result I was preparing supper much earlier and eating earlier and Joan was retiring earlier. Last night I unintentionally missed Joan's blood glucose monitoring. I turned off her bed lamp at 6:00 pm. At 8:00 pm she was up to urinate. At 10:00 pm she was up again and complained of being cold and not feeling well. I noticed she was undergoing short, convulsive-like shakes which were becoming a common occurrence in the last months except this time the episodes were much closer together. Since I had given her no insulin after supper I figured her shaking was not due to low blood sugar. To make certain though, I drew blood from Joan's finger and monitored it. It read 97 mg which was on the very low end of normal and much lower than Joan's usual count. Therefore, I gave her 2 oz. of orange juice and began rubbing her back and legs through the bed covers. After a half hour of that she seemed to feel much better and was soon asleep, much to my relief. It reminded me not ever to skip Joan's glucose reading after supper!

Later, not long after I had finally gotten back to sleep, I heard Joan moving around the bedroom in the dark. When I turned on the light she was reaching for the door to the hallway. When I asked her where she was going, she said she wanted to see her mother who was sleeping upstairs. I was able to talk Joan back to bed explaining that we were the only two people in our house and had been the only two all day. No one else was staying upstairs. Joan's notion that there are others in the house, sometimes an unnamed girl or woman sleeping in the bed next to her (where I slept) or staying upstairs, persisted and did not appear likely to change.

November 21, 2011

The convulsive-like episodes in the middle of the night had stopped as quickly as they had begun. The last three nights now Joan's pattern of getting up every two hours or so to urinate had re-established itself. It followed, I would guess, from not injecting Joan with any insulin after supper unless the glucose reading was especially high. Most nights now the readings range from 130-170. It appears that raising the morning insulin (Levemir) from 5 mg to 6 mg reduced the need for the short-term insulin (Novolog). That was just as well since Joan continued to resist the finger prick and injection routine to the point where I avoided it whenever I could safely do so. Only occasionally now did I monitor Joan's blood after lunch. Like everything else, keeping a sharp eye out for any abrupt change was mandatory.

Meanwhile Joan's reliance on me for even the most rudimentary tasks were growing. Getting her undressed at night and dressed in the morning was now SOP. She was unable to recall which items of clothing to take off and would just as soon sleep in her long johns (her duofold shirt and pants) rather than replace them with pajama tops and bottoms. Changing from day wear, mostly sweat pants and hooded sweat shirts, to night wear, her matching pajamas, made little sense to her and she would just as soon not be bothered. My evening routine had now expanded to leading her to the tub room to show her her toothbrush and tooth paste. Most of the time she asked me if it was right to put the paste (in this case, gel) on her toothbrush. Parenthetically, one of the great mysteries of late was what happened to Joan's lower bridge. I had left it to her to remove the bridge each night and place it in a small, white plastic container which she had been very good about doing. One night, though, she did something else with bridge for it was not in the usual container the next morning. I have looked everywhere for it, trying to imagine where she might have placed it. It had been three weeks now and still no luck.

Helping Joan to shower, like dressing and undressing, had also been SOP for sometime now. The problem was her resistance to showering was increasing. Her Sunday morning shower (two days ago) was the first in several weeks. It was not so much her indifference to personal hygiene, although that what was there, but her difficulty in climbing the steep stairs and climbing in and out of the tub which required an energy and strength she no longer felt she had. Every time I had urged Joan to shower, she answered that she did not feel well enough to try. I fear that physical weakness and feebleness were taking over, slowly robbing her of any ability to move and get around. Perhaps the time had come to bite the bullet and install a shower unit downstairs. The installation would be a major undertaking, complicated and expensive.

November 25, 2011

Two nights in a row Joan had gotten up hungry and wanted something to eat. It was not hard to see why since she ate so little at each meal. I disliked it because it required me to shake off my own need for sleep and made it almost impossible for me to get back to sleep later. Otherwise, though, it could be a pleasant interlude, talking and reading while she had some oatmeal and toast or in one case, hot chocolate. Another time, while Joan was absorbed in eating, I was able to get the kitchen stove cleaned and polished, something I had not managed to do during the day, so all was not lost except for my lack of sleep. With something in her stomach, Joan got back to sleep quickly and was a lot less restless for the remainder of the night. And that was always a good thing.

Yesterday was Thanksgiving. Joan's nephew, Randy Williams and his wife Lucie joined us for dinner along with their two children, Cassie and Zeb. Nora, our granddaughter joined us as well. We split the labor. I roasted the turkey and did the dressing and gravy. Lucie brought the potatoes and green beans and pumpkin pie. The arrangement worked out well except for the usual confusion at the last minute with everyone in the kitchen at the same time. How did Joan fare? She did okay, i.e., not completely overwhelmed by the extra company except that she drank more wine than I wanted her to and, of course, very much resented my effort to control her intake. I, on the hand, was surprised at how tired I became trying both to make certain Joan was taken care of and getting all the prep work done with the usual things like setting the table, cleaning the bathroom and the kitchen floor and vacuuming the dining room rug and surrounding area in the middle of which I needed to stop and fix an early lunch for Joan. The best Joan could do to help was to move to the front room to stay out of the way.

Appreciation

Appreciation, like gratitude, changes things.
What was hard to accept, takes on a certain grace,
enriching the moment with opportunity,
even the slightest shred of respect
softening despair's dark edge,
honing it bright with hope's stone wheel,
spinning out an old story in a new way,
humming a tune no one expected to hear.

Appreciation creates time for a second look,
a chance to peer beneath the surface of difference
to discover common ground and even
when unfound
leaves space down the way
for a further glance
and the possibilty of nobility
between, and among, enemies and lovers
in a world weary with dismay.

Appreciation wraps our lives in magic
seeing things we never expected to hear,
and hearing things we never thought we'd see
our eyes and ears open
to the other's special talents
as our hearts gear up for change

where there's no division in our vision
and the whole knows no hole
save where we, like the fox, hide,
every now and then,
to escape the demon hounds.

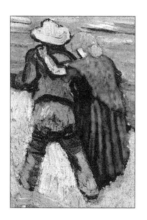

As I had mentioned before, one of the things which defined our household today was the absence of any division of labor. I was pleased to see that Joan recognized at one point the need to fill the seven water glasses at the table but then we could not find any pitcher which was light enough for her to carry. Lucie was always a great help, in this case, helping to load the dishwasher and Nora, equally helpful, moved in to get the second load of dishes and glasses ready. Even with all the help, though, I had plenty to do, putting food away and hand-cleaning the platter and serving dishes for storage, and soon stopped, with no energy left, to empty the dishwasher and begin the second load. Joan was tired and ready for bed at 5:00 pm. Nora, having travelled from California without much sleep, was crashing on the sofa early too. I was in bed, barely able to move, by 7:00 pm.

Now, sitting here writing at 5:45 am, I feel completely refreshed and ready once again to take on Joan and the world but I seriously doubted if I was going to try to entertain family or anyone else for Thanksgiving next year. It was strange because I never would believe I would get to the place where even the little bit of hospitality required of me was too much. Would I be foolish enough to try it again next Thanksgiving? Probably (unless Joan was less able to handle it which could very well be the case). A friend told me that they had made reservations for their family Thanksgiving meal at the Farmhouse Inn this year. My first reaction was envy.

November 28, 2011

I thought I was in for a long night last night. At 11:30 pm Joan awoke and as usual had to get to the bathroom. What was different (though not new) was the blank she drew. She stood, slipped into her slippers but had no idea where to go. I took her hand and led her to the bathroom. "Now what do I do?"she asked. I showed her how to lift the toilet lid, drop her pajama pants and had her sit down on the toilet seat. It was harder to explain how to urinate beyond trying to remove any anxiety about peeing in the toilet bowl. After some coaxing and running the water faucet nearby, she was successful and I led her back to bed. "Now what do I do?" she said. I described how to position herself on the bed, gave her to two small pillows, placing one between her knees and the other on her chest to support her right arm, and covered her, turning the electric blanket a couple of notches to number 5. Within a few minutes she wanted to get up again. I explained to her (as I had many times now) that it was not time to get up, it was sleep time, a time to stay in bed and relax and get rested for the day ahead. Joan remained quiet for a few minutes more, and then wanted to get up again. Since she seemed willing to take instruction, I told her she did not have to worry any longer when to get up. I would tell her when it was time. Much to my relief it worked and I relaxed and did not awaken again until Joan got up at 4:00 am to get to the bathroom. This time she found her way without assistance and positioned herself in bed without direction. The blank spaces Joan experienced, where not even her learned responses could save her , were both astounding and scary. I could not say they were becoming more frequent but I sure hated to see them whenever they occurred. I supposed I had to expect the frequency to increase and with it an upward shift in my caregiving role.

I did not look forward to it partly because I was not sure of my own ability to handle it, lack of patience continuing to be one of my many shortcomings. I could identify the source of the impatience but I was not certain that helped much. I wanted to keep writing. I needed the early morning hours to continue with this journal with an eye to publication down the road. But I also needed time during the day to write poetry which had become an extremely important part of my life. I had to struggle against Joan's need for attention to get any writing done which was difficult these days because she lacked any focus of her own. My laptop, opened up on the dining room table, was becoming an object of resentment so I tried to pick my times judiciously, when Joan was resting on the sofa, for example, but there was no denying the struggle to keep writing, to keep creating, in the context of caring for my beloved.

December 4, 2011

Whenever I mention to Joan that someone was stopping by or coming for lunch, Joan immediately begins worrying, constantly asking their names, the time of arrival, etc. It happened again when Beth (John's wife) phoned yesterday (Saturday) to say they wanted to have supper with us and would like to stay the night. John had already warned me weeks ago that they might be stopping by so I was prepared with my home-made pizza and pinto beans and ham. I began early in the afternoon to prepare the pizza sauce using some of my ground turkey from Thanksgiving. During the whole process Joan was bombarding me with the same questions: who was coming, when would they be here and, when the arrival time was near, she began guessing that they probably would not get here until much later if at all and that we should go ahead and eat. All this was said with a good deal of restlessness and agitation, i.e., lying down to rest on the dining room sofa and then getting back up again. Part of this behavior I directly related to failure to eat much at lunch so that an hour or so later she was hungry and started asking me questions related to food but lately would not consider a snack of any kind, all of which forced me to start supper preparation much earlier than I wanted.

What alarmed me on this particular Saturday afternoon had to do with the pizza sauce which I had left to cool in the big frying pan on our gas stove while I went outside to collect a wheelbarrow of firewood to set the fire in the Russian stove. After I had brought the firewood inside next to the firebox in the front room (now our bedroom), I went into the kitchen (for what reason I did not recall) to find the pizza sauce smoking and burning! I quickly turned off the gas (it was on high) and tried to salvage what I could from the skillet. Joan, of course, was concerned about what had happened but had no recollection that she had anything to do with it. I thought for a moment that perhaps I had left the gas on but under no circumstance would I had left the gas on high nor would I had put an undersized lid over the top of the sauce. I see this act on Joan's part as her effort to hurry the food along, stemming, I would imagine, from her own hunger. As it turned out we did not wait for John and Beth to arrive. Joan had to have something to eat NOW. John and Beth were running a little late so in reality it was a good thing, allowing me to give Joan her medications, including her insulin injection, and to help her into her pajamas and bed. She happily got up again when John and Beth arrived and even ate another small piece of pizza.

In effect the evening worked out well except for the burned pizza sauce, the smoke from the burning pizza sauce a clear signal that I now had something new to watch for and prevent. Joan was up several times during the course of the night per usual but with no episodes of confusion or disorientation. She made a direct line for the bathroom each time. By 3:00 am however I had been awakened enough that I knew it was useless to try to sleep and so quietly got dressed and wrote this section before going downstairs to start breakfast. John and Beth had to be on their way to SeaTac by 6:30

am to catch their plane to Baja. Muffins, fresh coffee and OJ should start them off on the right foot.

December 5, 2011

A recurrent theme in Joan's composition was her morning complaint, the series of notes quietly modulated with hints of pain and concern, as she made her way from bed to the dining room. Yesterday morning, with John and Beth at the table and Joan lying on the sofa, Joan kept saying she did not feel well and had to get to the doctor. I explained to her each time that it was Sunday and the doctor was not available. Eventually, with a blanket covering her, Joan slept while John and Beth finished eating and packed their belongings for the trip to SeaTac.

At no point did Joan seem either to recognize John and Beth or to be aware of their imminent departure. And just like that, without the usual hugs and goodbyes, John and Beth were gone and Joan slept on. Eventually, Joan joined me at the table for coffee and muffins and seemed her usual self, no complaints and no question about John and Beth's whereabouts. It was as if they had never been at our house overnight. Under normal circumstances, Joan would have been with me, standing by, waving our kids on to their next adventure in Baja. That Joan was disinterested and was sleeping instead on the sofa, indicated just how seriously ill she was, cognitively, and perhaps physically as well. Knowing as I did that no mother loved her children more than Joan, that no mother was more concerned for their welfare than Joan, made this overnight visit poignant and sad, extremely sad. How sad I felt for John, too, and his brothers and sister. They were losing their mother, had effectively lost her already.

December 6, 2011

Restless and nestless was the only way I could describe last night.
Joan slept well from the time she went to bed at 6:00 pm until 10:00
pm at which point she got up, put on her bathrobe and wanted
breakfast. It was hard to convince her that it was not morning and
time to get up. In any event she was hungry so I fixed her a small
bowl of oatmeal which she ate quietly. Once back in bed at 10:45
pm, she began every five minutes or so to ask "Is it time to get up
yet?" She could never articulate why she wanted to get up or where
she wanted to go but I observed she at least did not want to go
home to visit her mother. It may have amounted to the same thing
however, the yearning to be someplace else, offering a comfort and
security I did not seem able to provide. Finally, I rubbed her back
and legs for awhile, standing as usual next to the bed. I also gave her
a second Melatonex and finally she quieted down. I meanwhile had
developed a neck ache which was turning into a headache so I took
a couple of Ibuprofen. At 4:30 am Joan was again awake, wanting to
get dressed and on her way. She just knew she had to be someplace
this morning but she could not think where. I reassured her that we
had nothing planned and that she should stay in bed until I had my
shower, got dressed and did my usual exercise routine.

Contrary to her normal reaction, she thought an hour or so was
an awfully long time to remain in bed. Yesterday morning, Joan had
not gotten up to join me at the dining room table until 9:30 am.
This morning I could not keep her in bed. Even as I wrote I heard
her downstairs traipsing to the bathroom frequently. Between my
shower and exercises, I went downstairs and got Joan's promise that
she would stay put until 6:00 am. It was that time now, time for
me to descend and begin the day, baking a pile of fresh muffins for
Joan and neighbors which I never failed to look forward to. Baking

seemed such a magical art taking me from the liquid batter to a light delectable finish relished by all, especially the baker.

December 11, 2011

I was reminded again yesterday about just how much Joan's memory impairment seemed to be worsening. For the last week now I follow the same afternoon routine for setting the fire in the Russian fireplace, the firebox opening of which is located in what is now our downstairs bedroom. First I spread a small pad over the bedroom rug, then collect the firewood and place it on the pad. From there I stack the wood, piece by piece, in the firebox, finishing off the project with rolled newspaper and kindling. Joan had watched me each time, often helping by opening and closing the side door as I hauled in the firewood armful by armful. Yesterday afternoon she surprised me by saying, anger in her voice, that she hoped I was not going to leave that wood piled on the floor in the bedroom for her to trip over at night. I assured her that I was not going to leave the wood there, that I was soon going to stack it in the firebox for the night's fire. Right then, by way of illustration, I took what wood I had collected, and placed it in the firebox, thereby clearing the floor. She seemed satisfied.

Imagine my astonishment when, minutes later, I brought in the next armful of firewood and placed it on the floor and Joan repeated her fear of being tripped up at night! Not only was she unable to recall my routine of the last six days, she was unable to remember what I had explained and demonstrated to her just minutes earlier. I hid my shock by stacking the rest of the wood in the firebox. I knew by now nothing was gained by telling Joan I had already explained it all to her which served only to make her angry and feel bad. Slowly, I was becoming aware that living with Joan's increasingly severe memory loss became a whole lot easier when I get my own ego out of the way. At first, I took her failure to recall as a personal criticism. Early on, I would go to great pains to set the record straight, explaining in detail when and what I said, refusing to take the blame for her inability to remember. Now, I just let it go, a non-issue. Joan, I was sure, was frightened and upset enough as it was. Adding my ego to the mix only made it worse.

I have a hard time gauging exactly how disconcerting things are for Joan but I could not help but think that there must be some level of self awareness. I was thinking here particularly about the many times a day I had to remind Joan that her parents and brothers were all deceased. Why wasn't she told, she wanted to know. When I told her she was told and by whom and under what circumstances, she remained quiet, saddened I want to say, in response but seemed hardly convinced. Now, the image of a certain young woman was becoming more pronounced. Joan was unable to describe her exactly or provide a name but she was just sitting in that chair before supper, Joan pointed out last night, or she was just here yesterday afternoon. "I ought to know. I was talking with her," Joan insisted. Each time I could only say "Well, she may have been here but I didn't see her." Did my lack of confirmation, over time, carry any weight? I kept thinking it must to some degree but it may well be that I was woefully underestimating the commanding, swallowing up, take-over power, of Joan's impairment. Meanwhile her comfort and security remained my top priorities as I attempted to figure out what was going on and how best to cope.

December 16, 2011

I'd had a difficult time getting to sleep the other night- a United Farm Workers representative phoned me after I had gone to bed early and so when I did finally get to sleep. I slept hard and did not hear Joan make her way the bathroom. What woke me up was the panic in her voice when she shouted, "Bob, Bob!" I jumped up and rushed to the bathroom to find Joan slumped on the floor— just what I was afraid I would find, her body squeezed between the toilet bowl and the wash basin. Gently I began to lift her to a sitting position, testing each little movement for signs of broken bones. I was especially worried about a hip but I kept easing her to a standing position. Apparently, no permanent damage although her shoulder and tail bone took serious hits so that Joan was sore and could hardly move or sit. Back to bed she went with extra heat, both of us thankful that there were no broken bones. Later in the morning, I hurried to the drug store for some OTC pain relief and by the afternoon she was beginning to feel somewhat better.

Joan had no memory of falling down. I could only surmise that she must have had a dizzy spell or blacked out when she stood to pull up her pajama pants and simply fell to her left banging the bowl and wash stand on the way down.

Joan was getting less and less stable on her feet but she was not ready for a walker. I continued to notice on our walks that she stumbled or tripped frequently. Each time I had been holding her hand and realized the importance of continuing to do so. Viewers watching us walking down the street holding hands did not realize we did it to keep upright not so much as a romantic gesture, although to follow out the argument, keeping one another upright is itself an expression of love. And so, yes. It was not inaccurate to see us, an old couple holding hands as we made our way, as a walking Valentine, romance on the move, two people, after so many years, still in love.

But love with one partner being cognitively impaired was exhausting, the time table too often scrambled as it was last night.

Lately Joan had been ready for bed at 3:00 pm. The afternoon these days was frequently overcast and gray and no help, and Joan had little interest in eating the evening meal which I had been making a special deal of with lighted candles and soft meals. Last night we sat down to eat at 5:00 pm and she touched nothing on her plate except a bite of her dinner roll. She said she simply was not hungry. Soon after I helped her dress for bed, glad that I had been able to get the sheets laundered and could help her climb into clean pajamas. Two and a half hours later, after I had cleaned the kitchen and watched the news and was ready for bed, Guess what? Joan was up and hungry and wanted something to eat. There was nothing to be done but to return to the kitchen and warm up a meal for her, even relighting the candles. Surprisingly, as hungry as she must have been, she ate little and after a small dish of ice cream, was ready once again for bed. I tucked her in but by then I was wide awake again. I then stayed up another hour reading before I was relaxed and ready to sleep. Soon Joan started her normal schedule of bathroom trips every two hours. Sometimes she was unable to find her way so I walked with her to the bathroom and waited to walk her back. Each time Joan got up I was in full alert mode (except for the other night when she fell) and so getting back to sleep was not always successful. In such cases, I made use of a breathing technique I learned years ago in which I inhaled deeply, held it for a count of 8, and then slowly exhaled. Repeating the sequence for several minutes usually relaxed me enough to sleep until Joan's next move.

I realized, as I wrote this segment, that I had no way of preventing Joan from falling in the bathroom again unless I stood in the bathroom next to her as she sat on the toilet. Would it come to that? I would not be surprised.

December 20, 2011

The other night provided welcome relief. Joan slept without stirring from about 6:30 pm to midnight and again until 5:00 am. I cannot believe how much better I felt with a night of uninterrupted sleep. I have tried to recall what combination of things might have prompted Joan's night of solid sleep but I could not identify anything particularly. She took her regular sleep aides (Lorazepam, Melatonex and lately a pain killer for the recent fall) and she ate nothing unusual of the little bit she ate at meal time.

Needless to say, the normal sleep pattern returned the following nights with regular, sometimes hourly, trips to the bathroom. I continued each time to turn on the bed lamp and make sure she could find her way. Sometimes Joan seemed totally lost; other times she had no problem at all, a baffling phenomenon to me. Each time I tucked her in bed again, making sure the electric blanket was working. Once in a while she would sleep for two or three hours straight which was equally baffling and totally unpredictable.

I was reminded again that slowly Joan was becoming more dependent on me when on Sunday morning I finally convinced her it was necessary for hygienic reasons to take a shower. She would not believe her last shower had been fifteen days ago but I kept a record (as part of her daily glucose readings) and I was able to show her my last entry.

For the first time Joan was unable herself to turn on the water or adjust the flow and was unable to distinguish the shampoo from the bar of soap. She was using the shampoo to wash her body as well as her hair. She was okay once I pointed out the bar of soap in the soap holder mounted on the wall. Then, too, it was becoming more difficult for Joan to get in and out of the tub which I have mentioned before; this was forcing me now to get serious about replacing the tub with a shower stall. But how long would it be before Joan would not be able to use the stairs to get to the shower? This argued for replacing the jet tub downstairs which presents much more of a plumbing and design challenge not to mention what I would guess to be a substantial cost.

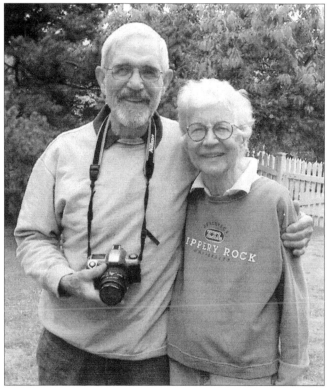

Bob and Joan, camera ready, in the side yard of their home. LaConner, 2005

A Piece of Peace

The holly halls echo with the words of Hallmark's
bards, "Peace on earth, goodwill toward men" one
greeting goes.

After all these years, centuries we should say, any
lasting peace eludes us, goodwill, yet another of our
common woes.

For many, born between the wars, the wish is much
too grand, the dream too big, to withstand its
strident foes.

Better to start smaller with a snippet of goodwill.
a piece of peace, king to king, maybe, or self to
other, suppose.

Would we not settle for picking up the peaces,
scattered though they be, piecing them, reaching
on our toes

together, as high as we can, gathering them, over
time, into a mosaic, peaces in pieces, forming,
who knows,

a spelling or a picture perhaps, giving credence to,
and celebrating, the piecemaker, blessed, like love's
other beaus?

December 27, 2011

Christmas had come and gone, whizzed by, it seemed, as I worked to complete the cycle of seasonal poems, wrote Christmas cards and remained a patient companion for Joan. Over the putting up of our small Christmas tree (4 1/2' high artificial with lights) to the exchange of gifts Christmas morning to Christmas dinner with Joan's nephew and his family, there seemed to be little glimmer of the special nature of the holiday. Joan enjoyed the lighted tree but did not miss the ceramic village we usually put up. I ordered the presents for both of us and she had difficulty remembering her connection with our dinner guests. Still, it was a productive time for me and pleasant enough but it was not without stress. Over the last two weeks I developed a certain breathlessness which seemed to lead to arrhythmic episodes, one lasting too long for me to dismiss. A visit with my doctor was reassuring and I had been fitted with a heart monitor (King of Hearts Express) for a month. So far the arrhythmic episodes had ceased altogether although I still experienced some breathlessness.

Yesterday, Boxing Day, found Joan unwilling to do much of anything. It was gray and windy with occasional rain so there was little incentive to walk and therefore to change into her daytime clothes. She opted to stay in her pajamas and bathrobe and lazed and slept on the dining room sofa most of the morning. When she was awake she was more confused than ever, unable to find her own way to the bathroom. Constantly asking why her mother had not notified us of her whereabouts or appeared for lunch was not new nor were the questions about her brothers. Joan was surprised and shocked all over again when I told her in as gentle terms possible that none of them were living.

I felt I made some domestic progress yesterday when I was able successfully to replace our 1987 RCA television with a new LG flat screen, a Christmas gift from our son David. I was amazed at the brighter colors and the clarity. Joan took no notice of the change and was not interested in the least in anything to do with television, her world reduced to sleeping and walking and the walking had suffered lately: there was less of it, and at a slower pace when she did walk. The following was the introduction to one of the poems I wrote over the holidays to convey my mindset:

Interlude, 1

The days between Christmas
and New Year's are a special time,
where faith's gift lingers,
regardless of a wet and wintery clime,
its healing hands and fingers,
kneading its warm promise into
the sinews of our mind and heart
even as we, as if to keep our distance,
shake free of such spiritual repast
to look ahead to a fresh start.
In the interlude the die is cast,
each year, the incarnation
melds with expectation,
the infant in the manger
and the infant new year
becoming figures of anticipation,
children to our hope.

December 28, 2011

Yesterday; my break away from home, found me traveling north up Interstate 5 to Fairhaven and there settling in at a table at the Village Books Cafe on the third floor overlooking Bellingham Bay. It had quickly become my favorite spot to write and browse and have lunch. Occasionally, a colleague from museum days joined me. On the way back I usually stopped at a store in Burlington and grabbed groceries and was back home by 3:00 pm. Joan seemed not even to miss me she so enjoyed the caregiver's company, thank goodness.

To make meal preparation easy during my day away, I picked up something from the store's Market Cafe to heat up in the oven (we had not updated our kitchen with a microwave yet). Last night it was a turkey pie which was quite good. Joan and I divided the single serving between us. She ate about half of hers which was about all I had come to expect anymore. Although still early, about 5:30 pm, Joan was tired and ready for bed. Between 6:00 pm and 9:00 pm she was only up once to pee. At around 11:00 pm the restlessness set in, beginning with her tossing and turning and stating repeatedly "I can't figure it out." She was obviously worried about something; I could never get her to tell me what it was but it was clear she was having a difficult time. My remedy was always the same and it worked again. I began rubbing Joan's back and legs, always gently, through the bed covers, and before long, maybe 20 minutes or so, she was relaxed and ready to sleep. Twenty minutes was about all I could handle at one time positioned as I was, standing next to her bed, with my right hand braced against the headboard, and leaning over to rub with my left hand. Had we the larger double bed or queen-size bed downstairs this would not present such a problem. I may yet make the change.

2012

January 1, 2012

A few nights ago Joan got up as usual but this time I could hear her making her way from one room to the other. I asked her what she was doing. She said she was looking for her mother. I did not say anymore and waited to see if she would try the stairs to the second floor. Much to my relief, she did not even venture into the hallway, a good sign.

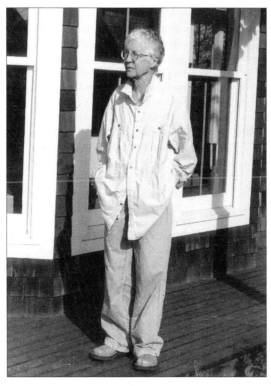

Joan at her most comfortable and casual. LaConner. April, 2003

Interlude, 2

So intent is Eos to celebrate the year's last day
that she surpasses yesterday's greeting,
the entire horizon ablaze, the fiery red
of it reaching up and out, diffusing the early blue
with a pink glow that touches each tree,
every house, the resting cars out front,
the porch and steps, facing east,
the neighbor's face
when she opens the door into the light,
all transformed for a moment as if blessed
by the gods. As the day turned out
our house was blessed, if you want
to call it that, but not by gods.
Rather by our neighbor, who in the spirit
of Eos' generous mood,
proposed buying our dinners from a most
elegant place, then joining us
around our dining table to enjoy
the taste of companionship and good food.

Last night, New Year's Eve, Joan retired early after having a New Year's dinner at our house which our next door neighbor provided. We ordered from the menu at Nell Thorn's Restaurant and the neighbor picked up the order and joined us for a lovely meal with candlelight and our best china.

The neighbor and I lasted a little while longer talking over a bottle of wine which he also provided. By 9:00 pm or so I called it a day, too tired to watch New Year's arrival in New York City. By 11:30 pm, Joan was awake wanting to get up and get dressed. In my stupor, I did not ask where she intended to go and soon convinced her to stay in bed. At 2:30 am I awoke surprised that I had managed to miss the fireworks and other noise as LaConner and the reservation celebrated the beginning of the new year. I was even more surprised that, to my knowledge, Joan had not gotten up even once to urinate. I awoke again at 4:30 am with Joan's concerned voice telling me we had to phone her mother. For awhile I played along, telling Joan we could not phone without a phone number, thinking maybe that would calm her down. It did not so finally I told Joan what I had told her many times before, namely, that her mother had died 28 years ago when we still lived in Vermont and how wonderful it was that she, Joan, had taken the time out of her busy schedule to fly out to Salina, KS. to see her just weeks before she died. Joan seemed to take in what I had said, saddened at the news, but then a short time later was talking again about finding some way to make contact with her mother who, she was afraid, was trying to make her way without a car. After walking around the downstairs Joan came back to bed and settled down to sleep some more. She would not, and probably could not, tell me why she toured the downstairs but I could guess: Joan was still looking for her elusive mother.

January 4, 2012

One of the more or less constant themes on Joan's journey was her morning complaint. She awoke most every morning saying she did not feel well which was usually accompanied with worry about getting to "school," although this morning she said something about feeling too bad to go to "college." What was different now was that Joan was actually looking like she said she felt. Her eyes were often red-rimmed, her complexion pale and drawn with puffiness under the eyes. Add to this picture, her general physical weakness, continued lack of appetite and need for sleep, and what appeared to me a heightened level of confusion during daylight hours and I wondered how much longer she could continue without a major breakdown. I kept expecting that most anytime now she would need emergency medical attention and there seemed to be no way to head it off.

Joan was adamant about not wanting to undergo what now were routine examinations. Once in a while her morning complaint actually pinpointed a problem: she pointed to the right side of her stomach. That was where I would start if I had a choice. But I did not. So I must be content to watch Joan's decline, providing whatever comfort and support I can. Under the circumstances, it seemed useless to insist (as I did) that Joan kept up her insulin therapy and took her prednisone and liquid vitamins and minerals daily.

I wrote in a letter recently that Joan was "in a tailspin and all I could do was make her landing as soft and graceful as possible." I was uncomfortable with that analogy. It was inadequate in some way. Joan was not exactly flying solo. She was not in a plane by herself because I was in the plane with her, her co-pilot maybe. Perhaps it was more accurate to describe her as being on a journey, a journey I was taking with her. It was something we were taking together, an ongoing experience in which I was intricately involved.

Yes, a "journey" was a much better way to describe what we were going through.

With all that was going on, surprises still occurred. I fixed an early dinner and by 5:30 pm Joan was in her pajamas and in bed. She asked me to come to bed with her. For several evenings now she had asked me to get in bed with her early in the evening and I had explained how it was much too early for me and that I still had a kitchen to clean up, laundry to do and things to write. Last night, however, I said I would get in bed with her for a little while but I would need to get up again. With that I went upstairs, got on my pajamas and came back down stairs to our dark bedroom. "Do you still want me to get in bed with you?" I asked, half expecting her to have fallen asleep while I was upstairs. "Yes," she said, obviously wide awake. So I climbed in beside her and within seconds we were in a passionate embrace, her strength and eagerness that of the young bride I remember. There followed a wonderful few minutes where we wildly stripped off our pajamas and forgot time and place, enjoying the moment. How could this be, two oldsters like us, Joan unwell?

Did I get up again? Yes, after holding each other for a short time, I got up to tend to the kitchen, pleased that Joan and I could hold and excite one another but vaguely dissatisfied too that the drugs I was taking prevented my full engagement. Is Cialis the answer? Take yet another drug to counter the effects of others? I so disliked the drug culture but here I was, a definite part of it, another of the many who were dependent on drugs to survive (i.e., to keep my prostate small, my blood pressure down and my cholesterol low).

January 6, 2012

For the last two nights now, Joan had awakened at around 11:30 pm and for the next two hours was restless, getting up to urinate frequently and when in bed unable to relax and get back to sleep. The night before last I was able to help by rubbing her back and legs through the bed covers until she began to breathe deeply but even then her sleep cycle was short-lived. I had gotten up at 3:00 am to shower and write. Just as I was getting into my clothes I heard a cry from Joan. I ran downstairs to find Joan crumpled on the floor in the doorway between the front bedroom and the piano room. I gently lifted her up to her feet. She was okay but said she felt weak at which point I helped her into her bathrobe and guided her to the dining room table. At 5:00 am she was eating hot oatmeal, toast and coffee but she could eat only a little of the cereal and none of the toast (the English muffin was too crisp and crunchy). With the house heating up, Joan opted to rest on the wicker sofa in the dining room while I baked my usual (and softer) morning muffins, taking time only to finish dressing. So began my day.

During the course of it I should mention that a professional caregiver now with Catholic Services, came to the house to meet Joan and our caregiver. I had initially met her at a friend's house and she seemed a good fit for the caregiving team I was slowly assembling to care for Joan and to fill in should something happen to me. The new caregiver would start coming to the house every Thursday afternoon from 2 pm to 5 pm next week and if that went well would expand her coverage to Monday and Friday afternoons as well at her rate of $16/ hour.

Last night, Joan again awoke at 11:30 pm to urinate and was up again at 11:44 pm and again at 12:01 am (I remember the times because I had a clock radio next to my bed). Each time I tucked her in bed, making sure the electric blanket was functioning but she could not settle down, lifting the bed covers, tossing and turning. Even after a 20-minute backrub, she was quiet for only a few minutes and then the tossing and turning started again. During a second rubdown

I concluded that the only thing that would work was another Lorazepam. Joan took it without hesitation and by the end of my second rubdown she was relaxed and had slept, without interruption, for the rest of the night (it was now 6:45 am and not a peep from our downstairs bedroom). It could well be that I would have to up her Lorazepam from 2 to 3 pills a day which I recalled was the original plan. The difference was that I would be giving her the third pill as needed at night rather than during the day. I would confer with our doctor but I was certain he would concur with the plan. No wonder drugs had become so much a part of our lives. They work!

January 15, 2012

I had just stepped out of the shower and into my boxer briefs when I heard a cry from Joan, panic in her voice like the last time when she had fallen. I raced down the stairs barefooted and shirtless. To my relief she was sitting up in bed. But the panic was real. In a quivering voice, fright in her eyes, she asked me to get her down. I was not certain of her meaning so I helped her out of bed and into slippers and robe. I checked the clock: 4:18 am. Holding her hand we walked through the downstairs rooms three or four times so she could recognize where she was. She kept looking for stairs to go down in spite of my insistence that we were already downstairs. Finally she seemed convinced enough at least to be willing to go back to bed until I got dressed and came back downstairs to start breakfast. I just checked on her at 5:10 am and she was sleeping soundly so I would continue to write. Nope. I guess not. I heard Joan moving around downstairs. A quick check. When I saw the relief in her face at my appearance, I realized that I needed to stay downstairs and get breakfast even though it was much too early. Oh well. So we would have an early Sunday breakfast!

January 16, 2012

The intervening days in early January (between 1/6 and 1/15) have been dominated by one notion: SLEEP. Most every afternoon after lunch, Joan began thinking it was much later in the day than it was and wanted to put on her pajamas and get to bed. That she was never very hungry and would easily forego supper most times did not help me to keep her up to her normal bedtime of 6:00 pm. One afternoon she retired at 3:30 pm. Last Saturday Joan reversed the order, getting up at 9:00 am, eating a muffin and going back to bed until after 12:30 pm. Neither extended sleep period had any effect on her sleep pattern through the night which was most always the same with frequent, sometimes hourly, trips to the bathroom. On nights like last night when Joan wanted to get up and get dressed to begin her day at 12:30 am I resorted to Lorazepam (once again) which did a good job of calming her down, allowing her to sleep until 6:00 am.

At our last consultation, incidentally, our doctor approved giving a third Lorazepam (.5 mg) to Joan at night as needed.

January 23, 2012

A major snowstorm and cold weather locked us in its grip for most of an entire week but we did okay with wood fires in the Russian stove and an ample supply of food. We missed the walks but for most of the time it was either too cold or too slippery. The week has gone by without comment because there is nothing new or different to report or to make a matter of record. I was thankful that Joan had not tried to get outside at night. A couple of times she had mistakenly opened the side door in the process of trying to find her way to the bathroom but in each case she had recognized her error and closed and even locked the door before trying another route.

I was also grateful for discovering the importance of giving Joan a third Lorazepam during the night. It has totally eliminated that period each night, usually between 9:30 pm and 1:30 am, of getting up frequently (varying from every 5 minutes to every half hour) to urinate which in turn allowed me to get much needed sleep. I really did not realize how sleep deprived I was until I began the nightly Lorazepam. Now my energy level was much higher and I have much more patience to deal with Joan's idiosyncrasies which continue unabated.

No matter how often I explained, Joan's mother was most always nearby as were her brothers, particularly Bill and Don. For awhile yesterday, she thought her sister Patti was sleeping upstairs and would soon join us for supper. The same was true with our own children. She frequently expected them to drop by for a meal. At least once a day, often more, I recited where our children were living now and the names of their spouses and children. Each time she was astounded that they were so far away and that I could keep track of them. Last night she wanted me to call up the stairs to tell anybody that might be up there that supper was ready. Joan continued to see herself wrapped around by family, surrounded by a mantel of warmth and familiarity which was obviously a source of comfort. I was much less concerned now to set the record straight.

The Year's First Snow

Always so welcome that first snow,
the large, white flakes, descending gently,
soundlessly, slow, soon covering the fir
trees' outstretched arms,
the broad, green-rich boughs, designed,
it seems. to catch nature's every pitch,
the gathering weight bending them down
until warmth and wind, nature's coaxing breath,
shake the boughs awake,
scattering the snow to the waiting ground below.
How wonderful if our own falls,
whatever they be, were as gentle and clean,
not cause for ouster or banishment under threat
as with Adam and Eve, but caught
by the limber arms of forgiveness
before dissolution claims us,
we circle, like snow's liquid heart,
free to find paradise,
and to live and fall again.

The two big struggles continued. Joan resisted, every time, my effort to keep track of her blood sugar and administer insulin, neither of which she saw as at all important. The other was the struggle to get her to take at least a shower once a week. She simply did not believe it when I told her it had been a week, sometimes two, since she had showered. She kept thinking she was still showering frequently, if not daily.

The only other important thing to note was Joan's weight loss. When she showered, I recorded her weight. It had dropped from a high of 93 pounds on December 18 to 89 pounds yesterday. It seemed that she was eating less at lunch and supper. I knew now it was not the food. No matter how good it tasted she could only eat a little of it, her stomach had shrunk so much. The exception: ice cream. She ate a small bowl of plain vanilla ice cream with great enjoyment after every lunch and supper, no matter her appetite otherwise. I was now totally grateful that she was eating at least that.

January 28, 2012

I was finding it difficult lately to get my morning writing done at my desktop (iMac) upstairs. Once, recently, I wrote a section of my Journal on my laptop downstairs in the form of an E-mail to myself and then transferred the copy to these pages. A round about way to do it but it worked. What was happening was that Joan was waking up earlier in the morning, feeling cold and hungry and ready to eat. Yesterday, for example she awoke at 4:40 am. I kept reminding her it was not time to get up. She kept repeating that she was cold and in fact would periodically shudder. It was so like the beginning of convulsions that it always really scared me. I turned up her electric blanket, piled on an extra blanket but still she complained of being cold. I checked her body. It felt warm, almost too warm, to be comfortable and yet she felt cold. The only conclusion I could draw was that she was not eating enough, not consuming enough calories to generate the inner heat she needed to stay warm. As a result, I encouraged Joan to get up, put on her bathrobe and eat a breakfast of oatmeal, toast and coffee. She managed to eat about half of a small bowl of it, a half slice of the toast and all the coffee. She immediately felt better and the shudders disappeared. She then rested on the sofa while I baked some muffins from scratch.

It turned out to be a beautiful sunny morning although a trifle cold. Joan had no interest in getting dressed and walking, preferring to rest and sleep on the sofa. Finally, just before lunch, she dressed and we got in our walk, picking up our mail at the post office and heading back home. Over lunch she complained about being housebound all morning and wanted to go for a walk. She had no memory of our earlier trip. I pointed out the pile of mail we had collected on the dining room table but she still could not believe it.

This morning Joan was again ready to get up at 4:45 am but was quite willing to go back to bed while I showered and dressed. There was no complaint of feeling cold or hungry. I hear her stirring downstairs now though, and so will stop here and get downstairs to begin breakfast. The time is 6:30 am.

January 31, 2012

Last evening just before Joan's bedtime (around 5:30 pm), we made an inspection of the house, room by room. During the day she had assumed various members of her family or our own children were around, most often upstairs. As she mentioned each person's name I would try to keep to reality, informing her when they passed away or in the case of our children, where they now resided, In each case, of course, she was surprised, having no memory to hark back to.

Last night, however, she insisted there were a couple of young girls in the house who we had just talked to a minute before. I told her that I had seen no such persons, that in fact there was no one else in the house, but the two of us. Thus the inspection. While walking upstairs to inspect the bedrooms, I noticed once again how difficult it was for Joan to climb them. She herself mentioned her difficulty, how weak she felt. It startled me all over again just how rapid had been Joan's physical deterioration. It was not all that long ago that Joan used to boast how often she climbed those 18 steps, so proud of the feat. Needless to say, we found no young women upstairs and so carefully descended to the first floor. I never had the feeling Joan was really convinced the young persons were not around but she said no more about it and was soon tucked in bed. Her last question to me before I turned out the light was no longer surprising. "What's your name?" she wanted to know. I told her my first name. "Hmmm," she said, "That's my husband's first name." She was, of course, puzzled to learn that I was her husband. But, I was glad to see, not displeased either.

Last night I was prepared for the pattern of the last two nights which was to get up on the hour for her trips to the "urination station" until around 2:30 am or after, at which point she would complain of being cold. After several rubdowns she would seem to fall asleep but would soon awaken and complain again of feeling cold when, all the time, her body was warm to the touch. As I had done previously, I got up and fixed her a hot breakfast. It worked. After eating she rested and slept on the sofa which gave me time to quickly run upstairs and get into my street clothes. I did not dare take the time to shower. I was so groggy though, that I had to sleep and persuaded Joan to sleep in her bed while I slept in mine. That worked for half an hour which was just enough rest to get me through the morning. Lack of routine sleep has seemed to catch up with me, leaving me feeling knocked out, unable to do much writing and requiring extra effort to remain patient with Joan.

I expected the same pattern to prevail last night. It started out the same with the hourly visits to the bathroom. At almost 2:30 am on the nose, Joan began to complain about feeling cold. After turning up the heat on the electric blanket, throwing on an extra blanket and giving her another slow, gentle rubdown through the bedcovers, I prepared for Joan to soon complain about feeling cold. I waited, fully resigned to getting up and preparing another early breakfast...I waited...and waited. It never happened. Joan awoke at 4:30 am and was quite agreeable to staying in bed while I got a shower and dressed. I was so glad for a more "normal" night. I was beginning to see the problem caregivers have over the long pull. I was feeling tired, not really rested, not quite as alert as I wanted to be although I was able to carry on, get through the day.

Getting a day away from the house like I do every Tuesday and Thursday for awhile helped, but it did not make up for the disrupted sleep. I had no idea what to do about that except to get more cat-naps during the day, rest when Joan rested and forget about chores and writing. I did not like the trade off.

February 3, 2012

The activity of the last two nights was beginning to reveal a way of dealing with Joan's nocturnal restlessness. I had mentioned before that I had begun to give Joan 3 Lorazepam (0.5 mg) each day, the first at 2:00 pm, the second at 6:00 pm. I find now if I gave Joan her third Lorazepam when she wakes up around 11:30 pm that she was able to sleep then until 4:00 am or so, thus avoiding that whole period when she wanted to get up and get dressed or experienced a bodily coldness beyond my ability to counter. I hoped this strategy would continue to work. Joan could certainly use that period of uninterrupted rest. There was no question that I could as well; in fact, it was essential if I was going to continue for any length of time in my role as caregiver.

Joan continued to enjoy her caregiver's companionship on Tuesdays and Thursdays. For three Thursday afternoons now, from 2:00 pm to 4:00 pm, the new caregiver had come to the house to provide some companionship as well. I noticed, happily, that Joan was beginning to accept her as another friend, someone who was going to be looking out for her. Last week Joan objected to her being here when she discovered that I was actually paying her for her time. "But she doesn't do anything!" Joan declared and was quite upset at the time. This week, though, Joan had not mentioned the issue presumably because she has not remembered anything about my financial arrangement with her friend.

During my two hour break yesterday, I visited with the new caregiver's patient who lived a block away and was a good friend of mine. She was dying from cancer and had only a short time to live.

The Hospice RN was there upon my arrival and she was able to direct me to the state's Medicaid program (COPES) to see if I might qualify for funds for home care. She was the same nurse who visited Joan and me a year or so ago on behalf of Hospice so it was good to make contact with her again.

February's Dance

We live in an old house on the hill
surrounded by fir trees to the south.
As my wife and I have gotten older,
the firs have gotten bolder
their growing limbs
now long enough to reach out
and touch our roof
and limber enough in a breeze
to wave at us
through our windows,
so intimate the gesture
it's hard not to wave back.

But this day
the waves became a dance.
A strong wind from the west,
bursting with energy,
power enough to
push away the clouds
and pull in the sun,
swirls wildly, this way and that,
whistling through the eaves.

Listening to the *Brandenburg Concerto*
on the radio, which of the six

I'm not sure, the waving limbs
and the sun's flicking light seem,
suddenly, to pick up the music's
clear, strong theme and beat,
the green-clad dancers so agile
and fluid they would, I'm convinced,
relish the chance to dance as well
to Ravel's *Bolero* or some other
hot Latin number but all I can do
is wonder, with a smile,
at the skill of the wind-blown
choreographer and his random,
upbeat style.

February 5, 2012

I was forced again yesterday morning to get up from bed early, forego a shower, and get Joan's breakfast. She was eating before 5:00 am. I provided her with muffins I had made earlier in the week and frozen so it was a simple matter of heating them up quickly in the oven. While she ate and sipped hot coffee I proceeded with my normal baking schedule. I may have given Joan the third Lorazepam a little early in the evening at 10:30 pm so last night tried a later time, perhaps too much later, at 2:30 am or so. I had wanted to try earlier but to my surprise Joan slept from 10:30 pm to 2:30 am without any sleep aids of any kind. I did not know what effect her lack of food played in the equation. Last evening at 4:00 pm while I was preparing an early meal at the stove per Joan's request, Joan, unknown to me, was sitting at the dining room table consuming a whole scone which I had packaged yesterday morning and set aside. Needless to say she was not hungry after that so I ate my dinner alone while Joan looked on. I had obviously made a mistake by leaving the scone in sight. I was learning not to put any food out until the last minute but since the scone was in a plastic bag I did not give it a second thought. This business of grabbing any food in sight and gobbling it down also suggested that I needed to find some snack for early afternoons that would appeal to Joan and ease her hunger pangs. So far though, the snacks I had provided such as milk and whole wheat cookies have not seemed to alleviate the need for an early supper.

Interruption. It is 5:00 am. Joan just called out my name from the bottom of the stairs. She wanted me to come downstairs and fix breakfast. She said she was hungry. I was not surprised with only a scone (and a small bowl of ice cream) for supper last night. So downstairs I would go. A hot cereal and muffins coming up!

February 8, 2012

The last two afternoons have ushered in startlingly new behavior from Joan. After 2:00 pm or so, Joan now became unusually agitated, wanting to go home which apparently was just down the street or just out of town, Joan was not certain where nor was she able to describe the house. The fact that she referred to the place "outside of town" made me think that she was thinking of her home on Old Scioto Trail in Portsmouth, Ohio but she kept denying it. I could not convince her either day that the house we have lived in for the last 25 years was our one and only home, that there was no "other house." She would just shake her head in bewilderment, saying in effect "How could this be?" and continued to worry about getting home. Sometimes she explained the urgency in terms of her children being there and worrying at her absence and wondering about their supper. Each time she mentioned the kids I explained that they all had their own homes now with their own families and were not worried at all about our whereabouts. They all know that we live here in our yellow house where we have lived all these years. As quickly as the agitation appeared, it left and Joan was calm and interested in plans for supper. The abruptness of the mood change surprised me but I welcomed it.

The primary caregiver who was with Joan from 9:00 am to 3:00 pm yesterday said she was concerned yesterday when Joan began to talk about getting to "her house." She actually walked with Joan down the street in search of it. Joan asked the first person she encountered, a neighbor who was walking her dog, where her house was. The neighbor pointed to our yellow house and said "That's your house." Joan obviously was not convinced, given her questions to me after the caregiver's departure.

Since I had just come off a night in which Joan had become

highly agitated, twisting around, throwing her bed covers off, saying repeatedly "I don't feel well," all after I had given her her third Lorazepam of the day, I concluded that perhaps the time had come to increase the pill's strength from 0.5 mg to 1.0 mg and I phoned the doctor yesterday for his opinion. He had already pointed out that Lorazepam loses its effectiveness after a time and dosage had to be increased which was the one thing he did not like about the drug and would explain his hesitancy in increasing the dosage unless absolutely necessary. Last night, by comparison, Joan's behavior was relatively normal. I would wait to see now how this afternoon went.

I should mention that last night at 6:00 pm or so as I was tucking Joan into bed, she asked me, as she often did these days, to come to bed with her. I did this time, stripping down to my boxers and crawling in beside her. I held her quietly for a half hour maybe and with only one light kiss she was soon breathing deeply. I then got up. put on my pajamas and bathrobe, finished cleaning up the kitchen and settled in to catch up on the primary election news, surprised at the Pennsylvania senator's victories in Missouri and Minnesota and strong showing in Colorado. But my mind was still on Joan. This seemed to be a time when Joan wanted, needed, close physical contact. What, I wondered, if anything, did this need for physical connection have to do with the urgency she felt in the last two afternoons to get to her house? Was she feeling the threat of disconnection, a loosening, a separation, from her known world which she would, understandably, be upset by? It made me want to reassure her with my presence more than ever, anything to lessen the frightening, even horrific, threat that Joan may be experiencing at this juncture.

February 9, 2012

What a relief to discover that the agitated behavior of the previous two afternoons and nights did not repeat itself yesterday! I was grati-fied as well to find that Joan had no trouble yesterday recognizing our yellow house. When we came around the corner and in sight of our house during the morning's walk, Joan was quick to identify "her" house and was relieved to get inside and enjoy the warmth and famil-iarity. I had asked our doctor's advice about increasing the Lorazepam dosage. His alternative was to continue with the 0.5 mg of Lorazepam three times a day and add the drug "Seroquel," one pill to be given before bedtime. Our pharmacist questioned the need for the jump from one class of drugs to another and took it upon herself (with my permission) to question the doctor. The upshot of the whole issue was that I was not going to make any changes at the present time. The pharmacist would return the drug "Seroquel" to the shelf and keep the prescription for such time that it may be necessary.

Last night was far more typical. I gave Joan her third Loraz-epam on schedule at about 10:00 pm. She slept straight through until about 2:30 am. At that point Joan awoke, slightly confused, not being able to find her way to the bathroom, for example, and carrying her two small side pillows with her to the bathroom and back, and then wanting to get up to begin the day. I persuaded her to go back to bed, but every few minutes she would sit up in bed, ready to get dressed and begin her day. Finally, I rubbed her back and legs through the bed covers (until I was too cold and stiff to continue), which was enough to relax her and allow her to sleep for awhile. Intermittently, Joan would wake up and I would tell her it was still too early, telling her the time on each occasion. Now, at 6:15 am, Joan seemed to be sleeping soundly enough for me to get this little bit of writing done. I did not feel that I had gotten much rest. My eyes were tired, a tell-tale sign for me that I needed more but I was happy to have even this little time to write. This morning, Thursday, the primary caregiver would be here to care for Joan so

I might be able to work at my next poem on "family." I had this wonderful picture of the entire Williams family (Joan's family) in their heyday and I wanted to include it in my next book *Side Show*. I had also to clear my desk and restore my study to some semblance of order. I had a hard time writing when the clutter got too bad, the pile of papers around me stacked too high.

February 11, 2012

The morning our caregiver was here to stay with Joan, I intended to spend some time in my study upstairs. When I told Joan that she should go ahead and take a walk, that I was going upstairs, she objected. She did not want me going upstairs while she was not here. Why not? Was she afraid I would steal something? No, not that exactly, it was just that I should not be wandering around the house when nobody else was here. I hastened to explain to Joan that I owned the house (along with her) and that I could well go where I wanted. That surprised her. She could not accept the fact that I was Bob Skeele, her husband and home owner. I did what I have done in the past pulling out my driver's license to prove my identity. As in the past it made no difference. Deep down she did not believe me but she seemed less worried about my staying behind as she and the caregiver departed for their walk.

Joan continued to spend a lot of time these days preoccupied with thoughts of her mother and other family members. Over the last two days I must have repeated the fact of her mother's death four or five times and how she, Joan, had responded so admirably to the news that her mother was ill and in the hospital (in Salina, Kansas) by closing her law office early on a Friday and flying out to see her and spending the entire weekend by her bedside, feeding her and tending her. Yet, this morning at 4:00 am when Joan returned to the bedroom after another trip to the bathroom, her only words to me were "Where's Mom?" "I don't know," I said. "All I know is that she was not here." Joan seemed content with that answer and appeared ready to sleep some more as I made my bed and slipped upstairs to shower and write.

With Valentine's Day coming up I decided to make a party of it, inviting my two former museum colleagues from Bellingham, to join a third colleague (our caregiver), Joan and me for lunch. We had gotten together before at our house on occasion. I would probably bake some rolls and do a dish from one of the recipes in the new cookbook I was beginning to put together. I would use the weekend to do some house cleaning and get the new curtains installed in the upstairs bathroom. I had spent a lot of my few free hours shopping for curtains at local stores. I was surprised to find so little selection to choose from. In the case of J. C. Penny, there was no choice at all except by catalogue. I ended up ordering the curtains online from Country Curtains. I also need to replace the curtains in my study and one of the bedrooms soon before the curtains disintegrate where they hang, so old and yellow. Joan used to enjoy selecting the material and making the curtains for the house. I would not want her to try it now and discouraged her when she offered.

February 13, 2012

Last night was the worst night yet in our journey and I have little time to write about it this morning. Joan got to sleep on schedule at 6:00 pm or so after taking her second Lorazepam of the day and her Melatonex but awoke again at 10:00 pm totally confused and upset. Sensing trouble, I quickly gave her the next scheduled Lorazepam but it had no impact whatsoever that I could tell. As happened twice last week, Joan wanted to go home, to her own house, because her mother would be worried and if I would not walk her there, just down the street, she would telephone her mother and have her pick her up or if not her, one of her brothers. You can imagine the ensuing conversation. I was trying constantly to acquaint Joan with present reality-her family is all deceased; there is no other house-and Joan was busy looking through the telephone directory trying to find her mother's telephone number. She found only our number, and wanted to call it as if that would do it. At midnight she still wanted to find a flashlight and walk to her mother's house. Finally, after two hours, she was tantalized by the offer of hot cereal and toast. By 1:00 am she was tucked back in bed and asleep. By 3:30 am, however, she was up again, restless, wanting to get dressed although she mentioned nothing about her earlier desire to get to her own home. I kept urging Joan to stay in bed which she would for a few minutes and then pop up again, unable to sleep and complaining of the cold. Finally, at 4:30 am I got up with Joan's promise to stay in bed until I showered and came back downstairs to prepare breakfast.

I was a little groggy for lack of sleep. I made the mistake of watching Masterpiece Theater last night, the one time in the week when I risk sleep deprivation, so much do I enjoy "Downton Abbey," but I was sure I would find a time during the day to catnap. I have also to think about the Valentine luncheon tomorrow. There was the kitchen floor to scrub, the downstairs to vacuum and bread and dessert to make for starters. I also needed time to finish installing the new upstairs bathroom curtains. Will Joan give me the time? She was willing yesterday to accompany me to the supermarket in Burlington but tired quickly, resting on a bench by the check-out counter without budging while I finished the last part of my shopping. Worrisome, though, knowing how easily she could wander off. But this time she did not, thank goodness, and I had the ingredients I needed for the entree tomorrow.

I will head downstairs now to begin my day, hoping that Joan is still resting. She always seemed to enjoy muffins, plain without chocolate or fruit filling. I will see what I can do.

February 15, 2012

It must often be the case that professional caregivers are constantly relieved that certain events do not recur. I was happy to report the incident referred to above did not continue the next two nights. Rather, Joan reverted to her more normal nightly routine of getting up on two-hour intervals to get the bathroom. What I noticed now was that her roughest time was the period between 2:30 am and 3:30 am. At that time she was at her worst, totally bewildered, often talking using unintelligible words and complaining of feeling bad and cold. During this period I usually spend some of the time standing by her bed, leaning over and rubbing her back and legs until she calmed down and in some cases fell asleep. This morning that strategy did not work although she elected to stay in bed while I got up (at 3:30 am) to turn up the heat and begin my day. Now that it was becoming clear that my day was most often going to begin at 2:30 am, I was making a point of retiring earlier (at 8:00 pm last night and about the same the previous day). Needless to say, Joan had no recollection of her nighttime activity. I was interested to hear her say on our morning walk yesterday something about her mother's house being nearby but when I pressed her on the matter she soon ended it by saying she "couldn't explain it."

The Valentine luncheon went well with everyone enjoying the fare. The Scandinavian Salmon Loaf and my mother's chocolate syrup recipe both won high praise and will undoubtedly appear in my proposed cookbook. Joan did not seem to enjoy the event particularly, often feeling left out of the conversation but that was her typical reaction anymore. I enjoyed every inch of it, on the other hand, but noticed how tired I was afterwards. Five or six people was about the max I wanted to prepare for these days. Right now at 5:45 am I was tired and found it hard to concentrate but needed to get down to Joan and the kitchen anyway.

Joan always liked the poem *Valentine Apple* so in the spirit of celebration and remembrance of all that was good about our life together, I included it here:

Valentine Apple

You say "I am the apple of your eye".
A sweet sentiment to be sure but now,
my dear, I want to know which one.
Which one?
Yes. Which apple.
You're pinning me down?
Yes.
Hmm. Let's see. Okay. How about a
Granny Smith?
On second thought that won't do. You're
a grandmother seven times over, to be sure,
but envious green doesn't play. It's the
wrong color for Valentine's Day.
Braeburn?
This apple speaks to your Welsh-Scots roots
and is a good baker all right but much too
noisy and juicy to eat in bed at night.
Fuji?
A wonderful apple but though the name be
short it represents a mountain much too big
for your small frame.
Gala?
With streaks of red and yellow, it's colorful
enough to attract many a fellow. You're lots
of fun to dance with and swirl but, happily,

you're no party girl.
Jonagold?
You're worth your weight in gold but in love's
Olympic race the silver in your undyed hair
and poetic tongue, in the end, wins first place.
Delicious?
Ah, yes. I have hit upon the apple of choice. It
is what I meant all along, you see. You're
delicious in every way, in taste, style and fashion.
And the color's right, the deep red of passion.

So let me say it again on this Valentine's Day.
"You are the Delicious apple of my eye!"
How does that sound? Are you satisfied now?

February 16, 2012

Things sometimes changed for the worse and, while expected, were not always prepared for. At least last night two changes occurred: Joan's paranoia and her resistance to my aid and instruction both increased. On the first issue, Joan had always been concerned that the house be properly secured, the doors and windows locked against home invasion. There's nothing wrong with that of course. It was natural enough particularly when you were older and felt more vulnerable and defenseless. Last night, however, was a new high, with Joan insisting on a room by room inspection of the doors and windows and even wanting me to close the interior doors, should the intruders break through the first barriers. It did not seem to matter that there are no locks on the interior doors. She also wanted curtains on the pair of side doors immediately, something she had not been concerned about for months. The second issue, resistance, had been building, notably in Joan's occasional refusal to let me administer her daily blood tests and insulin injections. Last night she was adamant about not taking her third Lorazepam pill at 11:00 pm. Without that pill, I was prepared for a long night. To my surprise Joan slept solidly to about 2:30 am, went to the bathroom and returned to bed with some persuasion, but at 4:00 am or so was up again, wandering around the first floor seeming to be looking for something but she was unable to explain what. At one point she gathered all her gloves together and wanted to take them to bed with her. At another, she was wondering how to get down to the first floor and had a difficult time understanding she was already on the first floor. All this time, I was urging Joan to come back to bed to get warm and sleep some more while I got up to shower and begin my day. Slowly she finally consented but she did not want me to touch her or her bed clothes and when I grabbed the velveteen side pillow to place between her knees which I always helped her with as I tucked her in, she pulled the pillow out of my hands as if I was going to take it, all done with a glare and frown, the complete opposite of her usual demeanor.

I noticed in general, too, an increase in her preoccupation with imaginary visitors in our house. Her mother and brothers were always around now as are some of our children and there were others to whom she had just talked that disappeared around the corner out of my sight, particularly a young girl and, once in a while, a young boy. On our walks lately, Joan had begun to tell me that she had until recently been working on First Street (the retail area of town) delivering packages and other items and worried that she had not told her employers that she had quit. Joan had fabricated another story of her recent employment in LaConner but I could not make out what she had been working at. It seemed to have something to do with writing or reporting, maybe working for the local paper. Joan's imaginary world continued to grow and expand. All I could do was listen and see if it gave me any clues that would help me do a better job of giving care. But, I confess, I was tiring some and was increasingly distracted and at this point seemed unable to get much thinking and writing done although I tried, grabbing an hour here or there while Joan napped and as I had the time between preparing meals, doing dishes and laundry and other household chores. It had been almost a week now since I had installed the upper set of new curtains in the upstairs bathroom but, believe it or not, could not seem to find the time to install the bottom half, so close did Joan want me at all times during the day. The minute she could not actually see me, she panicked.

And now at 6:30 am, it is time to get down to the kitchen.

February 19, 2012

After a few nights of relative calm in which I slept later than usual, getting up at 5:00 am or so and feeling more rested, last night was a return, a throwback to those terrible nights where Joan spent more time awake than asleep. She slept peacefully enough until about 11:15 pm but then refused to take her Lorazepam and could not sleep. At two different intervals over the next hour I stood by her bed and rubbed her back and legs until her breathing became slow and even but she would soon wake up. From then on, she was up every half hour or so, taking a trip to the bathroom. To make sure she could find her way back, I would per usual turn on the light each time and tuck her in, hoping that this time she would stay asleep. It never happened. The good thing about the terrible night was that at no time did Joan seem disoriented or lost until 4:15 am.

This time she made her bed, put on my robe and was ready to go "downstairs." She was not able to hear me say we were already downstairs so I let her walk around the first floor, listening carefully as she made her away looking for the down stairway. She was smart enough to find and identify the stairs that would take her upstairs—she went into the cold hallway three times as if to double check her findings—but did not seem able to figure out that the stairs up were also the stairs down. Eventually, Joan agreed to go back to bed with assurances from me that I would wake her up when breakfast was ready. Since being upstairs in the study writing these few lines, I heard the toilet flush twice, so Joan was still plying the shores between bed and toilet. It was 5:25 am.

I went downstairs to check on Joan. She had tucked herself in bed and seemed happy to stay there until I called her for breakfast later on. Even in the dark I could tell she had a smile on her face and was pleased to see me, a reassurance I guess that I was nearby and that my plan to wake her later was still in place. Okay, now back upstairs to get a few more sentences on paper. I was working as hard as I could on three different books, this one tracing Joan's journey into dementia the hardest to keep at on a regular basis because I did not have the early morning time to write. I was doing my poetry and the cookbook on my laptop downstairs late mornings and in the afternoons when I could grab the time but I felt I was falling behind schedule on the cookbook and losing my creative edge regarding my poetry. My work was much too flat these days. I kept thinking lack of sleep had something to do with the slowdown. I panicked at the thought that I may not be able to finish what I was doing.

I was pleased to discover that Joan's recent preoccupation with finding her own "home" had ceased. On the three previous afternoons Joan had agonized over how ill at ease she felt in our house, repeatedly stating that she did not like it here, that she did not intend to stay here another night and wanted to get to her own house right away. Never could I get her to tell me exactly what she did not like about our house. No matter my repeated attempts to convince her that the house she was standing in at this moment was our house, that we bought it and owned it and had lived in it for 25 years, my arguments made no dent. When I asked her where her house was, she said it was close by. I asked her if she would point it out to me so we went for a walk to find it. We looked on the next block, South Third Street, which was where she thought it might be but she could not find it. When we came up Benton Street and turned the corner in sight of our yellow house, I asked Joan if that looked like her house. "Yes", she said, "That's my house!" Joan's cognitive impairment being what it was, I expected her to raise the question about "her" house again but so far, she seemed to identify once more with our old yellow house, inside and out.

February 21, 2012

A most amazing walk yesterday made so by the conversation. Joan began it by asking about me, what my name was, where I grew up and went to school and where I lived now. This time, instead of protesting and divulging my name and my relationship to her, I just kept mum, answering her questions without embellishment. Her personal questions continued throughout the walk. At no point did she make a connection between me and her husband even when I told her I lived on South Fourth St. in La Conner in a yellow house. I would say now that for the most part Joan saw me more as a loyal caregiver than her husband of 60 years, but strangely I did not feel sad or bad about it partly because increasingly I saw myself as exactly that a "caregiver" which was the way I was identifying myself to Joan these days, someone who was never going to leave her which was one of her greatest fears and would always care for her. Writing these words made me realize I needed to put my commitment in more general terms because the day may well come when I had to relinquish my care for Joan to that of others. The literature on dementia I had been reading lately confirmed my suspicion and was no surprise: Joan's condition over time would get much worse and probably require a change of venue. Around the clock home care was prohibitively expensive.

I have now, incidentally, made my first contact with social agencies. A representative with the NW Council was helping me with my Medicaid application (called COPES in Washington State). Looking at my financial data, she was certain I would qualify for funding. It was now a matter of my getting all the pertinent information together to complete the application. I felt good knowing of the support out there from the NW Council and other professionals.

February 22, 2012

I cannot believe the amount of rest we both got last night. Had I stumbled on a way of giving us less interrupted sleep? Joan had gotten up to use the bathroom several times in the early hours. I got to bed about 8:30 pm. At 9:15 pm she was up again complaining of a headache. After thinking it over, I decided to give her a single Tylenol (acetaminophen) pill along with her Lorazepam. As a result (what else could it be?) she slept soundly, without once stirring, until 4:15 am! That was seven hours of uninterrupted sleep! For both of us! It actually felt strange to be sitting here at the computer this morning feeling so completely rested, no grogginess or tired eyes. Joan slept downstairs for a little while longer. It would be interesting to see if the extra rest would affect her attitude or behavior in any way. I heard the toilet flushing, so Joan was up and would be wondering where I was so signed off at 6:00 am to start breakfast, my favorite time, baking and listening to some good music from King 98.1 FM as the magic of transforming wet batter into light, edible muffins occurred before my expectant, and rested, eyes.

February 28, 2012

The three nights before last night were so disruptive I was lucky to get a shower let alone exercise or write. Getting up frequently was not new nor was Joan's insistence at a certain point, usually when the Lorazepam had worn off, i.e., after 2:00 am, on getting up to dress and begin her day while I kept urging her to stay in bed or rubbed her back and legs to the point where she fell back to sleep until I woke her up for breakfast at 6:30 am or so. These last three nights she had been unable to fall back to sleep and I finally got up with her at 4:30 am or so and began breakfast in my bathrobe and slippers which was not the way I preferred to start my day. But that was just the point. It was not just my day. It was becoming more and more her day, Joan's day. My routine of exercise and writing in the early morning had disappeared and I did not like it. I could sometimes write in the morning as Joan rested on the couch but exercise was out. The walks with Joan were becoming slower and of little value in terms of health maintenance.

Last night was a pleasant exception. Joan went to bed a little after 6:00 pm and although up frequently in the early hours while I was watching the news and doing dishes, she settled down about 9:30 pm when I came to bed and did not awaken until about 2:30 am. I then gave her her third Lorazepam for the night and she was still sleeping as I wrote at 6:00 am. which had given me a chance to shower and do my floor exercises at least.

Yesterday afternoon was another throwback, Joan insisting again that where she was was not her house and wanted to get to her own place. No amount of reminding her that we owned the house we were now in and had lived here for 25 years made any difference. She wanted to go to her house and at one point, without coat or hat, opened the side door and took off. I let her go for a few minutes to see if she would come back because of the cold but she did not. I followed her for a distance down the street and at one point when she had stopped, and was looking around at the different houses in bewilderment, I caught up with her. When she saw me her face lit up, so together, holding hands, we kept on walking around the block looking for her house. As we rounded the final corner and our yellow house came into view, Joan, just as before, recognized it as her house. There was no further discussion of the issue but I expected it would crop up again. Meanwhile Joan seemed increasingly unable to recognize or place me. When walking yesterday morning, she said she was embarrassed to have to ask my name but she wanted to know it. I told her but it didn't seem to register. There was nothing in her words or demeanor that connected us as husband and wife. All day long I would catch Joan looking at me quizzically as if trying to determine just who I was. Last night as I was helping her to get undressed for bed, she expressed concern that my bed might be taken by someone else, one of the several that might be staying overnight. I of course denied that possibility since no one else was visiting here and would have trouble getting in the house since I had all the doors locked. She was not as certain. I settled the matter by getting a blank sheet of paper and writing on it "This bed reserved for Bob Skeele" and placing it in the middle of my bed. Joan was satisfied.

Impersonation

To the strains of "Rocky Mountain High", I was drawn
outdoors to a live performance. The performer, Ted
Vigil, was bringing John Denver back to life in the
little town of Sedro -Woolley, in the rain, on a Saturday

afternoon. With the next song, "Take Me Home, Country
Road", I was taken in wholly. John Denver was right
there, his beat-up, wide-brimmed hat, dusty Levis and
worn cowboy boots, coating his familiar music with

authenticity as if in cahoots with truth, "Annie's Song"
keeping me dry, free of love's wrong, for a minute or
two, not quite ready to "Leave on a Jet Plane" until the
skies and my mind, breathing in the "forest's night",

have been cleared for flight. There have been other
successful impersonators. I think of Hal Holbrook
playing the part of Mark Twain, such a convincing
performance, a classic now, for other mimics to book.

...And who can forget Elvis and his legion of apers?
All these years and the King still controls his reign.
So here's my question: Of the many possible capers,
who would you impersonate? Mahatma Gandhi

would be hard and besides Ben Kingsley already
did that. Imitating Barbara Streisand might be fun.
She has acted in many roles and has an array of songs
to chose from. General George Patton was a good one

for the war buffs among us. Or would you pick a
more historical figure, Socrates, perhaps, or Jesus?
Who would I pick? I was afraid you would ask.
I would pick none of the above. I would pick a figure

more akin to my nature. I would pick Emmett Kelly.
Imagine, soaring through the air as a trapeze artist,
his first gig, and then becoming a white-faced clown,
trying to open a shelled nut with a sledge hammer to

everyone's glee and finally to portray "Weary Willie",
trying to sweep away the small circle of light shining
down on the sawdust floor, the epitome of life's sad
side. How remarkable, how special it would be, like

Emmett, to impersonate Life, its full spectrum of joy
and sadness, in the big tent's center ring, laughing
and crying with others, in unconscious salute to our
human condition, in so colorful and dramatic a way.

But wait a minute. Using the wrong tool and trying in
vain to collect the light, appearing the fool. We already
do that, don't we?

March 1, 2012

I skipped the early part of my morning routine (shower and exercise) so I could get right to my iMac but before I could get on my shoes I could hear Joan downstairs so in stocking feet I went back downstairs, tucked Joan back in bed with her promise that she would stay there until I had breakfast ready and called her.

I was happy to report that Joan had her first taste of Gentry House (an adult day care facility) yesterday. I made a big coffee cake for the adult guests and staff, about a dozen altogether, and told Joan I was baking it for the director who had invited us to her place. While the director appreciated my bringing a coffee cake what she really wanted was to meet Joan (pronounced "JoAnn"). Joan accepted my explanation and was quite happy to make the trip to Anacortes. "The Club" as the director called it, was located on 7th Street in Old Town. An older home, it was beautifully maintained, everything sparkling clean and comfortable with no steps to negotiate. Joan met the pleasant staff, and the director of course, and settled us down in the dining area as the other adults gathered for the first session which was coffee and tea and in this case my coffee cake. With only six other adults there, it made an easy, not overwhelming, group, as we started talking about the day's news and other topics of interest led by a staff member.

After a half hour or so we all moved into the living room for exercises seated at our chairs. The other staff member did a good job leading us through a series of exercises, designed by director herself to gently stretch and strengthen our upper bodies and legs, even using some light hand weights. The most fun was hitting the yellow balloon around the room which got everybody's full attention. The next part of the program featured a visit from five kindergartners from the nearby Montessori School. We all listened to nursery rhymes and sang children's songs together. It was a lively, lovely time, having the youngsters there. We next gathered in the dining room again to a light lunch of homemade bread, homemade soup and a light salad of mandarin oranges and kiwis with homemade cookies for dessert. At this point, after the leisurely lunch, Joan was tired and ready to go home.

We departed about 2:00 pm with Joan invited by the director to return Friday morning. I told her we would be there. From my observation, Joan's participation was minimal, mostly because she could not hear what was being said but she responded okay when addressed directly. I particularly noted that Joan did not follow the exercise instructions for the most part, appearing to think them silly, She turned to me, though, to answer questions about our family and the names of the children. Later I asked Joan how she enjoyed her visit. She said she had only a "vague" memory of the visit which meant she did not remember it at all. I will be interested to hear the director's assessment.

From the Senior Services' point of view the purpose of having Joan in the Gentry House program was to provide respite for me. It had nothing to do with Joan other than to make sure she was in a comfortable and safe place which Gentry House certainly seemed to be. I was impressed in all respects and was so glad—grateful is a more accurate word—to be able to report the same. Eventually, I would expect to be free on Wednesdays and Fridays from 11:00 am to 4:00 pm which I would use to get back into some sort of running/walking routine along with writing time. Weaning Joan from dependence on me while at the Gentry House was the next challenge.

March 2, 2012

Another one of those disruptive, disjointed nights when the Lorazepam seemed totally ineffective. It started out normal enough. I tucked Joan into bed around 7:00 pm (a little late for her) and she was quiet until about 10:00 pm or so while I finished the dishes and filled out forms in connection with Gentry House. I no sooner rolled into bed then Joan became restless, twisting her covers around, not able to get comfortable. It was time for her Lorazepam anyway so she took it without question and I spent the next 20 minutes rubbing her back and legs trying to get her to relax and sleep. It never happened. Instead, Joan became more anxious, wanting to get up every 5 minutes or so it seemed. At about midnight she said she was hungry. I could see why. I had tried making Pad Thai and she ate little of what was not a substantial dish to begin with so there was nothing else to do but get up and fix something. I decided on a quick oatmeal and with it some cornmeal muffins with jam. Joan obviously was hungry for she ate most of her small dish of cereal and 3 muffins. By 1:20 am I tucked Joan back in bed thinking that now she would rest soundly for the balance of the night. Wrong! She did all right until 3:20 am (2 hours exactly, oddly) but from that point on could not stay in bed and kept getting up, wanting to find her way downstairs. Finally she took one of our extra blankets with her and curled up on the small wicker couch in the dining room and slept there long enough for me to get a shower and begin writing. At 5:30 am she was up again. She was willing to go back to her own warm bed while I got the morning muffins baked. That was where she was now as I sneaked in a few more sentences before the timer sounded.

Joan was due to attend Gentry House again this morning. I so hoped this arrangement worked out. I planned to withdraw from her for a period today while she was there but would plant myself nearby at a restaurant where I could be quickly available should it be necessary, thanks to the good old cell phone.

March 3, 2012

The day went as planned. I dropped Joan at Gentry House at 11:00 am and parked myself at the Calico Cupboard in Anacortes, crossing my fingers and getting a lot of work done on the laptop. There was no emergency phone call asking me to pick up Joan early, much to my relief and surprise, so I arrived at the scheduled time of 3:00 pm. Joan seemed glad to see me. The acting director said she would phone me after 4:00pm with a rundown of Joan's day.

As I both feared and expected, the day apparently did not go well, that was to say, it went about the way it had been going at home. The acting director reported that Joan ate next to nothing for lunch; she did not like the peanut butter cookies for dessert so they substituted yogurt and banana and Joan took only a bite of the banana; she refused to participate in the chair exercises; wanted constantly to go home to be with her mother. When the acting director would say, "Bob will be here soon to pick you up" by way of reassuring her, Joan would ask "Who is Bob?" Joan carried around a handful of books the whole time, as if the books were a security blanket. One of them was a copy of my book "Whispering" which I had brought for the Gentry staff, (I tried to coax Joan into leaving the books behind when I picked her up but she clung to them for dear life). The acting director put as positive a spin on Joan's visit as she could saying that at least they did not have to call me and that she had seen clients who were more difficult to work with than Joan. She also thought that Joan's behavior might change as she became more familiar with the surroundings.

In any event I was to bring Joan to Gentry House next Wednesday as called for and to see how it went. The director would be on site then too, and would offer her assessment. So, it was unclear at this point whether Gentry House was going to be an answer for Joan or respite for me. As far as Joan was concerned, it seemed to make no difference. Several times I had asked Joan about her experience at Gentry House. She was unable to recall anything about it. It was hard to imagine going through an entire day in an entirely different setting with different people and not remember a single thing about it but that described Joan's state. I did not see how it could get any worse.

I was glad to see that Joan slept unusually well last night. Waking up at 1:00 am after her normal bedtime and after taking her third Lorazepam, going right back to sleep without waking or trips to the bathroom until after 6:00 am. Was there a connection between her full day at Gentry House with no rest periods and a good night's sleep last night?

Our son, John, and his wife Beth were due to arrive today for a short visit on their way from Baja, Mexico to Sitka, Alaska. It would be interesting to hear and see how Joan and the kids interact after a few months separation. I recalled when John was last here that Joan had difficulty recognizing him. There would be no reason to think that would have changed.

March 6, 2012

My guess was right. Joan seemed not to recognize her son, John, although there were times when Joan, after being reminded repeatedly, would look at John, grasp his arm or hand across the table and look at him adoringly as a mother would. Trying to explain to Joan who Beth was, not a daughter but a daughter-in-law, was too complex. Aside from the recognition issue, it had been good having John and Beth around and it gave some punch to my 85th birthday celebration. A successful birthday was measured by whether all your kids remembered and phoned, or failing that, sent a card. I was not disappointed. They all came through. The birthday meal itself was fantastic with fresh marlin, cooked by John himself, which he and Beth had caught in Mexico and brought with them. I contributed a chocolate cake from a recipe in the *Better Homes and Garden Cookbook* which will be in my new cookbook *The Poetry of Food*. Marsh (our grandson) joined us for the afternoon bringing some exotic cheeses and salami from Seattle where he had been living during the off-season. He would soon head back to Sitka to fish with John at least for the early part of the season.

One of Beth's birthday gifts was to stay with Joan while I took a long walk with a person I had never met before but had wanted to meet ever since his column *If I Ran The Zoo* began appearing in the local paper. Among other things, he was a talented writer and brought his world of film directing to La Conner which raised the quality of the paper to a whole new level. He had become a "bold presence" in a short space of time and, as I suspected, was a charming guy, wonderful to talk with. We talked a lot about dementia and what Joan was going through but as it turned out the subject of his next column was more about me! I did not really catch on until he wanted to take my picture to go with the column. The editor and he were obviously in cahoots. He phoned me just before departing for Los Angeles to assure me that he had finished the column and was happy with it and I would be too.

Joan had a small glass of wine to go with our birthday meal and that seemed to do her in. She said she wanted more than anything to go to bed and so by 2:30 pm or so she was in her pajamas and in bed where she stayed for the rest of the day but getting up frequently to make trips to the bathroom. I was worried she would be unable to sleep through the night but she surprised me, awaking only once, at 1:00 am, at which time I gave her her last Lorazepam and rubbed her back and legs until she regained her sleeping rhythm. The same thing happened last night though Joan did not retire until about 8:00 pm. I wished I could get her to stay up to that later hour every night but it seemed unlikely. John and Beth were up and showering so I needed to get down to the kitchen. It was now 6:30 am.

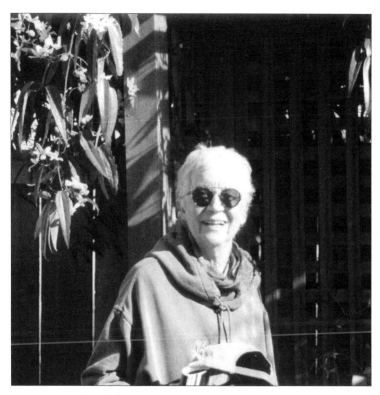

Joan, cap in hand, dares to stand under Bob's arbor and brave a smile.
LaConner, 2006

Plumbing

If you own an older house like my wife and I do,
you have to expect that things are going to wear

out or rust out. Seldom does a month go by that
I don't encounter a plumbing problem of one kind

or other. A couple of months ago tree roots clogged
the sewer line which was too big for me to handle so

I called in the professionals and they had the line
cleared within an hour. More recently I had to

replace the water lines beneath one of the bathroom
wash stands. The other night too many potato

peelings clogged the disposal which involved
dismantling most every drain pipe under the kitchen

sink but eventually I got it back together and
operating again. While I was waiting for the next

problem to bubble up I walked to the post office
to get the mail. When I opened the door to our

little mail box it was empty except for a large pink
card with an oversized word printed across its face.

OVERFLOW it said. How about that? Even our small post office box has a plumbing problem!

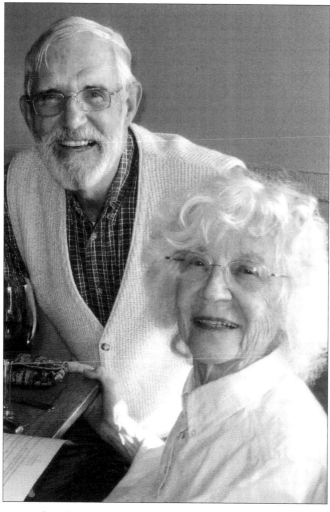

Bob and Joan celebrating their 59th wedding anniversary.
LaConner, September, 2010

March 8, 2012

I spent most of yesterday in Anacortes at the Calico Cupboard restaurant at my laptop trying to make some progress on my poem about Joan's family but did not make much headway despite the nice surroundings. I kept expecting that Gentry House would phone me to come fetch Joan but that did not happen. After doing some grocery shopping I showed up at "The Club" on schedule at 3:00 pm. Joan met me at the door, coat on and ready to get out of there. I had only time to get the director's impression of the day which was not promising. She said Joan was anxious, always looking for me and took a staff member's full time to be with her. I thought the director might call me later on the phone but she may have interpreted my parting words to her to be sufficient for the moment. I said I would see her again Friday and would bring along Joan's bottle of Lorazepam. The director thought the Lorazepam might reduce the anxiety level. My guess now was that having Joan at the Gentry House any length of time was not going to work out. I took one look at Joan when I picked her up and it was all I could do to choke back the tears. She looked so distraught, alarm and fear in her eyes, and so intent on escaping, to get out of there, that it was going to take a lot of will power on my part to return her to Gentry House tomorrow, Friday. In fact I would not even attempt it if it were not for the excellent staff of women who seemed to have a genuine affection for Joan and the other adult clients. My next call would probably be to Senior Services to consider the option of home care if that was an option.

March 14, 2012

On Monday I took the radical step, for me at least, of activating the doctor's prescription for Seroquel. It was the next level up in the drug world as the pharmacist had warned me earlier, an anti-psychotic drug not designed specifically for dementia patients but was becoming a more common antidote. Was this wise? The doctor thought it was the next logical step in the effort to maintain an acceptable "quality of life" versus a possibly longer one with all the agitation Joan was now experiencing. Starting now, Joan's medication would combine the Lorazepam and Seroquel: Lorazepam at 8 am, 12-2pm and 4-6pm and one-half tablet of Seroquel at 2 pm and at bedtime, around 8 pm.

I completed the first cycle of the new dosage last night and the change was noticeable with Joan sleeping through the night, waking only twice to urinate. This meant I was getting more rest for which I was most thankful and this morning felt more rested once I shook myself awake at 5:45 am. I had awakened at 4 am but decided I needed the sleep more than I needed to write at this point and rolled over for another two hours. Another noticeable effect of the Seroquel seemed to be that Joan had no desire to retire early and in fact stayed up until after 7 pm. The downside effects of the drug were several (and whether the changed dosage had anything to do with it was unclear) but yesterday morning she adamantly refused to allow me to prick her finger to draw the blood I needed to determine her glucose level or to administer her insulin. In contrast to past efforts, no amount of explaining the consequences made any difference so I could do nothing but let it go. She would not take the Seroquel either and I ended up both times burying the tiny half-pill in a small piece of chocolate truffle.

The other thing I noticed last evening was Joan's confused speech. I could make no sense of much of what she was trying to tell me mostly because she could not find the appropriate words, and when she could not find them, would wave her hands frantically.

My first reaction was that Joan might have had a mini-stroke. Often the sentences I did understand made no sense either, so much of it imaginary. It was important, for example, that we picked up our son, David, who was somewhere nearby waiting for a ride. At one point Joan wanted to get in our car and pick him up herself. At the same time there was a profusion of hallucinations occurring, "Didn't you see her, she was just sitting there in the chair?" she asked, pointing to the wicker chair in the dining room. Or as I was getting her undressed and ready for bed "Where's the young lady who's going to sleep with me?"

It was 7 am and I had so much more I wanted to report. It would just have to wait.

March 15, 2012

I could not be more relieved to report that Joan's experience at Gentry House yesterday was immensely improved! Joan still wouldn't eat anything for lunch except ice cream but otherwise there was some participation. At one point when I arrived to pick-up Joan at 3 pm when programs were still going on, one of the staff members made a point of telling me excitedly that Joan, at that very moment, was in the front room dancing to the music. Although Joan seemed anxious about some young children she saw outside (probably from the kindergarten nearby), she was obviously happier then on previous occasions. The director thought the drug Seroquel has been beneficial for Joan as it was for many other adult clients with whom she worked. Most of them were on Seroquel, she reported, which eased my mind. She also mentioned that the Lorazepam was working too. She saw firsthand Joan's reaction after taking her dosage. Before, Joan was getting anxious. A short time later the anxiety disappeared, smoothed out, and Joan appeared to be enjoying herself more. So, I continued on with the combination of drugs.

Back home, I noticed a big difference in Joan's behavior as well. She obviously had more energy and wanted to help me in the kitchen instead of curling up on the wicker sofa. Her appetite was much better last night but that may have been due to the good meal of tender strips of beef which I stir-fried with carrots and onions. She still wanted to retire early and did at around 6 pm. When she woke up at 8 pm I gave her the half-pill of Seroquel which she took without the slightest hesitation! I had the eerie feeling that Joan somehow knew that this strange little pink pill was good for her, was helping her to enjoy life more.

I know one thing: it was helping me to enjoy life more. The idea that she would be able to stay at Gentry House two days a week with most of the cost covered by Senior Services was a great boon for me as now I could begin to develop a balanced schedule of exercise and writing during those five hours, Wednesdays and Fridays. Right now the staying time was shorter, only four hours and this Friday, tomorrow, the director wanted me to pick-up Joan at 2 pm. This seemed to be the hour that Joan became anxious and apparently they would be short of staff. The intention and hope, over the long haul, was that Joan would come to enjoy Gentry House and would gladly stay, without any anxiety, the full time from 11 am to 4 pm. Wouldn't that be something!

As expected, Joan slept well last night, getting up to go to the bathroom only once! I had to help her find her way at 4 am and while she was in the bathroom I finished up the kitchen dishes and set-up for baking in a few hours. Did Seroquel create problems of orientation and confusion? I would have to do some more research but for now Joan certainly seemed better for taking it than not.

March 21, 2012

Driving from the Island Hospital in Anacortes to the Skagit Valley Hospital in Mount Vernon, with no interest in keeping up with the ambulance carrying Joan, I wondered at this dark hour, fifteen minutes into Saint Patrick's Day, if this marked the beginning of an accelerated spiral downward.

It certainly seemed like it. About 9 pm or so, St. Patrick's Day Eve, Joan complained of a growing headache, and then severe pain in the ears and along the jaw line into the neck and chest. After waiting awhile and determining that, if anything, the pain was increasing, we decided then and there to get to the emergency room and quickly phoned 911. Within minutes the local emergency unit arrived, followed by the two EMTs with Medic One. They gave Joan a quick but thorough exam, checking all vital signs, and rushed her by amulance to Island Hospital in Anacortes at my request. Island Hospital was my hospital of choice and her doctor's office was nearby.

The ER team quickly hooked up the monitors to Joan and started IV. After evaluating her condition, the ER doctor took me aside and said he was not certain any longer that Joan was having a heart attack and what, if any, precaution should be taken to prevent one. He therefore wanted Joan to have the benefit of the cardiologist at Skagit Valley Hospital to determine the next step, including the possibility of a catheter exploration of the heart. I consented to having Joan transferred to Skagit Valley Hospital, but after thinking about it on the drive over, decided against the use of a catheter. That procedure seemed much too invasive given Joan's age and small frame. When I finally met the doctor who would do the catheter procedure, he beat me to the punch by stating he had doubts that Joan had a heart problem. I told him whether she did or did not, I thought the procedure was much too invasive and would not permit it anyway. That settled, Joan was assigned a private room on the second floor where they wanted her to stay for overnight observation and longer if necessary.

Joan did not like hospitals; never had. Every minute she was in the emergency room she was struggling against the attached tubes that were on her finger, tabbed to her chest and imbedded in both arms. I kept trying to keep her from pulling the tubes loose until the nurse could calm her down some with a mild sedative. Nothing ever really worked and I earned her ire in my effort to limit her movement. It really got no better when Joan was moved to the second floor at Skagit Valley although the monitoring was limited to a portable heart monitor which the nurse tried to keep in Joan's shirt pocket.

When Joan was not fidgeting with the monitor, she was busy trying to get out of bed to go home. Fortunately, Skagit Valley Hospital now kept a handful of nurse assistants available for just such cases. Joan was one of three elderly patients who were restless and required constant watching. The first young woman assistant had a marvelously soothing effect on Joan. It was during her watch that I was finally able to snatch an hour's sleep in an upholstered chair next to Joan's bed. I did not know what I would have done without the assistant's presence. I had been awake since 4:30 am the previous morning and could barely lift my arms. I did not remember a time that I had been so desperate for sleep. When the assistant's duty hours were over, she was replaced immediately by a second young woman who had just completed the nursing program at Skagit Valley College. Joan kept insisting on going home and trying to get out of bed but the assistant was equal to the task, finding strategies to keep Joan in check. Joan was served breakfast and lunch but touched not one bite of food. I ate her bowl of cereal in the morning and half her white bread sandwich for lunch. Joan was discharged with no particular instructions. No heart problem had been detected. The nurse's last official act was to give Joan her 2 pm (12 1/2 mg) dose of Seroquel.

This writing was interrupted by a phone call from the director at Gentry House. Joan was too anxious, too concerned to get out of Gentry House, testing the doors etc. requiring constant watching. Best that I come fetch her, which was perfectly understandable. The director told me that Joan's dementia was well advanced and probably I needed to consider placement. Having caregivers in the home probably was not going to be adequate for the level of care Joan needed.

So Free

After such a long season, how wonderful, dear friend,
to see you still splitting wood to heat your house,
so free of the chaos of memory loss.
So free to let the chips fall where they may.
So free to let the strong downstroke carry the day.
So free to know the upstroke, too, is part of motion's play
and that even the still space, that brief moment
between the up and down, has a say
in the body's fluid grace for it's there, is it not,
in the middle of the swing, that the muscles coil
to spring and bring the axe head to bear?

In our lives of splitting would into could and should,
does the same hold true? Are there moments,
however brief, at the top of our swings,
when values coil and even collide, as we decide
and slam home our ideas, hoping to hit the mark,
letting the chips of other imperatives scatter
and fall away?

Yes, we say. But when you're memory-free,
the splitting takes a different turn. The split is real
but there's no longer a swing to mind, an axe to grind
nor ideas to hone, everything now is utterly gone.
So free now of the chaos that memory brings.

so free now of its endless stings
so free now to float like a bright balloon in Sandia's sky,
untethered, without any strings, subject only to the wind
and drifts of your own confusion, another of the gods'
questionable gifts.

So there you are, my beautiful lady, lavished with freedom
but even in the midst of others you stand so isolated,
wrenchingly alone, except for the figures you conjure up,
to keep you company, is it? The split from reality is true
but not complete for though you forget your husband's name
and give him space, you often remember his face and
in the end see him as a friend who helps you dress
and ties your shoes, baking muffins and over coffee
sharing the forgettable morning news.

Oh, if only we could split wood again like we used to,
in Vermont, me swinging the axe and you stacking,
or failing that, I could split would and you could stack,
carefully separating the coulds from the shoulds,
to keep promise free of morality's lack.

March 21, 2012

After our arrival home in La Conner, Joan was impossible to calm down. She wanted me to drive her home to her mother. Where was that home? In Portsmouth, Ohio. She was very clear about her destination as opposed to other times and would not take no for an answer. If I would not drive her, she would drive herself. To pacify her for the moment, I got her in the car and took her for a nice drive out into the countryside, eventually ending up where we began, at our own doorstep. I got her out of the car and pointed out our house and told her that she, in fact, created the yellow color of the exterior paint. "Old Yaller" she called it. Joan seemed momentarily satisfied that this really was her home.

In the process of getting lunch for Joan, I gave her a taste of ice cream with a dab of chocolate syrup and a Larazepam tablet. She was soon asleep on the living room sofa which gave me time to talk with Senior Services. The representative from there was going to apply to Catholic Services for a second caregiver which would provide 23 hours of support per month of which I would pay about $100 (the same financial arrangement I had with Gentry House). Senior Services was also willing to help with financing of a respite for me by placing Joan in a memory care facility for a three day stint sometime in the next few months. Meanwhile, I was going to continue my exploration of the memory care places that I have had recommended to me. Tomorrow I planned to visit Birchview in Sedro-Woolley and Josephine in Stanwood. Our caregiver was willing to take on the extra duty of caring for Joan from 9-12 am. So nothing had really changed in my general plan except to substitute home care for Gentry House and that I probably would have to place Joan in a memory care facility much earlier than expected, maybe even within weeks.

Meanwhile, in the midst of these deliberations, the nurse at our clinic reported that I should up the Seroquel to a full tablet (25 mg) twice a day for Joan. The problem the other night after returning home from the hospital when Joan would not, could not, sleep, was not too much Seroquel but too little.

By virtue of this most recent hospital experience I vowed never to subject Joan to it again, no matter how serious her problem. The whole event was simply too traumatic, too painful, too stressful, for Joan, this in spite of the fact that many skilled and caring people attended her.

March 25, 2012

I visited Birchview Memory Care facility in Sedro-Woolley on schedule and for the first time could visualize Joan being at home there. The building was large, big enough to handle 60 patients on two floors but the hallways were wide with good-sized rooms and numerous common rooms with dining on each floor. I particularly liked the large secured outdoor area where patients could walk at will, night or day. The site overlooked the Skagit River Park and playing fields. You got the feeling of spaciousness as compared to the previous two facilities I visited. Of course space was not the only measure. The staff and aides at all three places seemed friendly and competent in their care of the elderly, and then there was the question of cost. All are pricey. Homeplace costs $5600 per month or $67,200 per year. The director at Fidalgo never responded to my visit there so I lacked any specific cost figures. The outreach director at Birchview, said they needed to get a picture of my available cash resources which must be around $84,000 for the first two years. My resources would include, I assume, Medicaid funding plus anywhere from $500 to $1500 per month from the VA as well as availability of limited monthly support from the children, all of whom were quite agreeable to pitching in. I could also cash in my life insurance, if necessary, valued currently at $31,000.

After Joan's behavior the previous night and yesterday afternoon I was ready to throw in the towel. That night I got just two hours sleep with Joan up and restless and wanting to get home to her mother. Yesterday afternoon, however, was even worse with Joan insisting, even more stridently, that she wanted to get out of our house to her own, trying each of the exterior doors which required me, for the first time, to use physical restraint, pulling her back in the house, and locking the doors, during which time she was threatening me with lawsuits and at one point was intent upon phoning the police for assistance. I broke the impasse by piling Joan into the VW camper for a long drive along Skagit City Road which meandered along the river and through the flatlands. Sunny and windless, it was a perfect afternoon. By the time we returned home, Joan had quite forgotten her desire to get away and was happy to rest while I cooked an appealing meal of fried oysters with mashed potatoes (Idaho and sweet) and green peas.

Except for the Lorazepam at 8 am, I had not given Joan any medication until 7 pm when she took a whole Seroquel (25 mg). This soon settled Joan down for the night which meant we both got a sizeable amount of sleep. Joan willingly took another Lorazepam this morning, and after a walk, was resting on the couch beside me as I wrote. Reluctantly, Joan allowed me to prick her finger this morning. Her glucose read 233 mg but she refused to let me inject her with the usual 7 mg of Levemir, the last in a series of refusals. No amount of arguing was persuasive. Her health be damned, she was not going to allow me to do my job.

I continued to ponder the issue of placing Joan in a memory care facility. All of the children agreed that it was the next logical step and fully supported the move anytime I decided to make it. I was beginning to feel more comfortable with the prospect because I knew that I had limitations, one being my continued impatience. I just did not think I could handle caring for Joan much longer even with the two days of respite each week. The crux for me was to make sure she would be happy and well-cared for at Birchview or wherever. My greatest fear was that I would place Joan some place only to have her experience a certain loneliness or neglect. Level of care meant everything to me as I suppose it did to all spouses who had to make such an impossible choice. My professional advisors told me I would know when the time was right. Would I?

March 26, 2012

I thought I had hit on the proper dosage schedule with a Lorazepam at 8 am and noon with a half Seroquel at 2 pm and a whole pill at 7 pm. I was wrong. Joan was up much of the night wanting to get dressed to go home. At 1 am she was hungry so I made her a cup of hot milk with just a touch of chocolate and heated up two of my frozen muffins. She was surprised to learn that she had to return to bed but she did and slept for two hours, awakening at 4 am or so. I guided her to the bathroom and returned her to her bed and tucked her in but only after she had spent twenty minutes remaking her bed just so. She was completely deaf to the illogic of making her bed when she was going to sleep in it right away but I finally just let her walk from one side of her bed to the other until she was satisfied she had it made correctly. The next time Joan awoke was around 7 am as I was getting breakfast.

Today I would adjust the dosage: Lorazepam at 8 am and noon as usual but I will add a third Lorazepam at 4 pm. The Seroquel will remain the same. If this was not enough adjustment, I would probably up the Seroquel to one and a half at bedtime.

This week I planned to introduce Joan to the top three memory care facilities, starting with Homeplace, taking her there for lunch, presumably on Wednesday to see her reaction to the setting and food. I needed to do this in any event since the first responders, most likely, would need to have some place to move Joan temporarily should something happen to me. It also may give me some insight into long-term care possibilities.

Yesterday, Sunday, was fairly quiet. Joan slept some and we managed two walks but she complained of being exhausted in each case before we had completed the loop through downtown. Only once in the late afternoon did Joan want to go "home" but did not try to get out an exterior door. Referring to our house as the "yellow" house still seemed to carry some meaning for Joan, helping her to make the connection to where she was, cooling her ardor for a "home" elsewhere.

March 28, 2012

The most recent dosage as described above seemed to be doing the trick. For the second night now, Joan had slept most of the night, up just three times for trips to the bathroom.

There was one odd, unexpected, moment last night. Not long after I had put Joan to bed, I was listening to the evening news. Suddenly I heard the flush of the toilet. Joan had not walked past me downstairs so she had to have taken the bedroom door to the hallway and climbed the steep stairs to the upstairs bathroom! She had, all right. I walked carefully back down the stairs with her and explained again the danger in that route. It also reminded me to begin every day by moving the heavy side chair in the bedroom against the door so she could not escape my notice. I had, meanwhile, been to the hardware store and purchased brass door stoppers for the three exterior doors.

At noon Joan and I drove to Homeplace in Burlington. The marketing director walked us around the grounds. They had a small but adequate secured outdoor walking area with sidewalks and groomed grounds which allowed patients to roam freely in and out of any of the three bungalows at any hour. We had lunch with two residents, Lorraine and Richard, neither of whom uttered a word unless spoken to directly but they were mobile and could feed themselves. Joan was not talkative either but at one point she turned to Lorraine and emitted the sounds of a rooster crowing. For the first time, Lorraine opened her eyes wide and smiled. I told Lorraine that Joan often made that sound in answer to the rooster across the street and asked if she had had chickens. Oh yes, she said, we had had chickens. End of conversation.

After serving water and coffee to other patients (and us), the marketing director sat down with us and tried unsuccessfully to engage Joan in conversation. Joan did not eat much of the sweet and sour sauce and pork over rice and oriental veggies. I, on the other hand, was hungry and ate everything. The food was good if not quite hot enough. We did not stay long. Joan was anxious to get home. On the way out, I mentioned that we were next having lunch at Birchview Memory Care. The marketing director was quick to point out the disadvantage of Birchview: with 60 patients on two floors, it was much too big which I translated as not being able to deliver the more intimate personal level of care available at Homeplace. We would see. So far, I preferred Birchview with its larger grounds and easy access to Skagit River Park as well as its interior design with carpeting and multi common rooms and other amenities such as the hair salon, etc. I never got a sense that

Birchview was crowded. Far from it. But who knew. I expect to learn a lot more with our lunch visit next Monday.

Driving home I asked Joan if she enjoyed the visit at Homeplace. Oh yes, she said but you would never have known it. At another point Joan asked me if I was single or married. I said I was married and asked about her. Yes, she said, she was married to Bob Skeele and had four or six children, she could not remember which. Upon reflection, she thought four.

Tomorrow, an assessor with the Department of Social and Health Services, visits us which was part of Medicaid's two step process. As the assessor put it, "It takes two keys to start the car" His function, I guess, was to evaluate Joan's level of need. It should be interesting and vitally important, of course, to Joan's future care.

April 5, 2012

The assessor's visit was as pleasant as an official assessment process could be. He listened carefully and sympathetically, particularly when he had to ask Joan the hard questions: Do you know what day it is? The year? Do you know in what town you live at the present time? I'm happy to hear you have four children. Can you tell me their names? The answers to these and other similar questions were all negative, of course, but he hurried to reassure Joan that it was all right. The assessment interview lasted about one and a half hours.

The assessor called me that afternoon to inform me that based on his interview, we were entitled to 101 hours per month of in-home care or about 25 hours a week. I told the assessor at the time that I was thinking that home care was not going to be the long term answer and was pursuing placement for Joan at either Homeplace or Birchview memory care facilities. Meanwhile DSHS notified me that they needed March bank statements before they could complete the financial assessment. I submitted those directly to DSHS after Joan and I had lunched at Birchview.

To complete the Medicaid segment of this narrative, I received a phone call today, April 5, from the assessor stating that my application for Medicaid has been denied due to financial resources being about $2000 in excess of limit. I conferred with the financial assessor, who said it made perfect sense to reapply later during the second year of payments to Birchview. At a monthly cost of $4200, most of any resources I had would have been depleted. She would make a note on my file that we had conferred and this was the plan.

As implied, I had, as of yesterday, decided to place Joan in the Birchview memory care community beginning next Tuesday (after Easter Sunday). I completed all the paperwork this morning at Birchview. I realized that I was not capable of caring for Joan at home around the clock and that even occasional breaks would not really provide the rest and recharging I needed to continue. People who had experienced working with dementia patients and who had had a chance to observe Joan, said she would be a challenge to standard home care and at this point her dementia had developed to the point where she needed the care of professionals for her own safety. Furthermore, all expressed concern for my health over the long haul and noted more than once that often the family caregiver wore out before the patient.

The nighttime activity continued at one level or another. At a very minimum, Joan was up 3 or 4 times a night and these days most always needed my help to find her way to the bathroom and back. Now she was also beginning to be wary of objects on the floor: the dark green throw rug worried her (did she see it as a hole?) and several times now she had tried to pick up, or step over, the white triangle pattern in the oriental rug in the bedroom. The most noticeable change was in the level of hallucinations. Up until now most of the invisible figures had involved her family or our children. Now, however, she saw one or more persons sitting in our dining room chairs or moving across the room. Last Sunday was a perfect example of what I mean. Joan said she wanted to get "out of the house". I expected her to tell me it was to find her mother or to go to her mother's house but no, not this time. This time she wanted to get out of the house because there were a group of strangers standing around in the dining room. "No kidding," I said. I looked and, of course, saw no one. I turned to Joan and said "If I get rid of these people, will you stay in the house?"

"Yes," Joan said. So I went into the dining room and acted as if I were talking to the group, making the appropriate gestures and ushering them to the door, opening it and waving a final goodbye. I went back to Joan. "Okay?" I asked. She nodded that everything was fine and she would stay put. Five minutes later she went to the side door, looked out and reported that the people had not left after all. They were standing out in the yard next to the fence. I said, with great confidence now, that I would take care of it. So with all the assurance of a born thespian, I walked over to the fence and started gesturing again, indicating my displeasure and opening the gate to get rid of them. After I returned to the house, I asked Joan if she was satisfied. She looked at me quizzically. I said "What?" She said, "What were you doing out there waving your arms, talking to yourself?"

April 8, 2012

Last night was hectic and it looked like tonight would be also. The last few nights Joan had retired even earlier than she usually did, around 5:15 pm or so. With the change to Daylight Savings, the sun was still high and the downstairs bedroom, with two windows on the west side, was not conducive to sleep. Consequently, Joan had been up frequently to go to the bathroom which she could not find without my help these days or had questions to ask me about the whereabouts of her brothers, especially Bill for some reason. With her Seroquel at 8:00 pm or so, Joan quieted down for awhile but by 11:30 pm was up again. Last night she wanted to get dressed and "go home". The conversation never made much progress, Joan sitting up in her bed and me sitting on the edge of mine, making our points until we both became too exhausted to continue. Joan finally fell asleep and I turned off the bed lamp thinking maybe we would both sleep until daylight.

No such luck. A few hours later I awoke abruptly to discover Joan was not in her bed and that all the downstairs lights were on. I jumped up quickly, fully alert now, ran to the bathroom to see if Joan was there. She was not. I saw the hall lights were on as well and went to the bottom of the stairs and called Joan's name. She answered. I had failed to push the heavy chair against the hallway door so she climbed the steep stairway and now would not come back down. She was obviously afraid to come back down, even with me holding her and guiding her, and proceeded to crawl under the covers in our double bed in the front bedroom. I played along, turning off the lights and standing in the hallway. Soon, Joan was up and ready to have me help her down. Slowly, step by step, we made it back to the first floor and eventually back to her bed. Joan went immediately to sleep. It took me much longer and I felt the effects of it most of the day, finally getting a catnap as I watched the Master's Golf Tourney in Augusta, Georgia.

Most of Saturday (yesterday) was spent thinking about plans for Joan's admission to Birchview Memory Care next Tuesday noon. I wanted her room to feel as homelike as possible (even though she was not certain where her home was) so the caregiver and neighbors up the street, were going to step in after Joan and I departed for Birchview for lunch. They would direct volunteers from Senior Services about which pieces of bedroom furniture to pick up and haul to Birchview in our wake with the idea of getting the furniture placed by the Birchview staff before Joan saw her room for the first time. The conspiring neighbors joined us yesterday for lunch and saw for themselves the pieces of furniture I wanted moved: The twin bed and mattresses and bedclothes, the night table and lamp, the chest of drawers and the two green swivel chairs in the TV room.

Last night was every bit as bad as I expected, the previous night's scene repeating itself except this time Joan could not get to the stairway. Restless late in the afternoon, I made Joan an early dinner and she was in bed by 5:15 pm or so. She was up several times in the first hour. The Lorazepam (.5 mg) worked for a short spell but by 8 pm she was awake again worried about various members of her family. At that point I urged Joan to take her nightly Seroquel but she refused. Fifteen minutes later, I asked her again and this time she acquiesced, taking the equivalent of a full pill (25 mg).

Much to my surprise, the Seroquel seemed to have little effect on Joan beyond slurred speech and what appeared to be a slight drowsiness.

By 9:30 pm Joan was insisting (again) on going home and wanted me to go out in the dark and get the car warmed up for the trip. As I became more and more certain Joan did not have a specific home address in mind, I put the proposition to her: If she could tell me exactly where "home" was, I would drive her there. She could not tell me, of course, and after an hour or so she gave up. But not before I, in total exasperation, opened the side door for her so she could be on her way. With no moon the porch was pitch dark—and cold—and within seconds Joan was back inside. During the height of our discussion, Joan began to pull the bedcover and electric blanket from the bed thinking that she could wear them for her trip. At this point I had to physically restrain her and impress upon her that in any sort of physical contest I was going to be the winner and she knew it and at no point did she try to hit me. She used, rather, weapons of sarcasm and legal threats.

I had hoped that once Joan realized there was no way she was going to be driven home, that she finally would sleep. It never happened. She was up wandering around the first floor more than she slept and by 5 am she was up for good, seated at the dining room table waiting to be fed. I groggily complied, still in my pajamas, making coffee and pancakes, a Sunday morning favorite.

Getting up so early on Easter Sunday used to mean getting ready to attend a sunrise service, participating in the familiar liturgical response: "The Lord is risen ....The Lord is risen indeed." This time around, it was hard to focus on anything, the wealth and richness of the Christian tradition escaping me somehow as I struggled tiredly to come to terms with my decision to place Joan in others' care. It seemed as if the experiences of the last two nights were designed to put my mind at ease, to reassure me that my decision was the only option I had. I knew now absolutely that I could not continue to care for Joan under these current conditions, particularly without Medicaid and even that service would not be sufficient to match the need for more and more home care. The typical round the clock home care was running $300 per day or over $8000 per month. Birchview, as I have noted elsewhere, was half that and I suspect provided higher quality care.

Had I made the right decision? I answered with: Was there a better one? I was regrettably at the point where I simply did not have any other choice. For awhile I felt like I was abandoning Joan but I was not. I was putting her into the capable hands of others who could care for her better than I could. Moreover, I would still see and visit with Joan as often as it made sense to do so. So our life together was not ended, it had changed and the next chapter of our journey together was about to begin.

April 9, 2012

All our children phoned during the course of the sunny warm Easter day. To top it off, Nora Skeele, our granddaughter, joined us for a light Easter meal of sliced ham, yams, string beans and corn muffins. Nora, like her mother, was a tremendous help washing dishes and cleaning the kitchen afterwards and stayed around to take Joan for a walk. I was able to tell each of our kids of my decision to place Joan in Birchview this coming Tuesday. They all expressed their support for my decision. David, thinking ahead, asked if I had given any thought to selling the house and down-sizing. I told him I had but would not make any moves until the housing market picked up some. I had confidence that sensible alternatives would present themselves with the passage of time but, certainly, selling the house would be an additional way to finance Joan's stay at Birchview.

Umbrellas

Brightly clad, tightly rolled,
two new umbrellas,
the compact, telescoping kind,
rest, side by side,
very much alone
on an empty bench
on a busy sidewalk
on a sunny afternoon,
in April,
waiting patiently
for their owner's return
or, failing that,
for the rain's return,
to blossom at moisture's touch,
like thoughtful flowers,
unfolding in time
to keep their keepers dry,
whoever they turn out to be.

The string of terrible nights continued. Last night, Sunday, Joan was too tired to walk or do anything else but retire at 5 pm. I helped get her into her pajamas and settle her down. She seemed to rest, if not sleep, quietly for awhile, getting up to urinate once as I read and watched television. As I crawled into bed, around 9:30 pm Joan awoke and wanted to go downstairs. I tried several times to explain to her that we were already downstairs. At one point I walked her from one room to the other. At every step I pointed out the various objects and rooms that were part of our downstairs and got her verbal agreement. The piano would only be downstairs, right? The kitchen would not be upstairs, would it? It would be down stairs. Right? I would walk Joan back to bed thinking I had penetrated the fog that engulfed her but no, fifteen minutes later, Joan was up again wanting to go downstairs. So for a second time, I walked her through the downstairs rooms. She seemed convinced but only for a short period. Finally, at around 10:30 pm she became so agitated at not being able to get up and get dressed that I help her do just that.

Only when I had tied the last shoe lace did she seem calm and satisfied. So I got up with her, turned on all the lights, turn up the heat and prepared her a light snack of hot cereal and toast and jam. She ate only a small portion and just remained seated at the dining room table seemingly content to do nothing. I was tired and wanted to be in bed but instead I sat with her, working at my laptop. Finally, Joan, still fully clothed, laid down on the wicker sofa and was soon asleep. I let her sleep for a half hour but by 1 am I nudged her awake and led her to her bed and then piled into bed myself. By 3 am Joan was awake again and needed my help to find her way to the bathroom. I tucked her in bed again and she was soon asleep as was I. At 5 am or so Joan woke up again and kept wandering about downstairs. My offers to help her get back in bed were spurned and so I got up and start breakfast a little earlier than usual, feeling totally knocked out.

April 11, 2012

The date, April 10, 2012 was a date that would always be right up there with our birthdays, our children's birthdays and our wedding day. It was the day of THE MOVE, the day that Joan moved into Birchview Memory Care in Sedro-Woolley, a whole new world for her and because of our separation, a whole new world for me.

Because I did not think Joan would go willingly to her new home, I told Joan we were invited for lunch by the development director at Birchview as his guests and that we had to leave the house by 11:15 am. Shortly after our departure the volunteer crew from Senior Services was to arrive, pick up Joan's bed, the matching chest of drawers and the rest of the furniture and haul them to Birchview and get Joan's room set up before she ever saw it. It was touch and go. For one thing Joan chose this morning to drag her feet, saying she did not feel well and did nothing but sleep on the wicker sofa until almost 11 am. It was as if Joan sensed that something was afoot and wanted to delay it if not stop it altogether. Just as I was about to cancel the plan, Joan agreed to get up and get moving once she understood she had only to slip into her sweat pants and did not have to change from her pajama shirt and hooded sweater.

It was strange sitting in the dining room at Birchview eating lunch and watching the crew carry the pieces of familiar furniture into the building. With her back to the window, Joan did not see a thing. I wanted so much for Joan's first sight of her room to have some familiarity about it. Apparently that was what happened. The development director told me later that Joan walked into her room and sat down on one of the swivel chairs. She did not say anything but he said he could sense her pleasure. I liked to think the same would apply when Joan slipped into her own bed the first night between her own flannel sheets and with her head upon her own plaid pillow.

For that first hour at Birchview I was not sure how it was going to go. The development director had settled us down at a table in the dining room and departed to help the crew with the furniture. Joan was fidgety, ate very little and was anxious to leave. It did not help that a big guy in a walker who was seated with other male residents at a nearby table came to our table leaned over, kissed Joan and complimented her on her good looks, all before the food server pulled him back to his table. When I told the development director and the director, about the episode, they were visibly upset and looked into the matter immediately. It turned out the big guy was a new resident who had arrived the previous day, lived on the second floor and was not even supposed to be eating in that dining room. The three attendants assigned to the dining room were busy feeding three immobilized residents and had seen nothing. The director said they would alert the staff and make sure nothing like that happened again.

After I finished eating, I walked with Joan into the outdoor patio area, a pleasant place with a groomed walkway, budding trees and a nice view to the foothills and city park. While I was trying to slow our pace and get Joan to look around and enjoy the moment, she was pulling ahead of me, intent upon finding a door and getting out of there. Holding Joan's hand, I walked her back inside and proceeded down the spacious hallway, looking for the development director. He and my friend from Senior Services emerged from Joan's room, having just finished arranging the furniture. My friend immediately coaxed Joan into walking the grounds with her so the development director and I could unload the bedclothes and other items, i.e., medicines and toiletries, from the trunk of my car. The director and I then made up Joan's bed and I departed as prearranged, unsure at this point how Joan's residency at Birchview was going to work out. It certainly was not the beginning I had envisioned.

Driving back down Township Road and Ferry Street to Highway 20, I was struck with just how difficult this separation was for me. It was undoubtedly the worst experience in my entire life. As I drove down Highway 20, I was crying so hard I could barely see the road. Then I would stop sobbing for a moment, get my breath, and then start all over again. About the time I got to the La Conner turnoff, I received a telephone call from Birchview with the news that Joan was settling in nicely, that the caller had had a pleasant talk with her, and then the recreation director had taken her down to one of the common rooms and introduced her to others which Joan, much to my dismay, seemed to enjoy, patting people on the back in a friendly fashion and doing her share of socializing. The report could not have come at a better time. Wonder if it turned out that Joan really did enjoy her new life? How good would that be? I could not wish for anything better.

I had no sooner unlocked the door and stepped into the house then the phone began to ring. All four of our children telephoned me over the next couple of hours, offering me encouragement and support. I could only think how lucky I was as a father to have such devoted, caring children. In between their phone calls, I telephoned the caregiver to update her. She had been our primary caregiver for many months and helped me ready Joan for our trip to Birchview, staying behind to see to the furniture move and then staying to lock up. The next call was to our neighbors up the street, my first re-sponders, who helped as well to execute the furniture move. It was they who wanted me to dine with them last night at Nell Thorn's, the popular restaurant down the street I had mentioned before. The last call was to Senior Services, to thank them for providing the crew and van to move Joan's furniture and for their other timely services to me seeing, for example, that Joan could visit Gentry House.

Last evening I spent walking around the house getting used to the idea of my new, single life. Suddenly the house seemed much too large and I knew that I would eventually downsize. I also realized that I had now to completely restructure my mental processing. Until now every decision, every action, had been tied to Joan, things like letting her know every time I went upstairs to the study or outside to the car or up the street to deliver muffins. Last night I was going to use the disposal in the kitchen sink. Always before this evening I had to warn Joan to cover her sensitive ears before I flipped the switch and started the noisy grinding. Omitting reference to Joan in my own moves was going to take some time. This morning, returning from a walk and work out at the fitness center, I opened the door and almost yelled "I'm home" before I remembered that Joan was not here and was not going to be here again which brought on more giant sobs and a stream of tears. To overcome my sadness, I started my morning magic, creating muffins, which went well up to the point where I was pouring batter in the muffin tin. Always before this morning, the first three muffins were just for Joan, plain without chocolate or fruit. Now there was no need for the exception. That was too much to bear and I broke down again, with heavy, heaving sobs and blinding tears. After a few minutes, I was okay again ... until I was writing about the morning's experiences and suddenly, again, gigantic sobs and heaves and blurring tears. I expect this to go on for some time. It was, after all, a sad day, the first in a long series of sad days. A man in my Alzheimer's support group in Anacortes, said his wife had been in a memory care facility for a year and half and he was still grieving!

Separation's Grief

Grief arrives with little warning
and is slow to leave,
or so it seems, for
Grief follows me right out the door
of a memory care place
that April day with a trace
of spring in the air,
where I have just left my wife
of sixty years
in the care
of others,
at first dazed
and numb, without tears.

By the time I hit the highway home
though, there Grief is,
an unwelcome passenger,
obviously, content
and well fed,
blurring my vision, making it hard
to see the road ahead.

Not wanting me to walk into
an empty house alone,
Grief squeezed through the side door

with me, disappearing only
when I answer the phone
to hear my daughter's comforting words
and those of my three boys whose
calls soon follow,
the four calls together, along with
others, a network of concern,
a giant hand's hollow,
holding me, supporting me,
an old guy, a father and friend,
whose hapless vulnerability
wants to tumble me,
end over end.

And Grief has a field day,
drawing from me,
with every turn and touch,
wracking sobs, loud cries,
long, breath-sucking silences
exploding into gut-loaded wails.
Joan, memory-shot,
dead to me but still alive,
and never, ever, again to be
by my side,
in our own intimate space!
I can barely face the thought.
And might not have but for
the saving grace
of others who help me to lace
my world together,
to put it back in place.

Slowly, over the hours, Grief departs
leaving its thick shadow of sadness
for me to live with
and make something of.
And, surprisingly, I do!
Love seeps through,
reclaiming so clear, the wisdom I at first
couldn't hear:
I'm still a caregiver to my beloved,
and am now free,
blessedly free,
to be a better one.

April 12, 2012

I got through the loneliness of the afternoon and evening, beginning the task of cleaning out drawers of clothes Joan would never wear again and preparing to ship a selection of them to our daughter. The rest would go to Goodwill. After a small dinner of leftover ham and yams, I settled down to watch the Mariners beat Texas in the late innings. During the same time I viewed the video of Easter Service at First Community Church on my laptop. I was happy to see my friend was back in the choir after a heart attack last month. A stalwart, devoted soul, she. The sermon by the senior minister was relevant and lively. Don't come to FCC on Easter if you expect to have the Easter message explained to you. It won't happen. We come to church on Easter to sit beneath the story, to look up at it, to listen and watch in wonder (the last phrase mine). Reference was made to the story of Lazarus being raised from the dead (John 11:1-44) and Jesus' demand to remove the burial wrappings from his body, a metaphor for Easter: a time of unwrapping.

I was still feeling the weight of a profound sadness but so far today none of the wracking sobs and tears although at times I have come right to the edge, tears forming and then stopping, held at bay with the realization that I still had a lot of caregiving to do, visiting Joan at Birchview and participating with her in her world. In anticipation of my continued role, I today registered to take a series of six classes on "Taking Care of You: Powerful Tools for Caregiving" which would be conducted by the same person who leads our Alzheimer's support group and was knowledgeable and had been of immense help to me in these last weeks. In another hour I would be meeting with my neighbor up the street for lunch at the Waterfront Cafe. He and his wife would take the lead in caring for me and my affairs, should an emergency arise, until our son John could get here to take over as the legal executor.

It was the second morning in the revival of my exercise program. It felt good to again be running/walking and hitting the fitness center every day. I was starting slowly but expected to build up to my former speed and distance and weight levels within a few weeks but I had to be careful not to overdo it.

April 14, 2012

I skipped all exercising this morning partly because I was editing a recent poem and partly because I noticed some soreness in my shin bones and hips, a clear warning. I visited Birchview yesterday (Friday) to drop off more of Joan's clothes and copies of our three books.

I had a chance, while there, to talk with one of the caregivers who told me Joan was doing well, making friends, eating a good breakfast but not much lunch. She still wanted to "go home" so she needed more time to "transition" before I next see her.

Of course, Joan often wanted to "go home" when she was at home in La Conner so perhaps Joan's urge was simply a carryover. In any event, the staff there will let me know when it was time for my first contact. Meanwhile, they told me Joan was short of jogging pants so I spent most of Friday afternoon and evening searching for just the right size and style which, surprisingly were hard to find, particularly the hemmed cuffs. After trying Kohl's, Macy's, Target's and even Wal-Mart's, I ended up at Fred Meyer's, purchasing three pairs of Russell sportswear. By 8:30 pm I was on my way home to wash and dry them for delivery to Joan today. After that I headed to Eaglemont Golf Course for a commemoration service for a friend's husband who had died suddenly of a heart attack.

Joan's former caregiver and another good friend visited Joan and reported that Joan seemed to be doing well although she seemed preoccupied and was moving around a lot. She also reported that aides and other residents were waving to her and calling her by name. They both liked the pleasant building and surroundings, a lovely spot. They were also impressed, as I was, with the light, airy dining room. Both felt Joan was in the right place which was reassuring to me.

April 21, 2012

Even with all the phone calls from the staff and nurses at Birchview over the last week updating me on Joan's progress, consulting with me about medicines and Joan's food preferences, I was not prepared for my first sight of Joan yesterday after nine days absence. If it had not been for the striped polo shirt from LL Bean, I was not at all certain I would have recognized her. The attendants had corralled her hair, thank goodness, but otherwise she seemed so much smaller and bent over and when she lifted her pale, gaunt face I did not see any look of recognition in her red-rimmed eyes. I felt my heart break all over again.

I took her hand and we walked from the nurse's station where I had found her to the dining room at the other end of the hall. There a staff member provided us with glasses of refreshing fruit juice and left us to enjoy some privacy. I continued to hold Joan's hand most of the time as I attempted to get her to talk but for the most part her speech was too garbled and disconnected for me to understand. At one point she looked at me and gave me one of her dazzling, warm smiles, which I recalled with such fondness, and at another point she took my hand and brought it to her lips, gently kissing it. Moments of recognition? Maybe. I like to think so anyway.

The one word I did hear and understand was "go." This was the key word of my short visit so "go" we did, walking hand in hand outside in the garden area and then back through the halls and outside again. She would sit for only a few minutes with others in the parlor or the TV room and then want to go again. She had no interest in the television program or the old movie the staff was showing.

After a while she seemed tired so I took her to her room and helped her to lie down in her bed. I then began gently to rub her back and shoulders. Soon she was sound asleep. At that point I conferred with the nurses and aides. They were all concerned that Joan eat more and drink more. I mentioned her enjoyment of ice cream. They said they would give her ice cream with every meal. They have had a difficult time weighing Joan because their scale involved sitting in a chair which was wobbly and Joan felt too insecure.

I was still in shock from yesterday's visit. Joan had been slowly disappearing for months, losing strength and agility even though she had managed to keep her weight around 90 pounds. Now, in the first days at Birchview, she seemed to have diminished noticeably, shrinking, caving in … and giving up? I had no way of knowing her mind any more than she but I had to ask myself the question I had asked before: Was she slowly starving herself to death, the elderlys' secret weapon? I had come away from my first visit with two strong feelings: Joan could not be in a better place. She had plenty of competent, caring people looking out for her. Secondly, I was saddened, deeply saddened, by Joan's rapid decline. I felt I was going through the emotional turmoil of separation all over again. I just could not seem to get used to it. Her death seemed closer than ever.

Life in La Conner continued to be busy (thank goodness) using my time away from Joan writing and "thinning out" as a first step in down-sizing. This morning I continued the project of cleaning up the guest room. Happily I found a home for the old Sanyo phonograph and tape player and all the LP records and tapes at Birchview. The recreation director could already envision a musical activity involving the phonograph and residents. I had also cleaned out the sewing drawer in the sewing table and would take that and the portable sewing machine to Goodwill on my way to visit Joan again today.

My poem entitled "Separation's Grief" was published in the local paper this week and I got a number of warm responses. Several friends came up to me with tears in their eyes, embracing me. One teller at Key Bank, whose grandparents own and operate Tulip Town, presented me with a bunch of fresh tulips for Joan. She had read my poem and that was her response. To top it off her name was also Joann. I would soon head out to Birchview (Saturday), to visit Joan bearing gifts and one of her favorite baseball caps which was black cotton and bore the logo "Buns of Skeele." Oh, how I hoped to hear the good news that Joan had at least eaten her ice cream!

April 23, 2012

I arrived at Birchview on a sunny afternoon about 1 pm and began looking for Joan. I found her at the end of the long hall trying to get out the heavy doors into the secured courtyard, but she was having trouble. Holding the bunch of tulips and vase in my hands and her hat, I greeted her, pointing out the lovely tulips and giving her the hat. She took little notice, so intent was she to get out the door. I had the feeling she must be thinking of me as another resident or perhaps a staff member but in any event I pushed open the door and walked the full length of the courtyard with her, reentering the building at the dining room where I cut the tulip stems and placed them in the vase with water. With that done and hands free we continued walking, me holding her hand, making our way up the spacious hallway, greeting others and circling back through the courtyard until she seemed tired at which point I helped her into bed and softly rubbed her shoulders and back until she was asleep.

As one of the attendants let me out the secured door, I wondered whether this is to be the pattern: short visits with a lot of walking and then tucking her in bed. When I think about it, it was pretty much the pattern at our home. At least today, Joan looked a little better, standing straighter although no verbal communication or body language for that matter, that conveyed much except that she accepted my company and was quite willing to have me help her into bed. Did she remember that part of our former life together?

I was heading up to Fairhaven to have lunch and take in a dance performance at Western Washington University with a friend so visited Joan at Birchview in the morning at 10 am for the first time. I signed in, walked through the door and began looking for Joan. I checked her room first which was empty and then began my walk down the carpeted hall. I found her fast asleep in a cushioned lounge chair at the far end where it was quieter with less traffic, I knelt in front of her and softly called her name. Joan opened her eyes, cupped her hands around my face and smiled her loveliest smile. Recognition! Or so it seemed to me.

She happily got up, took my hand, and we began once again to walk the premises inside and out. This time around, she walked with me through the Parlor Room, a large space with a big, flat-screen TV but also big work tables with chairs and plenty of puzzles and games to play and in one corner a kitchen sink with ample counter space and cupboards. Along the same wall a free-standing commercial popcorn machine stood, inviting inspection. Joan and I each helped ourselves to some of the caramel corn inside. At another point I spied the weighing machine one of the nurses had told me about. Because you have to sit in a metal chair with a sling seat and back which though secure, feels unstable, Joan refused to sit in it. Therefore they had been unable to obtain Joan's weight. On a hunch, I asked Joan if she would sit on the contraption and she complied, just like that. I then pushed the "on" button on the display panel behind the seat and presto, her weight appeared moving between 86 and 87 pounds and settled at 86.2. If the scale was accurate Joan had lost some critical weight in the last couple of weeks.

At one point we encountered the duty nurse. When I told her how much better Joan looked today, the nurse mentioned that Joan had eaten more for breakfast that morning, drinking almost an entire protein-laden strawberry milkshake. She also thought Joan was just now beginning to settle in which always brings improvement in physical appearance. Having tucked Joan in bed and rubbed her to sleep, I signed out at 11 am, immensely relieved at the upturn in her condition. If she regained her weight I would know that things were changing for the better.

April 24, 2012

A warm, sunny day with the temperature at 70 degrees said the digital bank sign on Ferry Street in Sedro-Woolley. I entered the front door at Birchview to be greeted by the director, who just happened to be conferring with other staff members in the lobby. They all greeted me with smiles. The director said that he had just finished sitting with Joan on the davenport in the fireplace room and exclaimed again what a delight she was. I saw the back of Joan's silvered head as he spoke and was quickly sitting at her side. She recognized me immediately and as I sat down next to her, she put her head on my shoulder and her hand on my arm just as we so often did at home. We stayed in that position for some time, both of us content to rest in each other's presence, listening to the stereo that was softly playing a series of country ballads. It was all I could do to keep my tears in check.

Never had I felt such a strong urge to get up right then and there and take Joan home with me. Joan had made remarkable recovery even since yesterday, her speech clear as it had been before admission. I stayed with her for three hours, most of the time just walking, hand in hand. Joan often complained of feeling tired but was unable to stay still for any length of time. At one point, I got her to lie down on her bed but she could not relax, constantly stating there was something she had to get up and fix but was unable to state exactly what it was that needed fixing. I stayed until after 5 pm when the residents gathered for supper in the dining room entryway. As the nurse took Joan's hand to seat her, I excused myself on the pretext of having to use the men's room and quickly departed. I took one last look behind me to see Joan being led to her table and was overwhelmed by the separation and isolation I was exposing Joan to! She should be home with me! I should be preparing her supper!

It was strange. As Joan improved physically and was able to recognize me, I felt worse, finding it increasingly difficult to adjust to the New Reality. I cried, off and on, all the way home, as before, barely able to see where I was going. Last night as I ate and listened to the news, I was keenly aware of our separation and my loneliness. At some point in the early evening, a younger woman friend phoned to find how the weekend had gone. I reported the good news of Joan's recovery. Then she wanted to know how I was doing. I told her, not as well as Joan and described my experience of leaving Joan that day and how sad I felt.

My young friend was totally sympathetic and understood, this from a woman who herself was slowly dying of cancer with not much longer to live. When she hung up I racked up the tears again. Even as I wrote that day's segment, I had to stop frequently and catch my breath from the deep sobs that shook my body, getting up several times to get more tissue to blow my nose and wipe my eyes. I was not doing nearly as well as I thought I would be doing as I dealt with the double whammy of placing Joan's care in the hands of others in another location and as the sense of my own isolation hit me anew.

One thing would help in my adjustment. And that was the knowledge that Joan would not feel she had been abandoned, that she would greet my reappearance with pleasure each time as I tried to find ways to help her (and myself) to enjoy our new life apart. I would be visiting Joan again this afternoon. What would the visit reveal? My prayer today was to have the strength to keep my cool, not breakdown or cry, as I was doing now, in my beloved's presence. Today I would bring some framed pictures for the bare walls of her room including the Wave recruitment poster and the picture of her modeling a swimsuit.

Spring

The date tells me it's spring
but the early morning air
still has a nip to it.
Gloves and a stocking cap
aren't too much to wear
against dawn's brisk start.

It's more the sound
than a calendar
that gives time away.
The songbirds are out,
their full-throated whistles
stronger by the day,
warming up for summer.

I try to respond
with whistles of my own.
But puckering my lips,
pushing the air from my chest,
yields not the slightest trill.
Strange. I can't whistle
anymore.

But I can remember when I could.
and , most important of all,
I can still pucker

forming words,
singing about spring,
swearing at the dark,
Praising the light,
and now and then,
settling for a kiss.

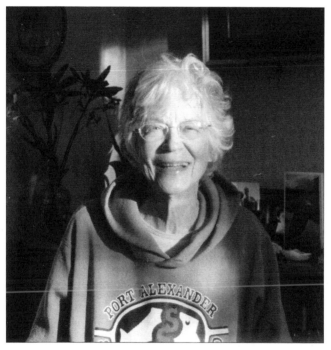

Joan, like spring, even in the down edge of winter. LaConner, 2008

April 26, 2012

The new pictures on the wall of Joan's room brought even more warmth and familiarity. Joan seemed happy enough and took my visit matter of factly, as if I had not just arrived. After a staff member and I installed the pictures and rearranged the swivel chairs and dresser, Joan and I went for a short walk but she soon tired so once again I tucked her in her bed and rubbed her back. I left her sleeping soundly after a few minutes, feeling reassured that Joan was where she needed to be.

I had driven the camper so that I could stop at Sam's Shine Shop and obtain an estimate on having it "detailed," i.e., washed, waxed and polished in preparation for selling it. Sam looked it over and we settled on $200 to make the camper once again presentable. The white paint was badly oxidized so I could see the amount of work involved. He would have to clean much of the window trim by hand as well.

My confidence that I had done the right thing grew even more during yesterday's visit. After hanging one larger picture (the painting of a young girl who looks much like our daughter sitting amid the flora on a summer's day) and placing the white floor lamp from Joan's study between the two swivel chairs, I went looking for Joan. I found her in the parlor, sitting with other residents most of whom were playing Bingo. Joan was not playing or paying much attention to anything. I watched her for awhile, listening to the activities director and an attendant, as they filled me in on Joan's behavior. The activities director reported that at one point in the parlor, she had reached down to pick up an object Joan had dropped but Joan had put her foot on the object and simultaneously slapped her in the face! At my surprise, the activities director just laughed and said it was par for the course. Joan had dementia. It was to be expected.

I was still shaking my head at Joan's behavior which led both she and attendant to talk about how they survived in this business and why they loved doing it. Why did they? Because they were Christians! In fact they both attended the same church. They both expressed the firm belief that they could not do this job, could not enjoy it, if it were not for their faith. Regardless of what others may think, they surmised, "we know, we know" (how important God was to their job) and as if to put an exclamation point on it, briefly embraced, and then departed for other tasks.

I went in the parlor to Joan who at this point wanted to lie down on the small bench she was sitting on. Another attendant and I finally encouraged her to get up and let me walk her back to her room. I had no sense at the time that she recognized me but she was tired and still wanted to lie down. Again I tucked her in bed and covered her with the blue throw I had just brought from home. Joan appeared to recognize the coverlet. Within a few minutes though, Joan said she had to get up to urinate. Once she had done that, she did not want to return to bed. Nor did she want to walk. She was quite happy to sit in one of the upholstered chairs in the Fireplace Room next to the entrance to the dining room with me holding her hand. For the next hour we sat there while others, mostly male residents, began to gather for supper. One of the men kept asking me where I lived, how long it took to drive here and if I was staying for supper. After a moment's anxiety (Was that what I detected?), Joan appeared to accept the fact that I would be leaving at dinner time and when one of the nurses, took Joan's hand to lead her into the dining room, she did not look back to me. At that point I left, letting myself out the secured entryway now that I had memorized the combination.

I met someone yesterday who had her husband in a nursing home. She knew of my situation and stressed the importance of keeping a journal mainly to remind yourself how much your spouse's condition varied from day to day. Yes, a point well taken for that was what I was seeing in just a short space. A few days ago, Joan notably more like her old self and today, paler, more withdrawn, even irritable, taking a swing at the activities director.

April 28, 2012

On the last visit, Joan did not want to walk at all. This time she wanted to do nothing but walk. Fortunately, the weather was good enough to make use of the courtyard as part of the route. Each time we came to a locked gate that led to the street, Joan would stop and try to push it open, stating that she wanted to get in the car and "go home" now. I explained to her that she was home now, that Birchview was her home and that she had special room, Room 108, which had all her own furniture in it. Joan was not buying it. At various points I tried to interest Joan in different things available in the parlor starting with some familiar 60s music from one of the LPs we donated. I wanted her to dance with me. She was not interested. I sat down on the sofa to look at a magazine and read something to her. She wanted to get up and walk. So walk we did.

Eventually, I stopped walking with her so I could talk to two of the attendants about Joan. They reassured me that Joan was doing fine, that she wandered most of the day like she was doing at that moment, stopping to talk to other residents. Because of Joan's renewed interest in leaving Birchview and "going home" I asked if it might be better if I came less often. Their opinion was unanimous: come as often as you want. Joan would not remember her urgency to leave. The nurse supervisor, with whom I checked today when I first arrived, had offered the opinion that Joan was settling in nicely. The two attendants confirmed it. Since it was supper time, One of the attendants ushered Joan into the dining room. Joan, distracted, did not look back and I left, letting myself out through the secured front door. I proceeded to cry my fool head off as I walked to the car. How damned sad it all was!

"Parting is such sweet sorrow" it was said. Maybe for young lovers but in my case there was nothing remotely "sweet" about it. Even as I wrote about it that morning, I broke into tears and sobbed some more! Would it never end? Others who had gone through what I was going through now had told me it never would end. You learn to tolerate the pain of it.

Dancing Heart

On Valentine's Day a dear friend gave me a big, red heart,
the shiny kind that's filled with helium and floats.
It quickly found a home in the corner
against the dining room ceiling,
its only control a long red ribbon dangling free.

Now, weeks later, the red heart, floating at eye level,
was less attractive and in the way.
Not wanting to deflate it, I pulled it into an open storage
space in the front hall beneath the stairs.

The next morning as I descended the stairs,
I was surprised to see the heart floating along, drawn,
I suppose, by the furnace's earlier stirrings, into
the narrow hall below me, its red tether trailing after.

To celebrate my arrival, the floating heart started bobbing,
dancing this way and that, to the lively current
of the forced-air as the furnace delivered,
through the floor vent, its newest wave of hot licks.

Some day the dancing heart, floating merrily now
at mid-level, still red and shiny, will run out of gas.
So will I.
Meanwhile, I'll keeping putting my heart to rest
each night with the highest of expectations
for tomorrow.

April 30, 2012

Some of us survive. Others of us thrive. I had hoped that Joan might thrive in her supportive environment at Birchview. I did not know why I should have expected that since she had not been thriving at home. Clearly, in my last two visits I had seen nothing in Joan's appearance and behavior that allowed me to think that Joan would ever thrive. I wondered now if she would even survive for much longer.

I encountered Joan yesterday walking with a new young attendant who was trying to fix her hair or at least trying to keep it out of her eyes. Every time they stopped, the attendant got one more swath of hair out of the way only to have Joan reach back and undo it. At that point I told the attendant I would walk with Joan for awhile. Joan did not recognize me but we walked hand in hand back and forth along the carpeted hallway for fifteen minutes or so. During one pass through the hallway, the nurse and two other staff were talking. I stopped with Joan and offered to serenade them with our song "Oh Honey," something Joan and I did often when we walked in La Conner. Joan did perk up a little to sing but her voice was weak and she could not remember several of the lines. The staff applauded, of course, and Joan broke into a slight smile. I was surprised, though, that Joan had forgotten so many of the words so soon. When all else failed, she could always recall the song's few simple lines. Not now. Oh, honey. My dear honey.

Several times I urged Joan to walk outside with me but she was cold and did not want to. Eventually, we ended up in the parlor room. Joan was obviously tired and wanted more than anything to sit on the large comfortable sofa and sleep. The RN on duty wanted to take Joan's weight on the chair scale but Joan waved her away. I urged Joan to come with me to the dining room for lunch but Joan would not do that either. The nurse suggested I bring lunch to her in the parlor room which I did. Over the next half hour I was able to get Joan to eat small bites from half of a melted cheese sandwich and a few spoonfuls of ice cream. After that Joan curled up on the sofa and was quickly asleep. The nurse said that for two nights now Joan had been up a lot, roaming the hall, which accounted for her behavior today. She was just tired, worn out from lack of rest. The nurse would try to get Joan's weight later. With Joan sound asleep on the sofa there was nothing more I could do so I kissed Joan on the cheek, signed out and headed home, discouraged. The nurse, on the other hand, thought Joan was settling in nicely, was generally much easier to work with, letting her give her her medications, for example, including the pricking of her finger to get a blood sample. Incidentally, Joan's blood sugar count was only 137 mg which was low for her. The nurse was happy with the count as well.

I wanted to be a good caregiver to Joan but it was unclear how to do that beyond what I was doing now which was to be with her a little bit each day, helping her to eat, getting her to walk, and advocating for her to the staff. Being around at meal time, lunch or supper, seemed to be helpful because the staff had its hands full with feeding some of the less mobile residents. It occurred to me also that Joan might eat a little more, as she did today, if I encouraged her to eat from a tray in her room or some other area outside the dining room.

May 2, 2012

Imagine my shock when I walked through the entry door into the Fireplace Room the next day when Joan, disheveled but standing straight, greeted me by name and embraced me much like her old self! As far as I could determine, nothing had changed: She had not slept any better during the night, still doing some roaming but perhaps not as much, no new drug had been introduced and she had not eaten any better. We walked the hall for awhile and then I helped her to put on a fresh yellow shirt under her cardigan and don socks and shoes. Apparently she had been fully dressed at the beginning of the day but for some reason had removed her shirt and socks and put on her slippers. I sat with Joan at the supper table encouraging her to eat some of the spaghetti dish and vegetables but she ate little, only a few small bites. I totally failed to understand her hesitancy to put food in her mouth for that was what it seemed to me: Less about appetite and more about the texture or feel of the food. I say this because she had no trouble eating most of the dessert, whipped cream over strawberry sauce, and pound cake.

After supper we went to her room and sat in our twin swivel chairs and talked quietly for a time as I tried to explain that we could not just get in our car and drive home now. During supper I had stated that she could not go home with me after we finished eating because Birchview was her new home now at which point her anger flared and she said, "I don't want to hear about it". Now, seated together in her room, there was no such angry reaction. She seemed to sense that she had to stay where she was but she did not ask me why. The answer, of course, was that I could no longer care for her adequately and was wearing out in the process.

Later in the conversation, Joan wanted me to go to bed with her. I told her I would like to (which was entirely true) but it was impossible in a semi-private room with a roommate to consider. Several times already, the roommate had expressed some unease at my being in the room and wanted to know if I did not have a room of my own. A private room was certainly to be preferred but there is the issue of additional cost ($600 extra per month); however, I told Joan I would look into it to find some way to have more privacy. After another stroll through the hallway as some of the residents were being attended to in preparation for bed, one of the many young, able attendants took over, distracting Joan so that I could make my exit. I disliked not saying a proper goodbye but that would only create a lot of unnecessary anxiety for Joan. A few minutes with the attendant and Joan would have forgotten all about me and our conversation. Sad, was it not, that distraction was the best way to say goodbye? But that was the way it was. Welcome to the world of dementia and the memory-impaired.

The next morning, May 1, I had a special May Day task. Get Joan to allow the hair stylist to trim her hair. This I knew would be a great challenge but I arrived early the next morning at around 9 o'clock armed with fresh muffins for the staff and the determination to use all the wiles in my possession to get Joan's long, wild hair trimmed and tamed. My main argument was the financial one. Her haircut was, in effect, free, already paid for in advance when Joan was admitted. Like any of us, Joan liked a bargain and so was willing enough to get in the barber's chair in the small beauty salon on Birchview's first floor. I sat in a chair next to Joan, trying to distract her with the story of my 90-year-old mother's weekly appointments at her salon in Ft. Lauderdale, Florida, while the stylist began cutting, wetting Joan's hair with a spray bottle every so often. Pretty soon though, Joan was complaining at the stylist's every move. The stylist, however, was very fast, and very good, and within a short time, Joan was transformed, against her wishes. If Joan had any lingering doubts about the wisdom of getting her hair cut, they soon disappeared for everyone who passed by Joan as she sat with me on the sofa in the fireplace room commented on how nice her hair looked. I looked on proudly like I had been the artist. I must say, I felt like it was a major accomplishment.

At one point I told Joan that I soon had to leave for an appointment in Fairhaven. Her look of anxiety told me she was not ready, and probably never would be ready, for a straightforward goodbye even when it was followed with the promise of return. Before long, the nurse saw my situation and immediately distracted Joan so I could get away to keep my appointment.

May 3, 2012

I arrived Wednesday noon at Birchview wondering how Joan would be today, "down" as she had been over the weekend or "up" as the last two days. As I started to enter the dining room I spotted Joan at a table for two talking with a fellow resident who I learned later was newer to Birchview than Joan. I watched them raise their fruit juice glasses to each other, clinking them in salute, and drinking the juice with gusto. I was so happy to see Joan talking and gesturing that I held off joining them at the table until the resident's brother joined them. At that point, I did too. Joan was definitely "up", animated and actually ate some of her vegetable soup and ham sandwich and most of the fruit cup.

The brother and I had a good conversation, talking a lot about his current pet, a black lab, and the daily walking the dog forced him to do, much to his betterment he was quick to admit. We got into a discussion of the value of walking and exercise generally because at some point his brother quit walking and soon lost his ability to get around. Now, with the aid of a walker, he was starting to walk the long hallway at Birchview and regaining his strength. As I told him, I had not thought of the long carpeted hallway at Birchview as an asset in that way before, but Joan and I had certainly made use of it. In fact, I spent a good deal of my time with Joan after lunch doing just that, walking the hallway and courtyard. With the spate of sunshine it was pleasant to get outside with Joan. For a few minutes Joan actually sat down on a bench outside while I gently rubbed her sore back but she was soon on the go again, wanting to get out of there and head home.

After my two-hour visit I was tired and soon left, pleased as punch by Joan's healthy turn. The only medical concern was a sore on the back of Joan's calf (I could not remember which leg now) which the nurse said was infected and would probably required antibiotics. Later that evening the afternoon RN phoned saying the doctor had prescribed a medication for the leg and wanted be sure I was notified. Joan was to begin the two week course of pills immediately.

Joan's nephew, Randy Williams and his wife Lucie, took me to dinner at Nell Thorn's restaurant. It was a wonderful occasion, getting caught up on the news over excellent food. I gave Randy and Lucie a copy of my long poem of the Williams family asking them to read it and get back to me with any objections or corrections. Randy had recorded enough songs for a second album of western songs. He was really talented. And Lucie, a medical doctor and currently a hospitalist at St. Joseph's Hospital in Bellingham is no less so, starting her own music career, learning to play the guitar.

May 4, 2012

I arrived later than intended at Birchview. Joan was already seated at the table for the evening meal, this time the attendants (I called them "the girls" by now, a super class of devoted women) had paired her with another resident, a tall friendly guy who was confined to a wheel chair. I watched them for awhile, not wanting to interfere with their conversation but soon ambled over and seated myself. Joan looked over and after a few seconds asked, "Are you Bob?" Immediate (almost) recognition! Her next statement was "I want to go home." I helped Joan eat her meal of barbecued pork and a

Mexican corn dish, both nicely seasoned with chocolate ice cream for dessert. After a half hour I got up to check with the RN about Joan's condition. They had started the antibiotics to treat the lesion on Joan's left calf. Looking again at Joan, still talking with her table mate, I departed for the day. I was working on the organization of this book dealing with Joan's journey and wanted to get back to it so I could get over to the printer in Anacortes tomorrow to create a few hard copies. As usual, I found it difficult to leave Joan without a goodnight kiss but realized that my romantic impulse would only make Joan anxious. She would want to get in the car and go home with me.

As it turned out, Joan did get in the car with me after all the next day, only it was not to go home but to the medical clinic in La Conner to see her doctor. The nurse in charge the next morning phoned to tell me Joan awoke with a swollen left leg and that the doctor wanted to see Joan that afternoon at 4:15 pm. I was not sure how Joan would react to her "freedom" but I need not have worried. Joan took no particular note of her surroundings during the trip and was quite happy, it seemed, to be back at Birchview. The girls had saved a hot plate of food for her and seated her with her old friend. I joined them to help Joan to eat another good meal of tilapia, mashed potatoes and peas, all of which were again pleasantly seasoned. At one point, I excused myself and went over to the attendants and nurse to thank them for seeing that Joan had on her nicest clothes (her gray corduroy pants and green wool, cable-stitch cardigan). On top of that they had managed to put waves in Joan's pretty silver hair. Needless to say, perhaps, but in my opinion, Joan could not be better cared for and looked after than at Birchview. I cannot sing the praises of the attendants staff highly enough, caregivers all. She was clearly in the right place.

That still did not mean she did not want to get out and go "home", a theme she kept repeating for the rest of our short time together after supper. I discovered that her table mate, too, wanted to get home. He told me at table that as soon as he was through eating he was going to hop in his truck and head south. Another resident, meanwhile, as we sat in the dining room, was periodically trying the exterior doors, shaking them, in the hope, apparently, that they might open and set her free. I asked the door-shaking resident where she wanted to go but I could get no clear answer from her. Like Joan she wanted to get out and go "home" but beyond that the destination was ill-defined and murky. After dancing with Joan in the parlor room to music from the Steely Dan LP and walking the hallway several times, I made my exit while one of the girls distracted her.

I worked on the book too long last night, had only four hours sleep, and was tired and had to get "home" myself but in my case I knew exactly what and where it was. At 7 pm with relatively little traffic, the drive home was pleasant enough. My only worry was Joan's swollen leg and the slight splitting of skin in the shin area and consequent seepage. The doctor and I were both surprised at how little swelling there actually was but what about the future? The swelling stems from lack of protein or albumen in the body apparently which, in Joan's case certainly, was a direct result of not eating enough. One of the girls mentioned that Joan seems to eat much better when I was with her which confirmed my conclusion that I should visit Joan around meal times.

May 5, 2012

I arrived at Birchview just in time to join Joan and her table mate for a Mexican style lunch in recognition of Cinco de Mayo which featured refried beans and a taco salad of hot ground beef and shredded cheese poured over lettuce, purple cabbage and small tortilla chips. I was watching Joan and her friend eat when the weekend chef offered me a salad, compliments of the house. I ate every scrap. Joan and friend did pretty well too. Joan even downed her entire glass of protein shake. When I took Joan in to the La Conner Medical Center yesterday she weighed in at a little over 88 pounds which was up a couple of pounds over what she weighed 3 weeks earlier. Joan said her swollen leg did not hurt or bother her in any way and the weekend nurse looked at Joan's leg wound and replaced the bandage. She checked to make sure she got her antibiotic. So everything looked good medically.

As usual, Joan kept wanting to get in our car and go home and I kept replying that that was not possible, that she had all her furniture in her room in Birchview now and had a lot of good friends among the staff who cared for her and wanted her to stay. We talked a little bit over small cups of ice cream one of the girls brought us after Joan said she was hungry (this just an hour after lunch) but mostly we walked hand-in-hand. At first Joan complained about the cold but with a hooded jacket and a cap and many laps back and forth along the courtyard pathway, she warmed up. At one point I suggested we jog. "No", she said, "I just want to jig." A few minutes later, I pointed to the clearing sky with the broken clouds. She wanted to know what was pretty about "broken cows." Finally, Joan was willing to sit still for a few minutes in front of the big stone fireplace. When I returned from the restroom, she was asleep. At that point one of the girls let me out a side door. I was there a little over two hours which was about my limit. The good thing was we got a lot of outdoor exercise even within the confines of the fenced area.

I will probably see Joan around supper time tomorrow to vary the hours. I needed the stretch of time Saturday night and Sunday to complete preparation for printing hard copies of my current project so that I and other readers can begin the task of critiquing and improving layout and text.

May 6, 2012

With the sun and warmth of a Sunday afternoon, the drive up Route 20 to Birchview was pleasant as was my greeting at the door. One of the younger attendants was standing there with Joan. She had seen me pull up in front and had located Joan and walked her to the front entry. She said Joan had been looking for me. Joan was obviously pleased to see me. She walked me over to the big sofa in front of the fireplace. We sat down and she immediately rested her head against my shoulder and gripped my arm. There we sat until called for supper, a half hour later. Joan, half asleep, did not want to rouse herself but after a short walk to her room to urinate and wash her hands, we proceeded to the dining room where the same attendant had a table set for us. Over a meal of breast of chicken, rice pilaf and green beans with chocolate cake for dessert, I encouraged Joan to eat, cutting up her chicken for her. She did pretty well. I was particularly glad to see her drink all of her health shake.

After the satisfying meal, I bundled Joan up in her down vest and wool cap (she complained of being cold all through the meal due partly to the cool air circulating in the dining room from the overhead venting system It bothered me too) and we began our walk up and down the long courtyard walkway. As usual it was hard to get Joan to slow down and enjoy the spring sun and birds flitting about. She wanted to get out of there and get home. I explained to her many times that Birchview was where she lived and again showed her her furniture and closet where her familiar clothes now hung which seemed to convince her for the moment.

While in her room I removed her shoes to redo the laces and took the time at that point to check out the swelling in her left leg. The swelling was obvious, made to look worse by the tight running sock hugging her ankle. The tear on her shin was also bleeding. At that point I pulled off both socks (her right leg showed some swelling too). I notified the duty nurse and she in turn noted it on her chart so the night nurse, who was just coming on duty, would check out Joan's legs and in turn notify the attendants to use softer, less tight socks of which there were several pairs in Joan's sock drawer. Meanwhile, I would find today some knee length socks with only slight elasticity. Perhaps that would help. The wound on the back of Joan's left leg had been checked daily and the antibiotic taken on schedule as expected.

Joan complained of back pain and was tiring so I suggested she lie down on her bed so that I could rub her back. She was agreeable and was soon sighing contentedly and within minutes was sound asleep. With a final check with the night nurse to inform her that Joan was now asleep and with a thanks to the young attendant and the others gathered in the nurse's station, I let myself out the front security door and as required jotted down my exit time on the guest register. It was 7:10 pm.

It seemed that my new role as caregiver was defining itself as we moved along: working with the staff to help Joan eat well, looking after her physical health and tracking her clothing needs. I also spent a few minutes reorganizing Joan's chest of drawers and getting the attendants to help me find one of Joan's missing slippers.

May 7, 2012

A short visit, arriving at Birchview at about noon and departing about an hour later. Joan recognized me immediately as I entered the fireplace room. Heading to the dining room, the lead server invited me to lunch, providing me with my own plate. Joan ate only a little of her sandwich and even less of her macaroni and cheese. I was not particularly hungry either but managed half a sandwich. I walked with Joan for awhile but Joan said she was tired so I had her rest in the parlor room on the big sofa while I rubbed her sore back. She was soon fast asleep. At that point I quietly exited, notifying the duty nurse of Joan's whereabouts on the way out.

May 8, 2012

Today I arrived at Birchview about 3:00 pm to attend the first of four classes on dementia. The nursing supervisor presented a well-organized and informative power point. Dementia is an umbrella term to cover all aspects of memory loss. Alzheimer's covers 70% of all dementia cases. Alzheimer's was a disease of the brain At death, an Alzheimer's brain deteriorates to the point where it weighs only one pound. A normal brain weighs three.

Following the class which lasted until 5:15 pm or so, I joined Joan in the dining room who was sitting with one of the other residents. Joan recognized me right away and her smile told me she was glad to see me. Joan, as usual, was eating little so I pitched in, eating her broccoli and a piece of the tender chicken which had been cooked in a nicely seasoned sauce with some bits of ham and a side of pasta. Really quite good. After a small cup of sherbet for dessert, I walked Joan back to her room to help her into her down vest and to find a cap for a walk in the courtyard, a standard ritual these days. She was wearing her leather, opened-toed sandals; a look in her closet told me why. She had only one shoe of each of her three pair. Before the evening was over, an attendant found the other slipper and soft cloth shoe but not the other New Balance running shoe. The attendants will all be searching for it in the course of their duties but no luck so far. Joan and I had a nice walk moving in a circle through the hallway and then outside and back inside. We stopped in the parlor room to dance to the Beatles for a few minutes but she quickly tired. I eventually led her back to her room and bed where she wanted to be but once in bed she could not relax. In spite of my gentle massage of her back and shoulders, she became restless, worried about whether her family, our kids, knew where she was but mainly she wanted to go home, to leave now and described her feeling at that moment as "very painful." At this point I called for help so I could get out of there. It was becoming much too painful for me as well. An attendant and the duty nurse, both intervened. The nurse explained to Joan that this was for just tonight and we could talk about it some more tomorrow. Joan said she did not want Bob to leave. The attendant said I had to leave to go into town to buy another pair of running shoes. With that, the attendant gave me the high sign and I quickly departed.

This little episode at the end of the day was obviously trying for Joan. It was trying for me as well. I so much wanted to get Joan dressed and take her home with me. I could not stand the pain. No sooner had I let myself out the door than I once more broke into the gulping sobs I thought I had overcome. Right there and then I was in as much pain as I have ever felt since our initial separation, April 10. Was it ever going to ease up? I had felt pretty much under control, my strength gathering. But here I was now as I recounted the separation last night, breaking into tears yet again! In the class today, the nursing supervisor referred to the last stages of Alzheimer's as "The Long Goodbye." Yes indeed. Given the difficulty of getting away this evening and on other past evenings as well, I was going to confine my visits to mornings or around the lunch hour at least for the time being. Maybe that would help both of us to cope.

Hello, Hello?

The public telephone, sheltered by
steel and plastic, stands lonely vigil,
at the marina's south basin,
its entry perpetually open
to catch people on the move.
Stiff with disuse, the black pay phone,
chrome trimmed, still works.
Put a quarter in and the dial tone
hums in expectation, waiting
for fingers,slow or eager, deliberate
or frantic, to jab the numbers
and make connection. But does anyone
whisper in its ear anymore?
Is there ever a voice now,
raised in passion, to right a wrong?
Does it ever hear these days,
of age's lament, Chronos' quick passing,
leaving its sad trail of obsolescence?
Is there ever an occasion, lately,
when a soothing valentine voice
from the phone's shelter protects us,
for a few moments, from the wind
and rain?

May 11, 2012

I shopped for and after second store found a pair of white NB training shoes for Joan in exactly her size. When I got to Birchview, I located Joan and we tried the new shoes and walked up and down the hallway. They seemed to fit. Of course, overnight somebody found Joan's other shoe that had gone missing earlier. Oh well, now she has two pair for walking. Today we did just that, walking, hand in hand, our usual route in and out of the building. The air had a slight nip to it, so the down jacket I had gotten Joan for Christmas came in handy. Right now I cannot find her gray polytech jacket with the faux fur collar and cuffs but suppose it will show up eventually. There always seemed to be something missing.

At 2:30 or so we sat at a dining room table with one of the other residents, while we enjoyed a glass of juice and a nutrition bar, two of many snacks served by the attendants as they wheeled the cart down the hall. A pleasant two hours with Joan. She remembered me throughout my visit and enjoyed, as I did, holding hands and sitting, for a few minutes here and there,, on one of the comfortable benches in the courtyard, snuggling close, exchanging love words, as birds whizzed by busy with feeding the young. One of the attendants took over walking with Joan and I departed feeling much better about the separation this time of day. But it still hurt and I broke into sobs as I got in the car and again, now, as I wrote about it. I could not believe the lack of control over my emotions.

I stopped to talk with the La Conner postmaster who had lost her husband last November. How did she handle it, I wanted to know. She did not, she replied. And then she described the experience of someone saying to her that she must have good days and bad days. "No," she said, "I have good moments and bad moments" within any given day. As she was saying this to me, her eyes filled with tears. Mine did, too. Grievers seemed to form their own unique club. That 'misery loves company' did not quite capture all that I was feeling at this point.

The next noonday I joined Joan for lunch. She was sitting across from her usual table mate, a nice fellow but like the others, quiet, but a good eater, finishing everything on his plate. Joan ate little, a few bites from her sandwich and maybe half the small bowl of soup. The lead server was happy to bring me half an egg salad sandwich and a few chips. A perfect lunch. Joan recognized me immediately which was becoming par for the course these last few days. Nice to be known and smiled at by your lover.

I had talked with the development director about venturing outside with Joan. He urged me to try it, making several suggestions. I ended up driving around town getting used to the lay of the land and stopped at Hal's Drive-In for an ice cream cone. Joan ate all of a double-dip of vanilla and seemed to enjoy the excursion. The next time we might travel farther afield, finding new places to walk perhaps even trying her old stomping grounds in La Conner. It would be more interesting for me, and I was sure for Joan as well, to consider outside options.

The other major departure from the usual routine was the surprising fact that not once on the visit this time did Joan mention wanting to go "home." Did getting outside and in the car have anything to do with the change? I am curious to see Joan's take on our next visit.

May 12, 2012

Yesterday, Friday, in the afternoon, Birchview celebrated Mother's Day with family members invited to enjoy a wonderful array of desserts and to listen to live entertainment from the development director's talented daughters playing violin and piano, followed by a professional balladeer who banged out some wonderful tunes with her music hall voice and electronic backup. Family members and staff could also buy plants for Mother's Day which were displayed in the sunny courtyard. All in all, a delightful occasion.

I arrived soon after the beginning of festivities and located Joan sleeping in the common room in a big lounge chair. She was sleeping so soundly that I did not have the heart to awaken her . As it turned out, Joan slept through the entire event which was probably just as well since she would not have enjoyed the noise and confusion. I left her still sleeping in the lounge chair for an hour or so. One of the attendants informed me that she and others had dressed Joan for bed by 8 pm last night but she was up again by 9 pm and soon settled on one of the soft lounge chairs in the common room (the same room where I found her today) and slept the night. I liked the way the girls handled it. They did not try to get Joan back in her bed but chose rather to let her sleep where she was, checking on her often, making sure she was safe and warm.

May 13, 2012

As usual, Joan and I lunched together in the dining room at Birchview. Joan did not eat much, a few bites of her ham and cheese sandwich and a couple of spoonfuls of soup. I was not particularly hungry and was happy with half a sandwich and a few potato chips. Joan always seemed to down her health shake which in the first days she would not do. Before I had finished, she was already to leave, the words I had hoped not to hear, I heard loud and clear: "Let's go. I want to get out of here. I want to go home."

Hoping she would settle for a drive, we got in our Saab and drove east on highway 20, planning to drive to Concrete, but after we were underway, I could see Joan was not particularly enjoying the ride and so settled for the town of Lyman only 8 miles away which I had never actually visited before. I thought I might find a small grocery store in the business center and possibly an ice cream of some kind for Joan. I found only a post office and an attractive city hall building which looked to be an older former home painted a brilliant white with stately, two-story columns along the front. Apparently the folks in Lyman got their groceries at the Mercantile Center nearby on highway 20. Joan was not interested at all in Lyman's architecture, or anything else for that matter. I wondered, in fact, whether she could even see. Not knowing what else to do that Joan might enjoy, I returned to Sedro-Woolley and to Hal's Drive-in for another ice cream. This time I got her two dips in a cup which she ate as we drove back to Birchview.

As we got out of the car and headed up the front entrance Joan hesitated. "I don't want to go in there." I thought "Oh no. Was this going to be a struggle?" but with my words of encouragement, we went through the doors and back into the fireplace room which Joan seemed to accept immediately as a familiar, welcoming place. There were no more words about going "home".

While we were walking the grounds. Joan got sidetracked by what another resident was doing. I explained she was just watering the flowers in the new greenhouse but Joan wanted to see more so at that point I went into the hallway and sat down to wait for her. After some time it occurred to me that this might be good time for me to depart and after checking with the nurse, did just that. The nurse reassured me that Joan would be fine. At that point I saw Joan through a window. She was walking outside in the courtyard and had by now probably forgotten that I had even been there, a realization I continued to find extremely hard to accept. Will I ever?

May 15, 2012

I have begun to think visiting Joan every day was too much and was now going to try every other day to see how that worked. I skipped yesterday, Monday, since I wanted to prepare for a luncheon on Tuesday noon which meant baking bread and the dessert and cooking the chicken for the vegetable soup. I debated going to see Joan late that afternoon but then neighbors were interested in buying our Eurovan camper and I had other shopping to do so did not. It may well be the case that I missed Joan more than she missed me. In any event I felt uncomfortable missing a day. The duty nurse called to say that there had been a slight incident. Joan apparently walked into a male resident's room and was promptly grabbed by the arm and escorted back out. Joan complained that his tight grip had hurt her arm. The nurse said there was no bruising and later on observed Joan talking pleasantly with the same resident. Generally speaking, the nurse thought Joan was doing quite well, sometimes walking alone, sometimes with others, seemed content and expressed no interest in going home. It was her opinion that visiting every other day made perfect sense under the circumstances.

Since I began classes on Caregiving this Wednesday for six weeks at the Burlington Senior Center, I will have to follow the Monday-Wednesday-Friday sequence. After six weeks I would revert to visiting every other day. I packed another box of Joan's many sweaters to send to Susan to wear. Almost all of them are pull-overs which Joan struggled with and would not wear again. The few cardigans were already in her closet at Birchview. I would have to do some more shopping soon for summer weight running pants with elastic cuffs.

May 16, 2012

Because I hosted a luncheon for three friends at my house to celebrate a friend's belated birthday. I did not get out to Birchview until 4 pm. I found Joan in a lounge chair in the common room where other residents were watching the Hallmark Channel and a replay of a *The Waltons* episode. She apparently had slept there most of the afternoon and was just waking up as I arrived. She seemed glad to see me, holding my hand and after a few minutes whispered that she loved me. I was struck by how pale, thin and unwell she looked, her eyes red-rimmed and without the customary eyes glasses. She said she was tired and wanted to know if I wanted to come to bed with her. I told her that that was a nice idea but it was much too early. She said it was getting dark outside until I pointed out the window at the sunny scene. I reminded her that she had not had supper yet which seemed to surprise her.

After sitting quietly with Joan for awhile watching *The Waltons*, she finally agreed to putting on her shoes and going for a walk with me "to work up an appetite". Pretty soon we sat down at our customary table. The staff invited me to a meal on the house but I declined. I was still trying to recover from the big luncheon I had prepared earlier. I did take a bite of Joan's chicken fried steak and mashed potatoes and gravy which were seasoned just right but Joan took only a few nibbles. She did drink all of her health shake which was something, of course, but no substitute for the food on her plate. All she could think about and talk about was the old, haunting theme: Going home.

Before long Joan grew restless, getting up and trying to open the heavy door in the dining room to the courtyard. I got up and helped her to push the door open and then walked with her up and down the courtyard pathway as she tried to find an open gate. I found the whole experience with Joan today to be totally depressing. Sometime later, after Joan and I had come back inside, she suddenly went rushing after another resident who was going out the courtyard door. At that point I made my own exit out the front entryway, asking an attendant who happened to be in the hallway to check on Joan in a few minutes. She said she would. One of the many things I liked about Birchview, as I had mentioned before, was the quality of the attendants, all of them certified with continuing on-site training. If the attendant said she would check on Joan, I was confident she would do just that.

Would the time ever come when Joan was satisfied and accepting of her new address at Birchview? I was beginning to doubt it. I must remember, though, that Joan had been residing there for only 35 days, slightly more than a month. So what would happen if I took Joan up on her wish and brought her home again? What would happen, undoubtedly, was that she would be doing the same thing, wanting to go home and looking for ways out. Two things would be different. Sleep deprived, I would soon wear out and, secondly, I could not provide the same level of ongoing professional care she now received even if I employed a home care agency. This was the nature of the ongoing debate I continued to have with myself as I drove back and forth between La Conner and Sedro-Woolley. Obviously, I had some accepting to do myself.

The Summer's First Rose

A rose is a woody perennial of the genus *Rosa*, within the family
Rosaceae. There are over 100 species. They form a group of erect
shrubs, and climbing or trailing plants, with stems that are often
armed with sharp prickles.

An accurate description is it not?
What would we do without the order science brings?
And yet, on this glorious summer morning
the sun's first rays
just beginning to wipe away the night's damp
from the delicate yellow petals,
I see nothing but this solitary rose,
surrounded, shoulder-high,
by its clustered leaves,
the contrast of the golden yellow
against the deep green,
the beauty
time-stopping,
riveting as Moses' fiery glimpse.
And as untouchable,
both flame and thorns
warding off invasion,
keeping our hands at bay
that our hearts may
hear

in the confirming silence
what Moses heard:
"I am."
I am able to behold beauty.
I am made to love it.
I am here to express it.

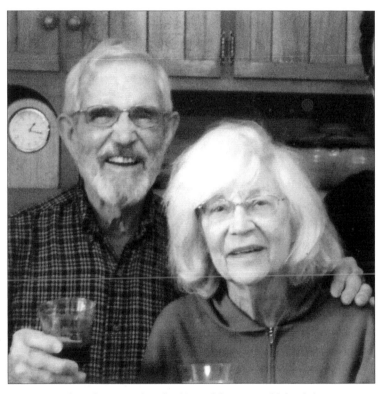

Bob and Joan in their kitchen, celebrating Bob's birthday.
LaConner, March, 2012

May 19, 2012

The debate ended yesterday. I had completely accepted the fact that Joan was best served where she now was. My mind was put at ease with the required 30 day evaluation I had with the supervisor of nursing. Based on her own observation and the observations from her nursing staff, Joan was settling in nicely even though she was moving constantly, unable to stay in anyone place for any length of time, including at the dining room table for meals.

The only major problem health-wise was Joan's weight loss. She had dropped from 90 pounds to 85 pounds in the five weeks which of course was the same problem I had at home. She did not eat much at any sitting. Surprisingly, Joan was not eating nearly as much ice cream at Birchview which was essential in my opinion to keeping the weight at 90 pounds. I relayed to the supervisor my experience the other day of buying Joan a double-scoop ice cream cone at Hal's Drive-in which I thought would be way too much for Joan to consume. Was I ever wrong. Within a short time Joan had eaten it all. The same was true the next time we stopped at Hal's, only this time she ate the two scoops from a plastic bowl with a plastic spoon. The supervisor concluded, as did I, that the reason Joan did not eat the ice cream at Birchview may have had to do with the small cup it was served in. That is, Joan may have not recognized it as ice cream. The supervisor placed an order with the chef to serve her bulk ice cream in a bowl to see if that worked.

I also alerted the supervisor to another observation I had sitting at lunch with Joan recently. Several times I noticed Joan trying to cut-up pieces of her barbecue beef with her fork but there was nothing there to cut. Same with scooping up pieces of food with the tip of her fork. She saw bits of food where there were none. There were bits of beef and roll on the plate but she missed them by an inch or so. So Joan's faulty vision was another factor in the equation. The supervisor took note.

During the course of the evaluation the activities director dropped by and described her experience of trying to get Joan interested in one project or another only to find within a short time that Joan would wander off to do something else. To the activities director Joan seemed very happy and content in her world, quite a "busy little lady" with lots of things to do. She was never sad, mopey or teary, she never complained, she was never angry. Seen against the community backdrop of dementia and other disabilities, Joan was adjusting well, in the director's opinion, and, except for the weight issue, there was no reason to worry.

On the question of reducing my visits from every day to every-other-day, they saw no problem as far as Joan was concerned. They were also adamant that I take care of myself and if that meant every other day then do it and do not feel guilty about it. Just enjoy Joan those times I did visit. On either schedule Joan would not be able to remember and at my departure would quickly move on to other things.

Joan, they both felt, was at a pretty low cognitive level by the time she arrived at Birchview and they were amazed that I had been able to manage at home for so long. As I looked back on the weeks leading up to admission, I was a little amazed too but I could not have stuck with it as long as I did without the support of the primary caregivers, and others at Senior Services and the leader of the Anacortes support group who spoke to me repeatedly about the importance of respite care for the caregiver, particularly when it was a spouse.

While finishing up the evaluation, I signed papers agreeing to the increased level of care required to tackle Joan's weight loss. The previous level of care had been calculated at $771 per month. The new level of care amounts to $1033 per month. The new monthly fee will now be around $4500. The supervisor pointed out, however, that the overall cost could go back down if they solved the weight loss problem and it no longer required the nurses' attention.

As I got up to leave I thought of one last thing: Joan's nails. Who takes care of grooming details like that. The supervisor explained that since Joan was a diabetic, the nurses were required to do all nail clipping, hands and feet. To find out where the nurses were on that issue, the supervisor used her two-way radio to call the RN on duty and get an immediate update. She had been able to clip two of Joan's fingernails at a time. After that, Joan objected. I had to laugh. I always had a difficult time, too, getting Joan to allow me to cut any of her nails.

I left the hour's meeting quite pleased (immensely relieved, more accurately), with the attention and care Joan was receiving at Birchview. Sure. I was paying a substantial amount of money (at least for me) each month but I knew I could be paying more money up front at home and still not get the quality of care Joan was receiving at Birchview.

I went in search of Joan for lunch. I found her sitting quietly on the sofa in front of the fireplace. The nurse took me aside and told me Joan had not been feeling well this morning, ate no breakfast and several times held her hands to her crotch as if in pain. Had she done that before at home? Pain in the lower stomach Joan has complained of from time to time but never the crotch area. With the Tylenol, Joan seemed to revive a little and ate a big meal, the most I had seen her eat for some time. On top of that she drank all of her strawberry health shake. After the pleasant lunch we retired to the TV room where Joan dropped into a big lounge chair and within minutes fell asleep. At that point I gave the nurses a high sign through the glass window at the nurse's station, and let myself out through the security door, for the first time not on the verge of tears. Given more time, maybe things will work out and I will feel comfortable with my decision.

May 21, 2012

Under my new schedule, visiting with Joan every other day, relieved the pressure, allowed me to get projects done at home and has the effect of making me look forward to seeing Joan. Saturday I had gotten some work done outdoors, weeding the butterfly garden and trimming and mowing the front yard, and indoors selecting and labeling some summer shirts and other items to take to Joan. Most of Joan's other belongings have been shipped to Susan since she was small enough to wear most of Joan's things. One closet and several drawers had now been emptied. The other bedroom closet was loaded with Joan's formal clothing, dresses, a few suits and coats, one with a fur collar and many pairs of handsome shoes, most in excellent condition. I was inclined to wait for Susan's next visit before deciding what to do. Meanwhile, consistent with my intention to downsize in a few years, I was looking to get rid of selected furniture items and probably the entire 12 place settings of Havilland and Co. china. Money from the sale of these items would be used, of course, to apply to Joan's ongoing care.

Saturday had been almost perfect weather-wise, cloudless, only the ghost of a breeze and sunshine. Sunday, by contrast, was mild enough but wet and windy, rain hitting my windshield off and on all the way to Sedro-Woolley. When I arrived at Birchview, Joan was already seated at her usual lunch table across from her usual table mate waiting to be served. Before joining Joan in the dining room, I checked with the nurse who said they were going to try serving Joan her food in different colored bowls with the thought that it might help her to see and identify her food a little better. It was reassuring to know the nursing staff was picking up on my observation that Joan was having trouble seeing her food and were willing to experiment. As it turned out, the food was served on a single plate but I was there to help her cut up her food and spike it for her so that she could bring it to her mouth. In this way she ate about half her serving which was much more than she normally consumed at lunchtime.

As had been the case recently, Joan recognized me immediately and held my hand at the lunch table. She quickly picked up on her old theme of wanting to go home. I said maybe we could do that but I would first need the permission of the director and he was not here on Sunday. I said what I could do was drive her out to the local Dairy Queen for an ice cream cone. She liked that idea so we wasted no time hopping in the car. Interestingly, Joan recognized the Saab and quickly pulled the safety belt over to fasten it as if she had been doing it every day. Joan preferred to sit in the car to eat the soft vanilla ice cream from a small plastic bowl. Incidentally, she almost did not get any. I reached in my back pocket for my wallet to pay for the order and it was not there. Fortunately, I had enough loose change in my front pocket to cover the cost (barely).

With that little sojourn we returned to Birchview which Joan did not recognize and had no enthusiasm for re-entering but she did. As we walked the first floor hallway, I got Joan to sit down with me at different locations but only for a few minutes and then she would be up again ready to go home. Finally at about 3 pm, I left Joan in one of the rest rooms and departed for home myself, alerting an attendant and the nurse of Joan's whereabouts. They both assured me they would check on her.

I did not know why I was so tired yesterday. On the way to Birchview, I stopped at the Goodwill store to drop off a few boxes and pulled into a parking space and slept soundly for a few minutes before continuing on. Perhaps it was the morning workout, first the floor exercises, then the 2 1/2 mile walk with a ten minute stop at the fitness center to pump iron but I do that most every day now that Joan was at Birchview. In the weekly class on caregiving, exercise was recommended as a way to manage stress. It seemed to help me.

June 4, 2012

Seeing Joan every other day usually in time to have lunch with her and to take her for a drive and an ice cream appeared to work as a general rule so far and it gave me the time I need to get things done at home. The real test for me came over the last weekend when I visited our son and his family in Sitka, Alaska and didn't visit Joan for four days.

Monday, when I next met Joan, it seemed no different than other times. She accepted me as a friend and perhaps more as the visit continued. As we sat in the Saab (her car actually, purchased with her own money a dozen years ago now) in the parking lot at the local Dairy Queen and I watched her eat, I was captivated again by her profile and reached over and with the back of my fingers gently brushed her left cheek four or five times. Joan stopped eating, closed her eyes, appearing to enjoy the brief moment of physical contact as much as I.

Joan ate very little for lunch, a few bites of a grilled hamburger which I had cut into small portions and a couple of French fries but I was glad to see she drank all of her health shake and two glasses of fruit drink. Later I thought to ask the nurse what Joan's weight was these days. She was happy to report that Joan was back up to over 88 pounds! The nurse and I both did a thumbs up to that bit of good news. Joan seemed tired, almost falling asleep at the dining table, as we waited for our lunch so when we returned from the drive, I took her into the parlor and while she lay on her left side I rubbed her back which often lulled her into a nap. Not today however. She had to get up and get going but where she was not sure. Walking down the hallway ahead of me allowed me to single one of the attendants who immediately stepped in and redirected Joan while I made my exit. I doubt I would ever become used to leaving Joan like that, without a proper farewell, but the staff kept reassuring that after a few minutes Joan would have forgotten I was ever there.

Over lunch I told Joan I had visited our son in Sitka, Alaska, mentioning all the family names. None of them rang a bell. Joan remained unresponsive and so I moved on to other topics. At one point in the conversation, she said she had to get to "school." I thought, "Oh, good. She is not thinking of getting "home" for a change." The hope was short-lived. After the ice cream, Joan wanted to stay in the car and head home then and there.

Speed Zones

Driving the Cascade Highway toward Sedro-Woolley
the speed zone changes from 30 mph to 50 mph just as
you pass the Skagit Adventist School.

On the return trip heading toward Burlington the speed
zone changes from 50 mph to 30 mph just as you pass
the Adventist Church.

Isn't that the way it's always been in the church's grand
intent? If you're living life in the slow lane, it urges you
to pick it up, to make something of yourself.

If, on the other hand, you're living life in the fast lane,
it urges you to slow down, to take time to smell the
roses, to find joy in every moment.

How about that? Is the metaphor apt? Can it possibly be
that the church, generally speaking, is not a speed trap
after all, trying to catch violators in their sins,

But a speed zone urging us, in our comings and goings,
to become something better, accelerating our service to
others in the slow, deliberate practice of love?

July 13, 2012

Although there is a big gap since my last entry, I had continued to visit Joan at Birchview on a regular basis, shifting recently back to daily visits. The change in schedule was prompted by my sense of change in Joan. Suddenly she recognized me, missed me and was desperate to keep me nearby, holding my hand, and frequently asking me to kiss her. I still tried to have lunch with Joan most days which seemed to help her to eat more and then stay for another hour or so, often taking her as before in the car for a small sundae at the local Dairy Queen. I had toyed with the idea of bringing Joan back to La Conner for a walk along First Street but it was a long drive and I was not sure what it would prove.

Father's Day brought two of our sons for a quick visit. Matt flew in from Vermont and David from Pennsylvania, meeting at SeaTac airport and driving north in a rental. They were both in fine spirits, met some of my friends and most important of all, had a good visit with their mother at Birchview. As expected Joan was not able to identify either of her boys by name but after lunch in the dining room as we walked along the corridor, she put her arm around each of her son's waists in turn, rested her head on their shoulders and smiled as only a proud and pleased mother could. At some fundamental level, I was convinced that Joan knew Matt and David to be her sons. They thought so too. It was nice to hear that they liked Birchview and thought their old man had made the right placement decision.

Just minutes before our arrival I had gotten a phone call on my cell phone from the duty nurse at Birchview, informing me that there had been an 'incident' last night. "Oh, no", I thought. Joan, it was reported, decided in the middle of the night to sleep in the hallway which was not as bad as it sounded since the hallway was nicely carpeted and frequently vacuumed. Later, while Joan lay sleeping a resident came by, saw Joan's prone body and nudged her with her foot. Joan took exception to the rude awakening, got up and socked the other resident! There was a slight note of pride in the nurse's voice. While not approving Joan's reaction, she was glad to see her feistiness and spunk. As I pulled into the parking area at Birchview, I reported the incident to the boys. None of us were quite sure what to expect as we entered the front door but, as conveyed above, the meeting was quite pleasant and as normal as could be expected, two of the boys and their mother united for a little while at least. Susan, our daughter, plans to visit sometime this summer and John, the other son, in October after fishing season.

I felt the pressure of visiting Joan every day. The 18 miles to Sedro-Woolley was not a long distance but the daily repetition made it seem longer. At this juncture, though, I would not have it any other way. After one of the young attendants told me she had found Joan crying one morning before breakfast, made me more determined than ever to be there regularly. Why Joan was crying was unknown but the fact that she was, filled me with sadness for what I could only construe as her loneliness. Even with daily trips, I had been able to get my next book of poetry and prose to the printing company and am beginning now to bring the book dealing with Joan's dementia into focus, so I was still able to do some of the things I wanted, needed, to do.

In response to our son, John's e-mail, I described this evening's visit with his mother: Just got back from a visit with Joan over supper at Birchview. Happy to see she ate well (Tilapia with cheese sauce and green beans) and recognized me right away and as we walked the grounds, told me she loved me followed by the wish to see her brother Bill and her mother who were somewhere nearby. I sat outside in a lounge chair with her until she decided to look for a way out and just got up and wandered down the enclosed side-walk. At that point I departed but will return tomorrow for lunch to greet her and say a silent goodbye again. Our daily visits seem to last about two hours, so sweet and so sad.

July 14, 2012

I arrived at Birchview in time to join Joan for lunch in the Dining Room. She was already seated with her usual meal partner. The staff had seen me coming and set a place for me. Slowly this place was becoming a second home, the residents, staff and attendants alike becoming good friends.

I had a chance again today to observe Joan's change in eating style. It took her about an hour and a half to get through her simple lunch of a half a ham sandwich, small bowl of soup and corn chips. She seemed not to want to place a typical spoonful or forkful of food in her mouth but instead would select a small portion and only sip or nibble at it. I have mentioned this before but it appeared to be getting worse, slower. The significant thing, though, was that she, in fact, ate most of her lunch (I gauged she ate 90% of her meal) but we were seated at the table long after the other residents had left the dining room. Joan resisted any attempt on my part to encourage her to take bigger bites. It is a puzzling phenomenon. I must do some research to see what was behind it. Obviously not characteristic of dementia or we would have had late company as Joan sat there nibbling away.

The other thing that got my attention this afternoon occurred when Joan declared she was finally done eating. The only other resident in the dining room was an older man who was sound asleep in his chair at the table next to ours. As we got up to leave, Joan went to him, patted his head affectionately and bent down in what looked like an attempt to kiss him. At this point one of the attendants came over quickly and moved Joan toward the exit stating to me that the resident sometimes reacted strongly, swinging his arm wildly, when awakened from his sleep. Though unintentional, Joan could have gotten hurt. I, of course, did not like the idea of Joan kissing anyone other than me but I had been told that this was just another one of those things I had to get used to. In the world of dementia, it was not surprising to find male and female residents displaying affection for one another, even sleeping together.

July 20, 2012

Joan continued to be on the move in the Birchview world including most nights. The nurse expressed her amazement that Joan could also manage to stay awake most of the day walking around and like many of the other residents, looking for a way to get "home".

It was the nurse who mentioned that Joan had sustained an ugly wound on her leg above the ankle. It alarmed her that her leg from the knee down had quickly turned red-purple even though the wound itself was healing properly. Tammy promptly reported the matter to Joan's new primary physician who recommended an anti-biotic ointment. I was much relieved to learn from others that Joan had injured her leg when she fell, slid off of, an upholstered recliner she favored and caught her leg on the foot-rest mechanism. Leg discoloration worried me as much as it did the nurse because of Joan's diabetes and the circulation issues that accompany it.

As energetic as Joan has been during the day, I found her sound asleep on the sofa in the fireplace room when I arrived at noon with my neighbor and good friend. He (and his wife) had agreed to be my first responders in case something happened to me and wanted to be acquainted with Birchview and its personnel. I introduced him to the director and the nurse supervisor and all the attendants who were around that day. He was given a tour by the development director. It was in the conversation with development director that the question was raised about Joan's care should I no longer be around. Would she be transferred elsewhere closer to one of the children? I intended to gather my children's opinion but I strongly felt she should stay at Birchview under any and all circumstances. I did not think that Joan could handle the move physically and in spite of all our previous moves she did not, or had not, adapted easily. My friend wanted me and the children to know he was quite willing to represent the children in their absence, visiting Joan, keeping tabs on her care just as I had been doing. It was a most generous offer and I had no doubt of his sincerity. Furthermore, He was entirely trustworthy and would feel his responsibility keenly.

My friend was impressed with Birchview and thought, too, it was a good choice for Joan. He was even accepting of the noon meal which in terms of Birchview's usual fare was a little on the skimpy, bland side: a slice of turkey roll on a slice of bread with a light gravy, sliced cooked carrots and a small cup of jellied cranberries. The dessert was a frugal Rice Krispies square. Fortunately, the gravy was nicely seasoned. Joan ate maybe 70% of it, one tiny bite at a time.

July 21, 2012

I arrived for lunch at Birchview to find Joan sleeping in one of the big recliners in the TV room. She seemed groggy and pale but she came willingly with me so I could change her footwear from slippers to running shoes. She kept falling asleep as I was changing shoes. I learned from the nurse, meanwhile, that Joan had a slight temperature (99.7 degrees) and was congested which I was now hearing for myself along with a lot of coughing. The upshot was to put Joan to bed with the help of one of the attendants, since Joan seemed much too tired to stand, walk to the dining room or to eat. The nurse consulted with the doctor and a round of antibiotics was prescribed to begin immediately. Joan had not had a cold like this for some time and it really worried me. She simply had no stamina to ward off infection. I stayed at Birchview for lunch and checked later to see how Joan was doing. She had gotten up to go the bathroom and returned to a soft chair next to her bed and was sound asleep. With that I departed but would visit again tomorrow at lunch time to see how she was doing.

July 22, 2012

I arrived just before lunchtime as planned to find Joan once again asleep in a soft recliner in the TV room. One of the new, young attendants, was with her coaxing her awake. Together we succeeded finally to walk her back to her room to find a pair of warm socks for her bare feet. Both the attendant and the duty nurse reported that Joan had been up most of the night (again) and was sleeping so soundly that the nurse had not been able give Joan her antibiotic medicine. Once at the table in the dining room Joan drank two glasses of juice and a glass and a half of her health shake but little else. The dining room hostess, heated some chicken soup but Joan ate little. The nurse and supervisor saw that she got her antibiotic. Joan said she felt too tired and wanted only to sleep. I, therefore, walked her to her room and helped her into bed. She was asleep in minutes. I stayed around awhile, checked Joan once again and departed for the day.

At one point the nursing supervisor mentioned that I was free to take Joan to the ER if I thought that best. On the way out the front door I stopped in the supervisor's office to tell her (and the nurse) that taking Joan to the ER was not an option. Joan did not respond well to the ER environment and service, was always agitated by it, and was much better off at Birchview where she was carefully monitored by the RN on duty and under the watchful eyes of the attendants. My last instruction was to continue doing what they had been doing, keeping an eye on Joan and letting the chips fall where they may. No hospitals. As I thought more about Joan's care, one option might be to bring Joan home to our house again under the care of Hospice. At this point I was deeply concerned, worried about Joan's weakened condition and seriously wondered if she would be able to snap out of it. The supervisor invited me to phone at any time to check on Joan's condition.

July 23, 2012

If body language was to be trusted, then our 60 year marriage unofficially ended last night. The dissolution did not stem from the illness described above. When I arrived at Birchview for supper last night about 5:15, Joan was already seated at her usual dining room table with her table mate across from her. I pulled up a chair and said hello. Joan smiled and asked my name. I told her. She responded by telling me her name and extended her hand for me to shake. She then went on to try to introduce her table mate but could not remember his name so I supplied it.

I was pleased to see how well Joan looked. She was alert, no longer pale and was trying to eat but as usual was not able to eat much. I tried to help her by cutting up some of the pasta dish but ended up eating most of it myself. She said she just was not hungry. I was, on the contrary. After I fetched her slippers and helped her put them on at the dining room table, I took her hand as I always do but she disengaged it to stop by her table mate who was just positioning his walker. Joan waited there for him to begin walking and then held onto the walker and walked with him out of the dining room and down the hallway without a backward glance.

After watching them a few minutes, I walked around them to the other end of the hallway to speak with the RN on duty. As I was conferring with her, Joan and her table mate walked slowly by. Joan looked right at me without a flicker of recognition. I watched them continue to the common room where Joan watched her new friend seat himself in a recliner and then sat down in the recliner next to his. At that point I departed for home wondering at the strange state of my life. My love for Joan required that I be happy with Joan's new interest. In the end, her happiness was the only thing that counted.

Even though I recognized we lived in completely different worlds now and that Joan was not the woman she once was, I did not like the change. On the other hand, it took the pressure off me, made me feel it was okay to visit less frequently than every day now that she had apparently found a companion and was presumably less lonely.

July 24, 2010

Concern about Joan's new love life has been superseded by the decline in her physical condition. I thought she was on the mend yesterday but when I arrived at 5:00 pm for supper she looked alarmingly bad, listless, pale, incoherent. While I was talking with Joan in a lounge chair in the hallway, the daughter of a resident and a RN, stopped to see how I was managing. She suggested that it might be time to consider bringing Hospice into the picture. She said Hospice had been tending her father at Birchview for the last several weeks and the special attention had helped immensely. After two hours with Joan tonight I was going to pursue the suggestion particularly when I learned that Joan's weight had dropped to 83 pounds, although it was slightly higher at the last reading, and the nurse reported there was still some congestion in the lungs. Since the first course of antibiotics was ending soon, the nurse was going to recommend to the doctor a second course of a different antibiotic.

Joan and I sat at the supper table with her table partner but she seemed too confused to do anything but concentrate on her plate of food. After nibbling at her meal for a few minutes, she indicated that she needed to get to the bathroom. I walked her to the one nearest the dining room. Once there, she was confused about how to position herself on the toilet and after she urinated kept tearing at her underpants. Finally I got her to stand and pull up her pants and wash her hands but by the time we got back to the table her plate of food had been removed since by this time the dining room was almost empty of diners and the attendants were cleaning up. One of them kindly brought Joan a warm, freshly served plate of food which looked good to me (I was hungry) but Joan just shook her head. No, she did not want it. After some time I convinced her to let me drive her to the DQ for ice cream. She seemed to enjoy the short ride down to the end of Township Rd but after we parked and I brought her a small hot fudge sundae (her favorite) she would not eat it because she had not had supper yet. I finally gave the untouched dessert to two young men who were standing by their car in the parking area nearby and drove back to Birchview. After we were back inside, I conferred with the nurse. She said I should talk with the other RN in the morning about Hospice which I intended to do. While Joan was preoccupied, I slipped out and headed for home and something to eat. It was about 7:00 pm.

July 26, 2012

I conferred with the day nurse before lunch about Joan's declining condition. She felt that Hospice was a fine agency and did a wonderful job but she suggested I hold off on contacting it until she and the doctor had more time to get Joan on the mend. For one thing, they had changed her antibiotics (to Cipro) and already her temperature was back to normal. In fact when I sat down with Joan (and her friend) at lunch, Joan already looked a lot better with some color in her cheeks. She ate none of the beef stew for lunch but she drank two glasses of a health shake and a glass of fruit juice. I noticed her frequent coughing, deep and prolonged on occasion, but it was loose (I could hear the congestion) and not dry. The important thing now, the nurse reiterated, was to make sure Joan kept enough fluids in her body. The nurse said she tried to get Joan to drink some water earlier, before lunch, but she refused saying she never drank water in the morning.

During the course of the meal, Joan reserved a few sweet smiles for her table mate but nothing more. When I took Joan's hand to go outside, there was no effort on Joan's part to stay at the table with him or to walk with him down the hall. Joan and I sat on an outdoor glider in the sun. The sun felt good but soon Joan wanted to walk, a sign of her return to better health. So walk we did but she soon tired so we sat in two of the recliners, side by side, in the common room. After a few minutes though, Joan was up again, wanting me to walk with her. I said "no" and she disappeared down the hall hand in hand with another resident who also does a lot of walking. After awhile, I left to get back home to my writing. I had to finish proofreading a hard copy of my new book and get my comments mailed off to the printing company by 4:30 pm.

July 28, 2012

Yesterday I arrived in time for lunch in the dining room but there was no space for me at the table. Whoever among the attendants had arranged seating, they had a resident at the next table which left no room for me and on the other side, Joan's friend insisted on having his walker against the table. Rather than make a fuss, I told Joan I would be back later and drove into town for lunch. The nurse had offered to place Joan and me at another table but I declined, not wanting to disrupt Joan's ritual of sitting at the same spot every meal. Was I over stressing the importance of ritual? I did not know. Maybe. My lunch consisted of a Cliff Bar from the Food Pavilion. Loaded with protein, it was just right.

When I returned, Joan had finished eating and happily accepted my offer to get in our car and drive to the Dairy Queen for a hot fudge sundae. Joan seemed to enjoy the short drive and managed to consumed about half the small double dip treat. Not too long ago she would have eaten it all. What she did eat, though, she seemed to enjoy. Joan often expressed surprise at returning to Birchview. Today was no exception but she walked through the front door without too much hesitation or resistance, giving me the impression that she was beginning to feel at home.

Once back I conferred briefly with the RN who told me Joan's doctor's vacation replacement visited with Joan, saw improvement and after seeing Joan's record of weight loss suggested that the nurses stop the insulin injections for awhile. I applauded her observation. It might very well be that with the weight loss, Joan could get along without the insulin which may in turn increase her appetite. I left Joan seated in a recliner in the TV room saying I would be back. I used the gentle deception to depart for home. It was 3:30 pm and I was tired.

Bull Trout

Rainbow, brown, cutthroat, lake, who hasn't heard of these,
    but bull trout?
Few left and protected, bull trout are most at home in the
    northwest, the deep
pools and cold, dark holes of streams and lakes, a mystery,
    seldom seen,
without difficulty, seldom caught, and since endangered,
    seldom kept.
Another mystery, from the beginning locked deep in the roil-
    ing waters of
creation's surging power, a word, in time, made flesh, some
    believe,
for all to see, a telling glance, a saving glimpse, perhaps, but
    still, only
a glimpse, no more.

The fly fishers, their wet flies going deep, pull, lug expec-
    tantly, their prize
to bay, the hues of the arctic char bring the mysteries to light,
    admired
and released, hoping, in good faith, to be thrilled again some-
    time by the
deep's brief yield.

The fishermen, of Galilee, catching no bull trout, no mystery in their

mended nets to acknowledge and release, are drawn land-ward instead,

casting their lot with, enraptured by, an old mystery in a new guise

to become fishers of men, the muted colors of the arctic char transformed,

brightened now by the fly fishers' very hope: to witness, to feel, the tug

of mystery. Like the fly fishers, the men fishers never quite knowing

what's at the other end, are thrilled by the prospect and live for it.

Today there was ample room at the round lunch table with Joan's friend on my right and Joan on my left. Joan looked healthy but as usual did not eat much, just a few spoonfuls of soup and a bite or two of her toasted cheese sandwich. The remainder of the sandwich she offered to the table mate. She did, however, drink her health shake and a couple of glasses of fruit juice. I walked with Joan outside and along the hallway inside, Joan constantly urging me to get the car and drive us home, finally settling for the sofa in the parlor room away from the traffic and TV. I rubbed Joan's back a few minutes and then we read some of a Time magazine. To my surprise, Joan began reading to me! And that was not the only surprise. At one point when she was urging me to get the car she elaborated stating that she wanted to get home to sleep in her bed "in the front room." She remembered! We had moved our twin beds downstairs to the front room (to avoid the steep stairway). Today, obviously, Joan was operating at a higher cognitive level. Who knew what her cognitive level would be tomorrow. Apparently it varied from day to day even as the general direction of the dementia was down.

I walked some more with Joan and at about 2:30 pm, did what I did yesterday: left Joan sitting in a recliner without any hint of my intent to depart and then did just that, walking out the front door of Birchview and, as usual, feeling terrible about it.

August 15, 2012

I kissed Joan one time too often, apparently because I came down with the same symptoms that had affected her, first a sore throat, then nasal congestion and then heavy congestion in the chest and a fever. Two and half weeks now and I still have a lingering cough but at least the fever is gone and the congestion. Except to fetch the mail and a few groceries I did not venture out of house. A neighbor fortified me with a big pot of homemade chicken soup which I devoured over the course of the first few days and I was sure sped my recovery. I did manage while inactive, however, to make strides in editing the book on dementia and was now getting my full second draft to my critical readers.

Yesterday I attended the last of four monthly classes on dementia being offered by the nursing supervisor and then had supper in the dining room with Joan and her table mate. Joan had no particular response that indicated her surprise to see me after my long absence. It was more like I was joining her for another meal. She was glad to see me, even then, smiling and reaching for my hand but all low key and matter-of-fact. She looked pale and unwell and I watched her eat maybe a total of one bite of her hot meal of spaghetti and delicate meat sauce and cooked vegetables. I urged her to take a walk with me outside and since she did not want to do that, offered a drive to DQ for a sundae but she did not want to do that either. She seemed to prefer just to sit at the table, mute and passive. After awhile I got up, checked with the duty RN, to report my concern about Joan's lack of appetite and called it a day and headed home to supper. An attendant had offered me a sumptuous plate of food at table but I declined. For some reason I wanted, my body craved, only fresh vegetables. Once home, I chowed down on a huge salad, much bigger than I thought I could eat.

Today Joan seemed only slightly better. Again she ate next to nothing, the equivalent maybe of one French fry and one small bite of battered fish and a few slivers of coleslaw and that was it. I urged her to eat more but you could just see the look on her face. The food on her plate was totally unappetizing whereas to me it was excellent fare. But then I was hungry. The duty nurse today told me that Joan's weight had actually improved to 84 pounds but she was concerned, too, and speculated that Joan's back was bothering her which may account for loss of appetite. She said she was going to consult with Joan's new doctor about starting Joan on a mild pain killer to see how that might help.

Joan was happy to move outside and sit in the hot sun (over 80 degrees) for a few minutes and when I saw her starting to doze, walked her down to the parlor room where I had her lie down on the sofa so I could rub her back. Within a few minutes, Joan was sound asleep. I departed for home at that point, concerned as ever about Joan's health. I honestly could not see how she survived.

I conferred briefly with the director, business manager and the nurse supervisor to make sure I got the documents I needed to complete the application for the VA's program on Aid and Attendance. Funds for Joan's support at Birchview were projected to run out by next July, so I was banking on the VA to fill the gap between the end of our funds and the time when Medicaid kicked in. I saw no reason why she would not qualify. But, in her present state, would she even be alive then? The question haunted me now as it did when we were still living at home in La Conner. I had to face the fact that Joan's dementia was progressive. It only got worse.

August 25, 2012

Except for the two days I missed when my car broke down right in downtown Sedro-Woolley last Tuesday (a broken idler pulley took out the timing belt), I had visited Joan most every day usually at noon time over lunch. I was just having a difficult time accepting Joan's downturn. I could not be more discouraged than I was now with today's visit.

Even with the nurse's update that Joan was as usual active most all night long and ate a good breakfast of scrambled eggs (with

cheese) and toast, I found her almost incapable of feeding herself.
At the same time she resisted my help. The best I could do was cut
up her food and mash it, in this case mixing canned pears and cot-
tage cheese, but it was still slow and laborious, her face only inches
from the plate. We must have spent almost an hour at table but she
left most of the food on the plate. Later I checked with the nurse
again to learn that Joan's weight seemed to be holding steady at
around 82 pounds. They wanted it to be higher, of course, and were
considering going to the next step of helping to feed her.

Several weeks ago now, the doctor decided to eliminate Joan's
daily insulin shots in the hope that it might increase Joan's weight.
Obviously it had not but Joan's blood sugar rate remained normal
without the insulin shots which meant one less traumatic thing Joan
had to undergo.

Joan talked little these days but sometimes uttered a word or two
I understood. Today she mentioned Cincinnati (Ohio) as a place
she wanted to get to. I had no idea what was behind that wish except that Cincinnati was down river from Portsmouth and she had
relatives who lived there. I walked the grounds with Joan for twenty
minutes following lunch and when she spoke of being tired, I led
her to her room, helped her into bed and rubbed her back. Within
minutes she was sound asleep. I signed out at 1:45 pm and headed
for home to complete some legal work connected with my durable
power of attorney status regarding sole ownership of our La Conner
home. The standard form I used, which I obtained online, did not
contain the power to make any property decisions independent of
Joan, so my lawyer had now to go through the courts to modify the
DPA document so I had sole authority. Such a modification was
required to be eligible for Medicare funding which I was applying
for down the road.

August 29, 2012

Joan's condition has varied over the last three days. One noon time I spent most of the time in the bathroom with her as she tried painfully to have a bowel movement. The nurses were puzzled because they had been working to solve that problem and the previous night she had had a large bowel movement. Finally, the duty nurse manually relieved the blockage and Joan was comfortable and content once again. By this time, however, we had both missed lunch, so one of the caretakers got Joan an ice cream with the promise of more food at snack time.

All the issues suddenly struck me as minor upon receiving a telephone call from the nurse this morning that Joan was experiencing terrible pain in the hip area and that she was being transferred to the nearby hospital by the medics for x-rays. An hour later the hospital phoned me directly to tell me the news I feared most: Joan had fractured her hip. The doctor agreed with my opinion that surgery was probably not a good idea. The trauma of a major operation might well prove too much for Joan at her age and frail condition. It was best to focus on Joan's comfort.

Further conversations with the Birchview nurse, director and the nurse supervisor followed, all deeply concerned to make Joan as comfortable as possible. We all agreed that the cause of the break likely had more to do with Joan's use of prednisone over the last 20 years rather than any kind of fall. The nurse suggested that this was an appropriate time to enlist the services of Hospice. I concurred. She would phone them to get the process rolling. The director was also going to try to do some rearranging so that Joan and I would have a private room where I could visit with Joan at length and perhaps stay overnight.

I had come away from the experience of Joan's hip fracture more thankful than ever that she was at Birchview in the hands of such caring people. I also came away worried about Joan's restlessness and whether she would be content to stay in the hospital bed Hospice was to provide. Trying to keep Joan in bed in a hospital setting had been a nightmare. Perhaps being in the more familiar setting of Birchview would make a difference. I hoped so.

August 30, 2012

I finally got to Birchview at 12:30 pm after an eye exam at North Cascades Eye Associates (to consider a partial corneal transplant to right eye) and stopping at the Hospice offices in Mt. Vernon to sign their consent form. As I was entering Birchview the Hospice nurse was leaving after making an assessment of Joan's needs. She was clearly in pain and so the nurse has prescribed a liquid morphine to make it easier to administer. The Hospice chaplain also stopped by later to confer and determine whether we needed any spiritual support. At my request he enveloped us both in a prayer signifying God's embracing love for Joan and me. Warm, personal, informal, sincere, this chaplain was the real McCoy. I was glad for his presence. Tomorrow the Hospice's social worker, would be making contact to discuss plans down the road.

When I saw Joan, so small and frail among the bed covers, she was resting comfortably with only occasional spasms of pain as her muscles contracted. I stayed by her bedside for an hour or so, stroking her head and talking to her. I think she recognized me. A lot of the time I was crying, the tears dropping to her pillow, as I studied her face. At several points it seemed that she stopped breathing, her face and lips turning pale white, but then the quiet breathing would begin again. She looked like I imagined she would look after she drew her final breath.

I was unbelievably sad as I considered the horrible, austere finality of our separation, Joan lost to me forever. I could do nothing but cry as I did upon Joan's initial placement at Birchview last April, huge, gulping, breath holding sobs, the tears streaming into my beard, interrupted at one point by my son Matt's phone call, his voice and words offering twin solace.

Grief's Second Time Around

Separation's grief visited once before,
a few months ago, Grief, all smiles,
sitting next to me on the drive home
and slipping in the door with me,
as, wailing, and flailing my arms,
I walked and stumbled, blind with tears,
from room to room, humbled at my loss.

Then I had placed my beloved
in the care of others; now her hip fracture
smothers most any hope for longevity,
Grief reappearing on the coattails of life's brevity,
more aggressive now, reaching into my very soul,
pulling me down, down
into a pond of despond, a small lake
of legion's tears, the murky water yielding nothing
but images of my beloved's face,
taken at times when she did not, could not,
remember me.

Occasionally, the power of others'
prayers loosened Grief's hold, lifting me to the
surface for a gulp of fresh air,
and then Grief grabs me again,
pulling me down, down

to view once more my beloved's blank faces,
an imagery that traces her memory's decline ,
and, at the same time, works to define
Grief's intent.

In the sea of tears he looks at me,
with his pal, Guilt, at his side and sneers,
spitting out his words:
This would never have happened,
you know, if she hadn't had to take prednisone
And she wouldn't have had to take prednisone

if she hadn't fractured her back
And she wouldn't have fractured her back
if she hadn't been in the boat with you.
The tears you're shedding aren't just for her!

So maybe this time, this second time, Grief remains,
never letting me forget what my beloved's
memory no longer retains.
But the power of others' collective prayer
is there, too, loosening Grief's hold,
lifting me to the surface, if only for a minute,
to gulp faith's bold and bracing air.

September 4, 2012

This will be my last entry. Joan died this afternoon at about 5:15 pm, an hour after my arrival at Birchview Memory Care. It was as if she had been waiting for me to say goodbye.

I had felt buoyed up by Joan's recent appetite. She was unable to communicate but she was beginning to eat some solid food, yogurt and a portion of her health shake. Yesterday, mid-morning, however, she began to fail, her breathing becoming difficult. At that point the duty nurse began giving her oxygen. When I walked in Joan's room at 4:15 pm, she looked different from previous days, more gaunt and angular, the labored breathing adding pain and discomfort to what I was seeing.

After consulting with the nursing supervisor and the nurse, I settled down on a small chair next to Joan, moistening her lips with a sponge and cooling her face with a damp wash cloth, telling her repeatedly of my love for her and how fortunate and privileged I was to be here with her now. Quietly, with my hand on her shoulder, I asked that she might be spared any further suffering, that she might experience the exit I so desperately wanted for her: a quiet, peaceful, graceful ending.

It seemed that my prayer was answered. Shortly thereafter, Joan's breathing began to change, the period between breaths becoming ever longer and drawn out. I kissed Joan on the forehead once more and then went hurriedly to consult with the nursing supervisor who, it turned out, was coming to see Joan. She quickly went to Joan's side to check her pulse. There was none. Just like that, Joan was gone. Six short days. The supervisor told me that they called it the "Old Folks Blessing." Even through my tears, it was easy to see why. Joan's suffering was quickly over. No more pain. Joan at rest, finally.

The supervisor and nurse both held me for awhile until I could catch my breath. The nurse then told me that she had brought her friend in to play the fiddle for Joan yesterday afternoon and I thought again what extraordinary people there are at Birchview. The nurse had done that entirely on her own without any prompting from me. I found great consolation in the fact that Joan's last days were ones surrounded by music and so much care and concern.

I also liked to think that what she envisioned about her future had actually come about. As she wrote in a letter to Horton Foote in 1996: *When I viewed the recent remarkable eclipse of the moon, I felt somehow a part of the universe, an infinitesimal speck, but nevertheless, I like to think that when I die, and gravity loses its grip on me, I will spin out to join all the other cosmic debris whirling out there and I will find rebirth in the stars.* (*Whittling*, page 251)

As previously planned, there was a party in the dining room at Birchview on that coming Sunday, September 9, to celebrate our 61st Wedding Anniversary. I provided the cake for the residents. Birchview provided the music, a lively guitarist and vocalist. I had heard her perform before at Birchview and she was exactly the right person for this special time. Joining with her and the others, I joyously sang the song Joan and I so often sang together as we walked along La Conner's streets: *Let me call you sweetheart, I'm in love with you. Let me hear you whisper that you love me too...*

Through the pain of loss, the searing finality of our separation, I found gratitude in two incidents, one at the beginning of our life together and the other at its end. I might never have renewed my acquaintance with Joan at the University had it not been for that empty seat next to her in the lecture hall. In a hall of 400-500 students what were the chances of ever seeing her again let alone striking up a conversation? So, I was grateful for an empty chair and my luck in finding it. I was equally grateful that I stayed home to write this love story on the morning preceding Joan's death on September 4. If I had traveled to Birchview in the forenoon as I usually did, I might well have missed being with her that afternoon, bathing her face, kissing her forehead and telling her of my love even as her breathing eased and she was cut loose from gravity's pull.

Love Is Like That: Reunion

As cliff-clinging trees are bent and twisted by years of
booming surf and hammering winds, so are the lovers
bent and shaped by time's silent and relentless power.

The Pacific weather systems come storming up and
down the coast, swirling counter-clockwise, to keep
the lovers guessing tomorrow's brightness.
Time, on the other hand, is just there, quietly clicking

off the days and nights, making the lovers time-smart in a
clock-wise world.
Counter or not, they come to know there is an end to love
and to all they are together.

The ebb and flow of yesterday is now giving over to neap
tide, moving, naturally, inevitably it seems, to where
there is no tide at all.

With their bodies bowing to the earth's pull, "gravitation"
and "grave" are no longer so dissimilar and their vow
to love "until death doth part" is of easy recall.

Together in their padded, dream-filled nightship,
his arthritic right hand soothing her sore right shoulder,
the two silver heads, as if in sleepy conspiracy against the
odds, whisper their surprising contentment,
their tidal past, six decades long, reeled in and settled,
more or less, by their future's short line.

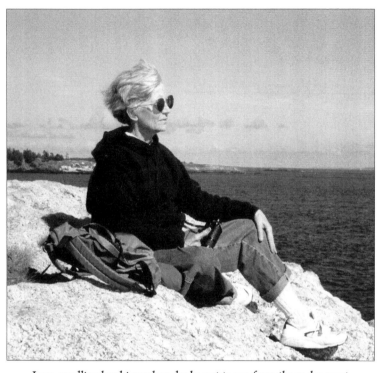

Joan, cradling her binoculars, looks out to sea from the rocky coast.
Near Blue Hill, Maine, 2000

Epilogue

The graveside service for Joan took place at the Pleasant Ridge Cemetery on Valentine Road east of La Conner on Monday afternoon, September 10, 2012, the day after our 61st wedding anniversary. It was one of Joan's final gifts, gathering her children, her nephew and me all together for a family farewell.

Graveside Service

Scripture sentences
Prayer
Psalm 23 and 90
John 14:1-3
Homily—The Rev. George Lockwood
Eulogy
Song—"When We Are Living"
Committal
Lowering of Urn
Military Honors
Lord's Prayer and Benediction

Reading—Annie Quest

She Is Not Gone

"I am standing upon the seashore. A ship at my side spreads her white sails to the morning breeze and starts for the blue ocean. She is an object of beauty and strength, and I stand and watch her until at length she hangs like a speck of white cloud just where the sea and sky come down to mingle with each other. Then someone at my side says "There! She's gone."

Gone where? Gone from sight...that is all. She is just as large in mast and hull and spar as she was when she left my side, and just as able to bear her load of living freight to the place of destination. Her diminished is in me, not in her, and just at the moment when someone at my side says "There! She is gone," there are other eyes watching her coming, and other voices ready to take up the glad shout, "There she comes!" And that is Dying." (Author unknown)

Reading—David Skeele

Excerpt from Joan's letter to Horton Foote

"I just want to comment on one more part of the article about you. I admire what you say about your wife, and I'm sorry you are without her. My husband and I have been married for forty-five years, and I know that after that much time how much a part of each other you become. Neither of us likes to think of the time when one of us will be without the other. But, of course, it will come. I have just finished reading *The Greenlanders* by Jane Smiley. In it, Margret, the main character, who lives, for Greenlanders, to a ripe old age of 62, says, when, I believe it is her daughter-in-law, asks her if she is hardening herself to her approaching death, that no, she tried to make herself into a hard ball, but instead she keeps becoming softer the older she gets, so that when death does come, it will be like the beginning of life instead of the end. When I viewed the recent remarkable eclipse of the moon, I felt somehow a part of the universe, an infinitesimal speck, but nonetheless, I like to think that when I die, and gravity loses its grip on me, I will spin out to join all the other cosmic debris whirling out there and I will find a rebirth in the stars."

Joan's Poem: On a Winter's Day

When on a velvet night
The pin-pricked brightness
Twinkles through,
I sometimes long to be
There,
Caught in weightlessness,
Forever fixed in
Eternity.

Reading—Randy Williams:

Excerpt from Joan's memoirs

"I must have been seventeen that summer, as, the following June, I too joined the service, enlisting in the WAVES, even though the age requirement was nineteen (the recruiting officer and I engaged in a conspiracy to pretend I was of eligible age)....Being at boot camp (Hunter College) wasn't bad, although the food was not great. We were seated at long tables with small swivel seats. We had only a short time to eat and before we knew it, the call came, "On your feet, shove in your seat, let's go!"As a result of this I always ate my dessert first, which was about the only decent part of the meal."

"One time when I was moving forward in the line that was entering the dining building, and another WAVE and I were talking and laughing about something, I was asked to step out of line. My first thought was, "I wonder what I have done wrong." But I was told to report outside in a grassy area, which I did. There, along with about twenty other WAVES, we were asked to sit down on the side of the small hill. Then, a man, the famous artist-photographer, Rockwell Kent, set up an easel upon which he began to draw funny faces on large sheets of newsprint. As we responded in laughter, he took pictures of us. It was only later that I learned that one of the photos became a recruiting poster. I now have the poster, framed, which was on display at the Skagit County Historical Museum during their year-long exhibit of World War II."

Recitation—Susan Skeele

Susan's poem: April Imperative

He arrived in an anorak and a floppy oilskin hat
Spoke in a voice of mud and pliant leaves
Through the window
spoke of following—

The path of pebbles rolled by torrents
Smoke steered by wind
Of climbing a small broken field
In order to turn around and
take in wholeness

I think I'll go with him
It's risky—
I might find the mould from older beds
and learn to
suck nourishment from longing
like dew from moss

Send to bed the unlived hours!
Loose the links in the chain called regret!
Unleash the habit of binding one splendour,
Over and over again to the same
thin householed air.

Go out and find wild loves!
In the unmet grass, the seed of footsteps is unknown
And the swallows laugh lovingly at all the seeming briars
erected into nests.

Go out, beyond the threshold made of human eyes
and navigate, with fiery nerves
the endless hollows and all
the subjugated walls.

October 5, 2012

Almost a month later, a hundred of Joan's friends met upstairs at La Conner Seafood from 5-8 pm to celebrate her rich life marked by raising four children, passing the bar at 59 years of age, opening her own law practice and writing poetry and prose.

I concluded the Celebration of Joan's life with one of her favorite benedictions, one we have used on many different occasions among family and friends. It was created by a dear friend, Dr. Roy Burkhart, who was the senior minister at my home church, the First Community Church in Columbus, Ohio. He conducted our wedding there in 1951:

Benediction

And now may
the courage of the early morning's dawning,
the strength of the eternal hills and deep valleys,
the peace of the evening's ending,
the love of God
and the fellowship of the holy spirit,
be yours,
now and forever.

Sympathy's Symphony

Over the weeks following Joan's death, I received a number of letters, e-mails and sympathy cards. Before putting the cards aside, I read each of them again and was struck by their thoughtfulness and beauty and decided, then and there, to try to capture their essence as best I could. *Sympathy's Symphony* was what I came up with. I included it here as a way of expressing my gratitude to those who had been so supportive to me in the early months but also to honor those among the readers who take the time to offer their support and comfort to others.

To create the symphony, I saw the card givers as individual musicians of the heart who were brought together for a single performance in the hall of imagination, a work of their own creation, a symphony of sympathy, the music they each performed rich with meaning, the high notes of hope and comfort and the low notes of separation and loss blending to perform a grand finale, which, like any good piece of music, was both moving and soothing, challenging and calming, eliciting tears of sadness and joy. Four themes swirled and curled around each other in this musical atmosphere, Death, God, Time and Memory all at home in the other's presence, cutting a new path into a receptive but crusty consciousness.

Death was given the respect it deserved, none of the musicians denying the devastating power it carried for the one who remained to face the future alone. The unspoken assumption flowing through all the lyrics was that the deceased was okay. She was home and safe. One musician's solo sentiment captured it all: Don't think of her as gone away—her journey's just begun, life holds so many facets—this earth is only one/ Just think of her as resting from the sorrows and the tears in a place of warmth and comfort where there are no days and years/ Think how she must be wishing that we could know today how nothing but our sadness can really pass away... (Hallmark) The violinists and violists, their upper bodies bent to the task, manage to soften death's sharp edge, coming in behind the solo with flare, stressing in a series of high notes, the immortal nature of both love and spirit. "Unable are the loved to die. Love is immortality."(Emily Dickinson); Never the spirit is born/ The spirit will cease to be never/ Never the time when it was not/ End and beginning are dreams/ Birthless and deathless and changeless/ Remains the spirit forever/ Death has not changed it at all/ Dead though the house of it seems. (Indian prayer of Passing)

God's name was invoked explicitly a number of times in *Sympathy's Symphony*, as it often is, in the face of death's final claim. Several percussionists, their arms moving methodically among the brass cymbals and tight drumheads, providing the beat, barely noticed, that runs under the melody, holding the orchestra together. In syncopation lies survival, the music wants us to know. Look to the heart, it insists. Pulse is everything. May God, who watches over us and hears us when we pray/Be very near to give you strength and comfort you today/May he bless and keep you within his loving care/And may it help you just to know that He is always there. (Tender Thoughts Greetings) May God's loving compassion surround you and give you strength in the days ahead. (Papyrus) And from a member of the orchestra's Chancel Choir: May God walk with you and bless you as you walk the journey of mourning. (MH, Minnesota) As mourners compelled to reach deeply, God was often the only source to satisfy the unease, if even for a moment.

For others, God's name was not used but implied as a source of consolation and strength: May the gifts of Earth touch our hearts. May we be filled with kindness for ourselves, for our planet and for all beings. May we have the courage to change. (Raventalk) What an incredible journey you have been on. Your faith, love and caring are evident and have been a bulwark for you. I hope they continue to support you tenfold as you continue your life without your wonderful partner. (GB, Pennsylvania) Thinking of you. May the concern and sympathy of those who care help you through this difficult time. (Hallmark)

Time's music was rendered most gracefully by the many flutists whose firm lips and sure fingers, holding the oldest of all musical instruments, create sounds, intricate and subtle, haunting and playful, stirring us to the core, as they weave in and out of the harmonies of others, adding vitality and color to the symphony's glorious mix, soothing and mending us all. With profound sorrow and deep sentiment I read in the local paper about Joan's departure from this world like a gentle rain the sun has dried out but left behind a rainbow of sweet memories of a dear friend never to be forgotten. Peace be with you, Bob. Time heals everything from a wounded bird to a wounded heart. Believe me, it happens. (AG, Washington) Beyond the acceptance of death as a natural process comes the unacceptable loss of loved one. We can't bear it but we do. (SB, Vermont) Someone once said to me what I wish for you: It hurts so much in this difficult time, but then, it is often followed by light. I wish this for you. (LC, Vermont)

Memory, time's closest friend and ally, takes up the reed section, the silver and brass instruments glistening from the overhead lights, the licorice sticks no less obvious, as their reedy sounds, sometimes voice-like and far-ranging, run with the melody, enriching the listeners on the way, shoring up any faint hearts with the liveliness and vibrancy of their offering: Let us remember the smiling, the laughing, the talking, the sharing, the caring, and all the loving. Let us remember the good times—always. (American Greetings) Long after a rainbow has faded from the sky, its beauty is remembered by all those it touched. (Gartner Greetings). Memories to treasure/ They will always be with you whatever you do and wherever you go/For now may caring thoughts from others help you through as time passes little reminders of your loved one will touch your heart. (Unmarked card) Oh, how our days are forever charmed by loving memories of you and Joan, walking, swinging arms and hands, and even serenading us on our way to Nell Thorn. We are truly saddened by Joan's passing. We share in your loss... Every blessing for a consoled and gentle journey... (CS/SS, La Conner) Cherish the memories/Hold on to hope/Rest when you're weary/Take time to grieve/Let your heart mend/Thinking of you. (Hallmark)

We do survive every moment after all, except the last.

(John Updike)